3C

B
C

D1341750

St Vincent's Hospital
1834–1994
An Historical and Social Portrait

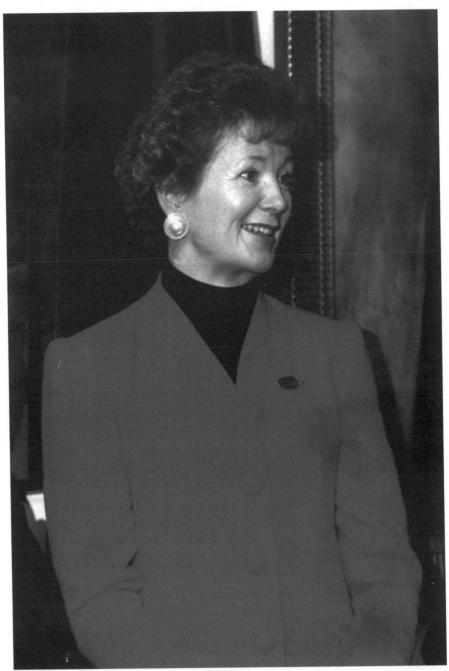

President of Ireland, Mary Robinson, visited the hospital at Elm Park on 23 January 1995 to unveil a plaque commemorating the 25th anniversary of the admission of patients to the new hospital.

ST VINCENT'S HOSPITAL 1834–1994

An Historical and Social Portrait

F.O.C. Meenan

Gill & Macmillan

Gill & Macmillan Ltd
Goldenbridge
Dublin 8
with associated companies throughout the world

© F.O.C. Meenan 1995
0 7171 2151 8

Index compiled by
Helen Litton

Design and print origination by
O'K Graphic Design, Dublin

Printed by
ColourBooks Ltd, Dublin

A catalogue record is available for this book from the British Library.

1   3   5   4   2

For Liobhain and the family

I long to provide a hospital wherein the sick in need can receive every remedy that the physician has to offer and every comfort that the Sister of Charity can bring.
MARY AIKENHEAD

CONTENTS

Preface	xi
Acknowledgments	xiii
Prologue	1
1. Background	3
2. Mary Aikenhead	8
3. The Foundation of the Hospital	13
4. Expansion	21
5. A Teaching Hospital	32
6. New Generation	39
7. The Medical Board	51
8. The End of the Century	60
9. New Spirit	72
10. The War Years	81
11. The Twenties	94
12. Annus Mirabilis	105
13. The Emergency Years	116
14. The Community	123
15. The Nursing School	134
16. The Winds of Change	151
17. Women Doctors	159
18. Last Years on the Green	164
19. Memories	173
20. The Road to Elm Park	185
21. The Move to Elm Park	194
22. Bright Morning	207
23. Consolidation	223
24. The Difficult Eighties	232
25. Towards the Millennium	241
Epilogue	256

Appendixes   258

  1 Mothers General   258

  2 Superiors of St Vincent's Hospital 1834–1993   258

  3 Members of the Board of Management 1972,
     1989, 1993   259

  4 Members of the Executive of the Medical Board
     1993   261

  5 Secretary Managers   261

  6 Chairmen and Secretaries of the Medical Board   262

  7 Consultant Medical Staff   263

  8 Mary Aikenhead School of Nursing   271

  9 Lady Presidents of Financial Aid Committee
     since 1957   272

  10 Past Students of St Vincent's Hospital 1834–1909   273

  11 Medical Examinations Medal and Prizewinners   287

  12 Nursing Examinations Medal and Prizewinners   296

  13 Some Current Research Projects in the Hospital   298

  14 Poem, 'Sister of Charity'   303

References   305

Bibliography   312

Index   315

PREFACE

When, on the suggestion of Dr E.A. Martin, Sister Mary Magdalen, the Secretary Manager of St Vincent's Hospital, invited me to write a history of the hospital, I was highly honoured. My pleasure was tinged with a certain amount of trepidation, for to write a history of St Vincent's was a formidable but necessary task.

It is now almost twenty-five years since 'Vincent's on the Green in Dublin' moved out to Elm Park. Naturally, the number of those who worked in the Green is fast diminishing. There is a danger that the labours and achievements of the old hospital might be forgotten. *A Century of Service*, compiled by Alice Curtayne and William Doolin in Centenary Year 1934, linked us to the early days of the hospital and recounted the struggle of Mary Aikenhead and her sisters with her medical advisors to build St Vincent's on sure foundations. It is now the task of our generation before it also disappears to carry forward the story of St Vincent's achievements and its subsequent transfer to more spacious surroundings at Elm Park.

There are other reasons why the history of the hospital must not be forgotten. In the early years of the last century, it was customary for nuns to remain in their convents. Mary Aikenhead and her sisters, clad in their distinctive black habit with pectoral cross, created considerable interest as they walked through the streets to visit the homes of the sick and the poor in all parts of the city, bringing succour and relief. The formal name of the congregation is the Religious Sisters of Charity, but to generations they have been known as the Irish Sisters of Charity, and it is by this name they will be called for the purpose of the book. St Vincent's Hospital itself was a unique institution. It was the first hospital founded and run by women in these islands, and the first teaching hospital of Newman's medical school. Many of the most eminent men and women of the early-Victorian era climbed the steep stairs of the old Georgian mansion to Mrs Aikenhead's office, there to seek advice and assistance. The fame of the hospital spread far beyond these islands, even to the Antipodes. Former students of the hospital could be found practising their art in every part of the world.

PREFACE

Writing the history of a hospital presents its own particular problems. It cannot be reviewed in isolation; it reflects the ever changing political and social mores of the times. This is especially true of St Vincent's. Over the last 160 years, it has carried out many changes, not for the sake of change itself, but for the welfare of the hospital and its patients. In 1970 it successfully organised the transfer of the whole hospital to another site. The political upheavals; the improvement in public health and social welfare; the rapid advance in medical science and technology, all play their part in shaping the work of the hospital. It is in many ways a synthesis of scientific departments working together for its primary object, the care of ill patients. Each department plays a vital role. As far as possible the life of the hospital has been described from contemporary sources—newspapers, journals and historical works.

It is difficult to pay adequate tribute to all who have worked in St Vincent's. Some records may be inadequate, because members of the staff are of course more concerned with their contemporary problems than the curiosity of future generations. Thus the labour of many people who have given great service to the hospital must go unchronicled. Perhaps they may take some consolation from the fact that they have played a significant role in the work of a hospital which has a proud place in Irish history.

Si Monumentum Requiris Circumspice

ACKNOWLEDGMENTS

There are many people who helped me in the preparation of this book and have been most generous of their time and knowledge. Firstly I must thank Liobhain, Frances, Charles, John, Anita and Helen for their constant and crucial support. They have read innumerable drafts of the book and tactfully but firmly recommended alterations in the script when they thought it was necessary. I owe an enormous debt of gratitude to my secretary Patricia Cunningham for her infinite patience in preparing the script and photographs. She also spent many long hours in helping to compile the lists of members of staff.

The members of the community helped me in every possible way. Sister Mary Magdalen, Sister Joseph Cyril and Sister Teresa of Avila made sure that I received all available documentation. Sister Baptist, Sister Lorcan, Sister Manus and Sister Carmel Mary also provided me with important records. Sister Marie John took a great interest in the preparation of the history and assisted me; I am sad that she did not live to see its publication. Sister Canisius and Sister Paula with their vast experience had a wealth of information on the history and administration of St Vincent's. The Principal Nursing Officer, Sister Agnes, and her staff from the department of nursing and Sister Anne from the nursing school also guided me. I thank Geraldine McSweeney of the School of Nursing for allowing me to quote from her excellent article on the history of nursing in the hospital; and Charles Lysaght who gave me access to Moira Lysaght's memories of her experiences as a young probationer in the hospital during the 1920s. J.P. McMullin gave me much important material on the history of the building of Elm Park Hospital. I also thank T.J. McKenna for recounting the establishment of the Education and Research Centre, in which project he played a vital role.

Many of my colleagues and friends gave me invaluable information and photographic material. They include John Blake, Charles Coyle and the *Irish Independent*, Morgan Crowe, Ray Davys, Frank Duff, Muiris FitzGerald, Oliver FitzGerald, John Fleetwood, Sean Galvin, Brian Hourihane, Nicholas Jermyn, Dan Kelly, Brian Keogh, Sean Love, J.B. Lyons, Donal MacErlaine,

ACKNOWLEDGEMENTS

John Mackey, Edward A. Martin, Brian Maurer, Declan Meagher, Winifred Meagher, Patrick N. Meenan, Eileen Monahan, J. McAuliffe Curtin, Eugene McCague, Oliver McCullen, Nancy McDermott, Gerry Noone, Dermot O'Donoghue, Denis K. O'Donovan, Niall O'Higgins, Seamus O Riain, William Quinlan, Robert Towers and many others. John Fitzpatrick of Leeson Lane has been a fund of reminiscences of life in the Lane.

Mairead Markey, secretary to the executive of the hospital, in spite of her busy schedule spared no effort to assist me and I appreciate her ever willing and efficient help. Eimear Couse and Alison Galbraith of the Medical Board Office were always ready to provide data from the records of the Medical Board. I would also like to thank Brian Fallon from Records for guarding carefully the old ledgers and records of St Vincent's.

I have been very fortunate in being able to enjoy the fruits of the first class reference library built up by the hospital librarian, Hylda Beckett; Beatrice Doran and Mary O'Doherty of the Mercer Library are an unfailing source of knowledge; and what more can one say of the staff of the National Library beyond the fact that they are as helpful and efficient as ever.

A book like this must rely heavily on photographic material. I have been blessed with good fortune to be able to avail of the services of our hospital photographer, Stephen O'Connor. He has taken innumerable photographs of all aspects of life in St Vincent's and is always most willing to take more. He has improved skilfully the definition of older pictures which though of historical importance were of poor quality. I am also fortunate in being able to reproduce several photographs taken by Tom Nolan.

Michael Gill and Deirdre Rennison Kunz of Gill & Macmillan have guided me again safely through the problems of writing a book. Finally I am sure that it is a happy omen that this history of St Vincent's Hospital has been published by the same firm that published the definitive history of Mary Aikenhead over one hundred years ago.

F.O.C. Meenan
28 Fitzwilliam Square
Dublin 2
January 1995

CHRONOLOGY

1787	January—Birth of Mary Aikenhead
1808	Mary Aikenhead's first visit to Dublin
1809	November—Dr Murray appointed coadjutor bishop of Dublin
1812	June—Mary Aikenhead and Alicia Walsh enter Bar Convent York
1815	First convent established North William Street Dublin
1815	Formal establishment of Congregation of Sisters of Charity
1816	September—Sisters begin visiting the sick poor in their homes
1817	September—Father Kenney S.J. preaches at Clothing Ceremony. Text of sermon 'Caritas Christi Urget Nos'
1833–4	Three sisters go to Paris to train as nurses
1834	January—Earl of Meath's House 56 St Stephen's Green purchased on behalf of the Sisters of Charity
1834	23 January—Sisters take formal possession of house. J.M. O'Ferrall appointed First Physician
1835	April—St Vincent's Hospital opens with beds for twelve female patients
1836	O'Bryan Bellingham appointed Second Physician
1841	57 St Stephen's Green purchased. House collapses during alterations
1845	September—Mary Aikenhead takes up residence in Harold's Cross
1852	February—Death of Dr Murray
1852	August—Florence Nightingale visits hospital
1855	Founding of Catholic University School of Medicine
1857	Death of Bellingham
1858	July—Death of Mary Aikenhead
1858	Passing of Medical Act, instituting a General Medical Council empowered to keep a register of qualified medical practitioners

1868	December—Death of O'Ferrall
1879	55 St Stephen's Green purchased for £1,300
1879	Establishment of the Royal University of Ireland
1884	Celebration of Golden Jubilee
1885	Foundation of hospital's football club
1886	Medical Act passed, enacting that a person should not be registered under the Medical Acts unless he has passed a qualifying examination in surgery, medicine and midwifery
1888	58 & 59 St Stephen's Green purchased
1892	Training school for nurses opened
1897	96 & 97 Lower Leeson Street opened as private home
1908	August—Passing of Irish University Act, establishing National University of Ireland
1910	Nurses' home built
1910	May—First conferring of medical degrees of National University of Ireland
1912	94 Lower Leeson Street converted into semi-private nursing home
1917	60 St Stephen's Green becomes semi-private nursing home
1919	Nurses Registration (Ireland) Act passed
1930	November—Hospital participates in Hospitals Sweeps for first time
1934	January—Centenary celebrations
1934	July—Lands at Elm Park purchased for new hospital for £25,000
1947	New building committee established
1948	November—Permission to build a 450-bed hospital for £1,350,000 granted
1950	Bord Altranais established
1955	June—Blessing of the site of new hospital
1956	January—First sod turned on site of new hospital
1956	First tender signed for site development
1957	University departments of medicine and surgery established in St Vincent's Stephen's Green
1958	First tender completed and all work ceases
1958	New residency built
1958	Pembroke nursing home purchased
1960	Permission granted for 250-bed hospital for £1,500,000
1964	Work on superstructure of all the main building started
1965	December—Permission granted for 450-bed hospital
1965	June/July—Annual General Meeting of the Irish Medical Association held in St Vincent's Hospital

1968	January—Commissioning of the new hospital begins
1968	July—Messrs Llewelyn-Davies, Weeks, Forestier-Walker & Bor appointed to advise on commissioning of hospital
1968	September—Mother Canisius O'Keeffe appointed first Rectress of the hospital
1968	October—Community take possession of St Vincent's Hospital Elm Park
1969	January—Three-quarters of the department of pathology moves out to Elm Park
1969	July—Nurses' home completed
1970	January—First patients admitted to Elm Park from St Stephen's Green
1970	October—First operation carried out
1970	1 November—St Vincent's Stephen's Green moves completely to St Vincent's Elm Park
1970	27 November—Official opening of St Vincent's Hospital Elm Park by Minister for Health Mr Erskine Childers
1970	Establishment of Comhairle na nOspidéal
1972	Board of Management established
1974	May—Private nursing home opened
1978	January—New day-care/five day unit opened
1984	Jan./May—Celebration of sesquicentenary of hospital
1989	Education and Research Centre completed
1992	Commissioning of Liver Unit
1992	May—Celebration of centenary of school of nursing
1995	23 January—Visit of Her Excellency the President of Ireland Mrs Mary Robinson to unveil a plaque commemorating the 25th anniversary of the first admission of patients to St Vincent's Hospital Elm Park

PROLOGUE

arly on a fine spring morning in 1834, Mr Henry Inglis, an English traveller, crossed the bay of Dublin and entered Kingstown Harbour a little after sunrise. He made his way swiftly to the centre of Dublin and reported what he observed in the capital city of Ireland. 'In walking through the streets, strange and striking contrasts are presented between grandeur and poverty. In Merrion Square, St Stephen's Green, and elsewhere, the ragged wretches that are sitting on the steps, contrast strongly with the splendour of the houses and the magnificent equipages that wait without.'

Mr Inglis took up residence in a house in Kildare Street opposite Leinster House where the Royal Dublin Society was holding a cattle show.

> It was very favourably situated for observing among the crowd collected some of those little traits which throw light upon character and condition. I remember in particular, the great eagerness of every one to get a little employment, and earn a penny or two. I observed another less equivocal proof of low condition. After the cattle had been fed, the half eaten turnips became the perquisite of the crowd of ragged boys and girls without. Many and fierce were the scrambles for these precious relics; and a half gnawed turnip, when once secured, was guarded with the most vigilant jealousy and was lent for a mouthful to another longing tatterdemalion, as if the root had been a pineapple.

After travelling around the country Mr Inglis summarised his observations on Ireland.

> I Henry David Inglis . . . report that the destitute, infirm and aged form a large body of the population of the cities, towns and villages of Ireland: that in the judgement of those best qualified to know the truth, three-fourth part of their number die through the effects of

1

destitution, either by the decay of nature, accelerated, or through disease induced by scanty and unwholesome food—or else by the attack of epidemic, rendered more fatal from the same causes. That the present condition of this large class, is shocking for humanity to contemplate and beyond the efforts of private beneficence to relieve; and is a reproach to any civilized and christian country.

From his writings, Mr Inglis would appear to have been a man of feeling and compassion. However, there is no evidence that we can attribute to him the gift of prescience. During his perambulations through the centre of the city he must have noticed the Earl of Meath's home on Stephen's Green, but would not have known that in the building—and quite possibly at this very time—a gallant band of sisters under the banner *Caritas Christi Urget Nos* were planning to found a hospital to combat the scourges of illness and poverty which he had noticed to be so prevalent in the city.[1]

CHAPTER 1

BACKGROUND

The first three decades of the nineteenth century were a time of great social and economic distress in Ireland. The Act of Union in 1800 did not bring the hoped-for era of peace and prosperity. Catholics had to wait almost thirty years before they were allowed to sit in parliament and be appointed to the higher positions in the judiciary, following the Catholic Emancipation Act in 1829. It has been pointed out that in spite of the Union, the government of Ireland carried on very much as before.[1] The Viceroy was still in his castle and together with his Chief Secretary and officials he still governed the country. Little seemed to have changed.

In spite of the fact that by the terms of the Act of Union Ireland had to pay an unduly large amount of the national debt of the United Kingdom, the country remained fairly prosperous till the end of the Napoleonic wars. Up to 1815 farmers were paid a good price for their agricultural produce but with the restoration of peace there was a disastrous slump in the price of grain and other crops. Farmers changed from tillage to pasture. Many of the unemployed agricultural labourers flocked to the overcrowded cities.

The woollen and cotton trades which had flourished in small country towns fared no better. Protective tariffs which had been brought into force after the Act of Union were abolished by 1824 and the trades had to compete with the flow of cheap textiles from industrial England. Moreover, England had the advantage of an abundant source of cheap energy in its coal fields. A steady influx of English manufactured goods swept away the small Irish industries. Against this deteriorating background the population of Ireland was heading for eight million in the mid-1830s. The main cities were affected by the slump in agriculture and the textile industry. In addition, Dublin, the capital city, had its own particular problems.

Up to the Act of Union Dublin was recognised as the second city of the Empire, and its development had reflected this position. The second half of the eighteenth century and the early years of the nineteenth were an Augustan era of expansion in Dublin. Many of the city's finest buildings date back to this period. Majestic administrative edifices such as the Four Courts

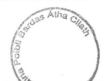

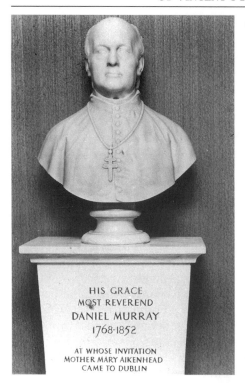

Archbishop Murray

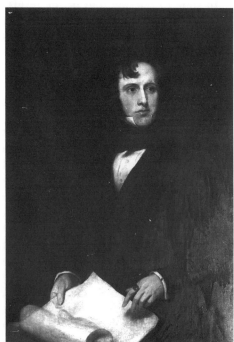

Joseph M. O'Ferrall

and the Custom House altered the sky line of the city. Suitable dwelling houses had to be constructed for those who carried on the affairs of State. The three main Georgian squares, Merrion, Mountjoy and Fitzwilliam, appeared from the 1750s onwards. Their handsome brick houses were designed as residences for the members of the Lords and Commons of Ireland.

Following the Act of Union the status of Dublin was reduced to that of a provincial city. The legislators fled to London, and only passed briefly through Dublin on the way to their country estates. Many of the houses in the Squares were left empty and in due course, over the next half-century, they were taken over by the professional classes.[2] There was no shortage of doctors and lawyers in nineteenth century Dublin. They were probably more interesting and stimulating than their aristocratic predecessors, but lacked their wealth. This in turn caused a decline in employment among builders, plasterers and ancillary trades. Meanwhile, many of the older houses in the city were rapidly turning into slums. In 1818 the population of Dublin was approximately one hundred and seventy-five thousand and the conditions under which great numbers of the population lived have been graphically described. The findings were very similar to those of Henry Inglis nearly twenty years later.

> The Liberties contain a population of 50,000 individuals, by far the greater part of whom are in the lowest stage of human wretchedness: they for the most part inhabit narrow lanes where the insalubrity of the air usual in such places is increased to pernicious degree by the effluvia of putrid offals constantly accumulating both in front and rear; the houses are very high and the numerous apartments swarm with inhabitants. It is not infrequent for one family or individual to rent a room and let a portion of it by the week or night to any accidental occupant, each person paying for that portion of the floor which his extended body occupies. In this way it will not appear incredible that 108 individuals have been reckoned in one building and that seven persons were found lying in a fever on the floor at one time out of twelve that occupied the small apartment.[3]

There is not one covered sewer in that populous portion of the Liberty south of the street called the Coombe.' They described the conditions around St Stephen's Green, 'In extent first in the British Empire . . . has in its present neglected state little else but its magnitude to recommend it. Of 124 houses that surround it about half are modern and substantially built, of the remainder, the greater part verging on decay. The proprietors also of these houses are as might be expected of all degrees, from the inhabitant of the Dram Shop and Porterhouse to that of the Nobleman's Palace.' There was a gravel path around the Green separated from the middle by a ditch containing stagnant water and animal bodies. Although from about 1815 onwards efforts were made to clear up the Green it was inevitable that under such conditions famine and pestilence could not be far away.[4]

There were many outbreaks of fever and famine in Dublin and throughout the country before the Great Famine. In 1805, 1,024 persons suffering from fever were admitted to the newly-built Cork Street Fever Hospital: of these 1 in 10 died. In 1815, 3,785 were admitted of whom 1 in 19 died. There were particularly severe epidemics of fever in 1817–18 and 1826–27. Added to these was a major epidemic of cholera in Dublin in 1832–33. As a sea port Dublin was particularly vulnerable to visitation by cholera and there were to be many more epidemics during the century.

Life expectancy for the citizens of Dublin was poor. The more prosperous one was, the longer one lived. In the decade 1831–41, the average age at death of a prosperous businessman or merchant was fifty-five to sixty years; that of a tailor was thirty-five to forty years and of a dressmaker thirty years. Less than 10 per cent of the mercantile class died of epidemic fevers; over 40 per cent of washerwomen died of respiratory disease while 23 per cent succumbed to epidemics.[5] Few measures could be taken to combat illness and hunger in the city; those that were taken were ineffective. The practice of medicine was in a primitive state. Health services consisted of a hotchpotch of medical and social institutions. They included voluntary hospitals, county hospitals and infirmaries, workhouses, special dispensaries and labour schemes.[6]

There were many voluntary hospitals founded in the eighteenth century for the relief of the sick poor. Among these were Dr Steevens' (1733); the Charitable Infirmary in Jervis Street (1728), the Rotunda Hospital (1765) for the care of lying-in women, the Royal Hospital for Incurables (1744) in Donnybrook and St Patrick's Hospital (1747) for the mad, founded by Dean Swift. These hospitals usually had their origin in the coming together of a group of charitable gentlemen who wished to provide hospital support for the sick and destitute. They were supported principally by voluntary subscriptions. Members of the medical staff of the voluntary hospitals had honorary status and gave their services freely to the patients.

As voluntary hospitals developed they also took on other functions such as the teaching of medical students and nurses and the advancement of knowledge through research. By the very nature of the times, the founders of these hospitals would be Protestant and the ethos of the hospitals would be Protestant. Other hospitals founded around this time were Grangegorman Hospital (1815) for mad people, which had its origin in the Richmond Asylum, and the Fever Hospital and House of Recovery in Cork Street (1798). The Meath Hospital was founded as a voluntary hospital in the middle of the eighteenth century; it subsequently became the County Dublin Infirmary and received public funds.

As the eighteenth century progressed many of the voluntary hospitals received financial assistance from the State, the amount varying from one hospital to the other. On the basis of an Act passed in 1765, the government established county hospitals and infirmaries throughout the country. Special dispensaries and various workhouses were also established, but the workhouse system did not come into effective operation until the passing of the Poor Law Act of 1838. By the terms of the Poor Law Act, the country was divided up into Unions and each Union had a workhouse. Dublin had two Unions: one based at the Richmond Hospital on the northside and one on the southside at James's Street, site of the Foundling Hospital and an old workhouse. The destitute poor were admitted to the workhouses. Families sought entrance as a last resort as on admission to the workhouse they were immediately broken up and separated. Most of the institutions worked as effectively as they could in the light of the medical knowledge and social standards of the time. However, no matter how devotedly the staffs of the various hospitals laboured, they could do little to assuage the misery that was the lot of the greater part of the population of early nineteenth century Dublin.

CHAPTER 2

MARY AIKENHEAD

Mary Aikenhead was born in Cork city on 19 January 1787. Her father Dr David Aikenhead, a medical practitioner, came from a Scottish Protestant family who had settled in Ireland about the middle of the eighteenth century. Her mother was Mary Stacpole, a member of an old Irish Catholic family. Dr Aikenhead allowed his wife to practise her own religion, but Mary the first born in the family was baptised a Protestant. She was fostered out to Mary and John Rorke, who were Catholics and described as being of unusual piety. Mary Aikenhead as a child attended Mass with her foster-parents every Sunday. In her seventh year she returned to her parents' house. Mary Rorke came with her to mind her and the other three children who had been added to the family in the meantime. John was also given a post in the doctor's service.

During the next few years Mary Aikenhead often visited her grandmother, Mrs Stacpole, and accompanied her to evening devotions. Dr Aikenhead died in 1801; he had become a Catholic on his death bed. It would appear that Mary inherited much of her father's common sense and directness, attributes which would be of great assistance to her in her future work. Mary herself became a Catholic in her sixteenth year, in 1802, and for the next few years she engaged in social life in Cork.

In 1807, at the religious profession of their sister, she met two young Dublin women, Mrs John O'Brien, married to a wealthy Dublin businessman, and her sister, Fanny Ball. She was invited to visit them in Dublin in their home in the newly-built Mountjoy Square. This invitation was accepted and Mary travelled to the capital city in 1808 to stay with the O'Briens. It was a visit which was to have momentous consequences.

When in Dublin she became friendly with Fr Daniel Murray, curate at St Mary's, Liffey Street, the parish church of the O'Briens. At this period Fr Murray, although not yet forty, was becoming a leading Churchman. He was born in Arklow in 1768. He was educated in Dublin at the school run by the famous Jesuit priest Fr Thomas Betagh. A curate in Arklow, he had a narrow escape from death during the Rising of 1798. In St Mary's parish, Fr Murray

Mother Mary Aikenhead

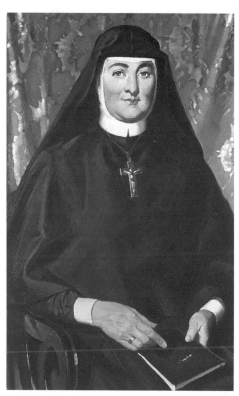

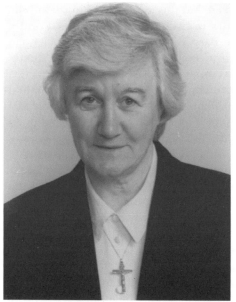

Sr Francis Ignatius Fahy,
Superior General

was well acquainted with the problems experienced by the Catholic population and laboured ceaselessly to alleviate the misery of the poor in his parish. Mary confided in Fr Murray that she felt her vocation in life was to assist the sick poor. Soon after her return to Cork her mother died suddenly and her sisters became boarders in the Ursuline Convent in Cork. She visited Dublin again in 1809.

By now Fr Murray had been consecrated coadjutor bishop of Dublin to assist the ageing Archbishop Troy. At the consecration of Bishop Murray, Fr Betagh preached the sermon—and it was only on his insistence that Fr Murray had accepted his new post. He well knew the problems that lay ahead. Surveying the widespread dilapidation and misery of his flock he realised the need for an order of nuns who would care for the sick poor in their own homes. He felt that he had in Mary Aikenhead the ideal leader of a new congregation of nuns who would carry out this mission. Mary accepted the task with diffidence and foreboding.

It was decided that she should undergo a period of noviceship to prepare herself for the work that lay ahead. The Convent of the Institute of the Blessed Virgin Mary at Micklegate Bar, York—the Bar Convent—was chosen as a suitable school for her training. The Bar Convent had been in existence for 200 years, a part of which time was spent on the continent. The nuns were known as 'English Virgins', or 'English nuns'. The Bar Convent played a significant role in the development of the religious orders in Ireland during the nineteenth century. Fanny Ball, sister of Mrs O'Brien, was educated there. She subsequently introduced the Loreto nuns to Ireland and established their first foundation at Rathfarnham. A few years later Mother Ball was to open a school for girls near the newly-established St Vincent's Hospital at St Stephen's Green, but this was for the future. In June 1812, after putting her family affairs in order, Mary Aikenhead and a companion Alicia Walsh entered the Bar Convent. While in York she had lengthy correspondence with Dr Murray concerning the rules that should govern the new congregation to be known as the Irish Sisters of Charity.

In August 1815, the two sisters returned to Dublin. Dr Murray had arranged for them to take over an orphanage in North William Street as a residence, on condition that they would look after the children committed to the care of the orphanage. Over the next few years under his guidance and that of Fr Peter Kenney S.J. (a distinguished Jesuit and first Rector of Clongowes Wood College), the Congregation of the Irish Sisters of Charity was established. The rules of the Bar Convent at York were considered the most suitable for the new congregation. Another Jesuit, Fr St Leger, drew up the rules and constitutions of the congregation which were approved by Rome in 1833. From its earliest days the congregation had a happy relationship with the Society of Jesus.

In September 1816, Mary Aikenhead, in religion Sister Mary Augustine (now the Mother General), and her companion Alicia Walsh (Sister Mary Catherine) began visiting the sick poor in their own homes. This was a completely new development in the role of religious orders of women in Ireland. Up to then congregations of nuns were confined to their convents and did not undertake work outside. It is difficult at this remove in time to appreciate the interest that the appearance of nuns, on the streets and visiting the sick poor in their homes, raised amongst the population. In September 1817 the congregation had its first clothing ceremony. A plain black habit was adopted and all the sisters wore the well-known solid broad brass cross. Fr Kenney S.J. preached the sermon taking as his text *Caritas Christi Urget Nos* (Charity of Christ urges us on)—a text which was to be the guiding motto of the congregation.

In putting on the habit the Sisters of Charity did not relinquish their surnames. Up to quite recent times many of the senior nuns in the community were called 'Mrs'. The reason is obscure. One explanation is that it dates back to the French Revolution and to penal times in Ireland when religious titles were abolished so the appellation 'Mrs' was used instead. Sarah Atkinson the biographer of Mary Aikenhead does not give this explanation.

> Outside the convent they were called Mrs Aikenhead, Mrs Walsh and so on with the rest.
>
> In the community the foundress was never called Mother Augustine, for from first to last she was invariably the Reverend Mother. Mother Catherine indeed was only for a short time known to the world in general as Mrs Walsh. The poor, owing perhaps to the singular motherliness of her countenance and manner, caught at the title and spoke of her and addressed her only as Mother Catherine. In the end rich and poor alike called her by no other name and in common parlance it was curious enough to hear the associated names of Mrs Aikenhead and Mother Catherine.

Over the next seventeen years the congregation expanded rapidly. In 1819 a house in Stanhope Street was purchased for the novitiate. Houses were subsequently founded in Cork (1826), Upper Gardiner Street (1830), Sandymount (1831) and Donnybrook (1833). In all her work Mary Aikenhead was supported by the ever faithful Mrs O'Brien who helped the new congregation in many material ways. Another supporter was Nicholas Ball, a brother of Mrs O'Brien. Nicholas Ball was the second Catholic raised to the judiciary after Catholic Emancipation. He became a Justice of the Common Pleas.

While the work of visitation of the sick poor was progressing satisfactorily, Mother Aikenhead had realised for many years from personal experience that there was something fundamentally lacking in the services that the nuns could offer. She felt that Dublin hospital services were inadequate for the demands made on them; she had learned from experience that many patients died from sheer want and neglect. She was also worried that in the public hospitals many poor Catholics died without religious support. Her ambition was to found her own hospital in which the best medical care and the consolation of religion could be provided.

Cholera broke out in Dublin in 1832. The overcrowded city, lacking most sanitary facilities and with inadequate hospital services, was particularly vulnerable to the ravages of the disease. Grangegorman penitentiary was turned into a fever hospital and the sisters were invited by the public authorities to visit it daily and care for the patients. Fortunately none of the Sisters of Charity succumbed to cholera. In 1833 there was another major outbreak of cholera in Dublin; the population of Ringsend and Sandymount was particularly affected. The congregation set up a small temporary hospital where the victims of cholera could be nursed. Writing to Mother de Chantal in Cork, one of her senior colleagues, she stated: 'It certainly will be less injurious to our Sisters than going about from one dirty hovel to another,' and again some weeks later: 'No hospitals are open except this poor thing of twelve beds for the parish and a small one in Townsend Street for that parish.' In the same year a government Commission to inquire into the state of the Irish poor was established and Mother Aikenhead was invited to submit her views. At this time she was resident in her Sandymount convent. She took the opportunity to describe the dreadful conditions under which the poor lived in Sandymount, Ballsbridge, Irishtown and Ringsend, and the remedies that could be taken to improve their lot:

> When the poor are confined to bed by fever, they frequently fall victims to the want of medical aid and most frequently relapse for want of proper food when in a convalescent state . . . the poor are obliged to buy even the water that they drink . . . the poor have no bedclothes. We have often seen them expire on dirty straw and are frequently obliged to furnish them with covering before we can approach to administer to their wants . . . We are at all times ready to lend our assistance in superintending hospitals or administering relief to the sick at their own dwellings in fever or cholera morbus . . . We most sincerely deplore that we have not the means to erect a hospital where our care of the sick might be attended with more beneficial results than any we can possibly effect amid the desolation of their wretched homes.

CHAPTER 3

THE FOUNDATION
OF THE HOSPITAL

In spite of her statement to the Commission that she lacked the means to fund a hospital for relief of the sick poor, Mrs Aikenhead had for some time been laying plans to achieve her ambition to establish such a hospital. It was inevitable that in undertaking such a major project she would be exposed to considerable criticism. The main criticism was that she should not commence such a project without having first secured a regular source of funds for its maintenance. She countered this argument in a letter to Mother de Chantal on 3 February 1834: 'Did anyone point out to me, any one of our Catholic institutions which had a fund to commence with?' Writing to a friend, she said that her only resource was the 'Bank of Divine Providence'.

She set about her task in a typically-methodical fashion.[1] A new member of the congregation, Sister Francis Teresa O'Farrell, on the occasion of her profession presented Mrs Aikenhead with £3,000 for the purchase of a suitable house. Another problem to be resolved was the appointment of a competent medical advisor to run the hospital. This was of paramount importance. In the 1830s there were not many adequately-qualified Catholic doctors who would undertake such a task. However, about 1830 Mrs Aikenhead developed a chronic spinal condition which made movement difficult and painful. It has been suggested that she was suffering from spinal tuberculosis.[2] Her doctor's treatment of the condition was not successful and she was recommended to change her medical advisor. On the advice of Fr Whelan, a Carmelite, who subsequently became Archbishop of Bombay, Dr Joseph Michael O'Ferrall was called in and his treatment proved relatively successful.

Mrs Aikenhead realised that she had a suitable candidate for the position of medical advisor for her proposed hospital. She made a good choice. O'Ferrall was one of the few successful Catholic doctors of the period. He had a background typical of his class and creed. His mother was described as 'a lady of superior refinement and great beauty'. She had been brought up a Protestant, but secretly became a Catholic after instruction by the Carmelite priests in St Teresa's, Clarendon Street. When the aunt and uncle who had brought her up discovered this she was literally cast out of the family without a penny. With the encouragement of the Carmelite priests she married a young man in the neighbourhood called Farrell, a barber by trade. There were three children of the marriage: Joseph Michael, the future doctor; another son who became a distinguished barrister and was called to the English Bar; and a daughter.

The future doctor was educated at Samuel Whyte's famous school in Grafton Street. This school had a reputation for producing distinguished men. The Duke of Wellington and his brother, Richard Brinsley Sheridan, Thomas Moore and Robert Emmet had received their early education in the Academy. After school O'Ferrall worked as a clerk in Blackpitts Distillery to make money for his medical education. He commenced the study of medicine at the age of twenty-four. He was apprenticed to the famous Richard Carmichael of the Richmond Hospital and also worked with another well-known surgeon of the time, C.H. Todd. After five years at the Richmond, O'Ferrall passed the Licentiate examination of the Royal College of Surgeons in 1821 and was elected a member two years later. His name in the register of the period was given as 'Farrell', but he subsequently liked to be called 'O'Ferrall' to rhyme with 'Overall'. He had been very attached to his mother and this insistence on the pronunciation of his name was probably designed to rehabilitate his mother's status. It was in an age when social standing was of paramount importance. O'Ferrall was to show a singular determination on many occasions during his career. When over seventy years of age he sat for the Licentiate of the College of Physicians. He was appointed to the Maison de Santé in Charlemont Street.

The famous William Stokes described him as a master of diagnosis. Residing at 15 Merrion Square North he developed a large practice and made many valuable contributions to the literature of the times. He never married and his sister kept house for him. He nearly achieved eponymous fame in medical history by his description of what he believed was a hitherto undescribed capsule in the eye. Unfortunately it was subsequently discovered that three continental surgeons had alluded to it some years previously.

O'Ferrall was appointed first medical advisor in ordinary to the hospital.[3] Having chosen her first medical advisor Mary Aikenhead set about staffing her hospital with properly-trained personnel. In April 1833 she had sent three sisters, Sisters M. Ignatius, M. Camillus and F. de Sales, to Paris to learn hospital administration. The system chosen to study was that of the Hospitalières of St Thomas of Villanova, who administered the hospital of Notre Dame de Pitiè. The hospital had seventeen wards, the smallest of them 140 feet long and 40 feet wide. There were always 600 patients in the hospital. There was obviously no lack of clinical material for the sisters' studies. During their stay in Paris one of them also worked in the Children's

Hospital. Already at this stage Mrs Aikenhead apparently planned to open a children's ward in her new hospital. The sisters returned to Dublin in June 1834.[4] Sister M. Camillus was to play an important role in the development of the new hospital and—possibly more important—became the archivist of the congregation. Her name was Isabel Sallinave. She had also been educated at the Bar Convent in York.

The next step in the project was of course the purchase of a house which would be suitable for conversion into a hospital. The final choice was the house belonging to the Earl of Meath situated at 56 St Stephen's Green East. This was a large Georgian house rising four storeys over basement. It had been built in 1760 by Usher St George. He left it to his daughter Amelia Olivia, wife of the second Duke of Leinster, in 1775 and it was subsequently sold to Anthony, eighth Earl of Meath.[5]

The house was noted for its exuberant plasterwork. The staircase from the ground floor which ascended from the back of the main hall to the first floor (subsequently St Joseph's ward) was famous for its rococo style.

'The decoration is crowded with birds, flowers, musical instruments and swirling plaster, and there are three groups of figures, two of them enclosed in elegant Berainesque frames. The whole composition is unique in that there is no cornice, and the decoration continues uninterrupted from wall to ceiling.' The plasterer and architect was most likely Robert West. 'The work at St Vincent's is one of the last examples of Dublin Rococo, which was finally killed by the fashion for the geometrical "Adam" ceiling.'[6]

Like many other big houses in Dublin, 56 St Stephen's Green had been unoccupied since the Act of Union. It was ideal for Mary Aikenhead's purpose. 'On the 3rd of January 1834 no. 56 St Stephen's Green East, the Earl of Meath's noble mansion having a frontage of 90 feet with extensive gardens and rere extending backwards to Leeson Lane was conveyed by John, tenth Earl of Meath to Thomas Trant Simpson Esq. Solicitor, who bought it in trust for the Sisters of Charity.' The price paid was £3,000. On 23 January 1834 the Sisters of Charity took formal possession of the house and it was named after St Vincent de Paul.[7] The Marchioness of Wellesley, the wife of the Viceroy, was a supporter of the sisters; uniquely for the times, she was a Catholic. Through her good offices Mrs Aikenhead endeavoured to obtain the patronage of Queen Adelaide, Consort of William IV, for her hospital. This was not forthcoming.

The work of adapting the house to the needs of a hospital was now undertaken. Mrs Aikenhead had decided that the main rooms of the building should be used for wards and that the community could occupy the top storey. As these rooms were small Dr Murray insisted that the roof should be raised to make the rooms more airy and suitable for the community. This work took several months and delayed the admission of patients to the hospital. In October, she and three sisters took up residence in the hospital to supervise the organisation of the various departments. Three rooms were habitable. The best room became an oratory, another the

PROSPECTUS

OF AN

INSTITUTION

INTENDÉD TO BE ESTABLISHED,

In Stephen's-Green, Dublin,

BY THE

SISTERS OF CHARITY.

WITH THE CONCURRENCE OF THEIR FOUNDER,

THE MOST REVEREND DOCTOR MURRAY,

CATHOLIC ARCHBISHOP OF DUBLIN.

———

DUBLIN:

JOHN S. FOLDS, 5, BACHELOR'S-WALK.

1834.

First Prospectus of the hospital

offices of the Reverend Mother and the other became a community room.

The opening of the hospital attracted much interest amongst the general public as it was the first hospital organised and staffed by women to open in these islands. A prospectus of the new hospital was drawn up, printed and circulated. It was headed 'Prospectus of an Institution':

Intended to be established in Stephen's Green Dublin by the Sisters of Charity with the concurrence of their founder the Most Reverend Dr Murray, Catholic Archbishop of Dublin. The Hospitalières and Sisters of Charity of France have for centuries continued to provide the utility of placing public hospitals under their immediate care. From the period of their foundation, they have had the charge of all the hospitals under the various dynasties, which have successively held the reins of government in France and every new administration has equally confided in their zeal and ability for promoting the public good.

The Sisters of Charity in Ireland commenced their efforts in 1815. The many public charities of which they have accepted the charge have since occupied a great portion of their time; but the experience which they have thus acquired of the characters, habits and wants of the indigent sick of this country have only strengthened their conviction of the necessity of completing their original design. They have been in fact for nineteen years visiting a class of sick persons who will not go to common hospitals; and they have constantly had the painful trial of witnessing their best exertions, though aided by occasional advice from medical gentlemen, defeated by the unpropitious circumstances of their patients, the want of wholesome air and of those comforts and accommodation which are strangers to the abode of the poor.

The Sisters of Charity therefore propose to found an establishment to which they could remove persons of better feelings or habits, leaving to the common hospital those who may be labouring under infectious complaints. With this view a large and airy house has been purchased in which the plans and comforts of the hospitals in France, Notre Dame de la Pitiè, l'Hôpital des Enfans Malade etc. etc. and of the great hospital of Havre de Grace are intended to be introduced. Some of the Sisters of Charity of Ireland have been for the last year residing in the above named hospitals for the purpose of acquiring such additional information as shall enable them to conduct the establishment on the most useful and economic plan.

In this way, it is expected that an institution will be formed in which every friend of humanity will feel an interest and the benefit of which will be so much the more widely extended, as its regulations will present to individuals of every sect and every creed equal advantages and equal attention.

The Sisters of Charity feel certain that they incur no risk in thus fearlessly commencing an undertaking naturally attended with considerable expense. They recollect that they have already been made ministers of the charity and benevolence of individuals to a very considerable amount, and they cannot think it presumptuous to hope that in their arduous endeavours to enlarge the sphere of their usefulness, they will be cheered on by a still more liberal share of public confidence and support. They cannot for a moment doubt that while they make a great and expensive effort to meet some of the more pressing claims of human misery by opening a door to receive the poor wounded wayfarer there will be many good Samaritans found anxious to convey him to their care and to supply them with the means of pouring oil into his wounds and accomplishing his cure.[8]

In reply to the prospectus subscriptions came in from many parts of Ireland, England and Scotland. High on the list was the Marchioness of Wellesley with a donation of £20. Unfortunately her friend Mrs O'Brien had gone bankrupt at this time and could not give the £100 she had promised. Charity sermons were preached in aid of the new hospital. Begging letters at Christmas raised £36.18s.4d. A subsequent gift to the hospital was unusual. A sailor grateful for services rendered to him in St Vincent's presented Mrs Aikenhead with a parrot. She kept it in her office. The parrot remained silent however, until one day a sister tripped over a mat and fell to the floor, whereupon the parrot uttered some uncomplimentary words. He was immediately raffled and brought in £60 for the hospital. In April 1835 the alterations were complete and twelve female patients were admitted to St Joseph's ward. They were looked after by two nursing sisters and one doctor.

The question must be asked: what role did hospitals play and how effective were they in the treatment of illness in the first half of the nineteenth century? Many of the treatments used in the management of disease at this time had been in vogue for several centuries. Blood letting was the main form of medical treatment. This was accomplished by cupping, the use of the lancet and the application of leeches. Many of these practices lasted well into the twentieth century. Here and there, shafts of scientific light were piercing the intellectual gloom, but there had been no real advances in the understanding and treatment of most diseases.

The *Dublin Journal of Medical Science* for January 1834, the month in which St Vincent's was bought, illustrates the state of medical science at the time. The contents were a mixture of primitive medicine and the glimpse of a scientific approach to illness. In a typically scholarly article Robert Graves, the physician to the Meath Hospital, defined pneumothorax (air in the pleural sac) as a definite entity. He observed, 'rare diseases should not be looked upon as mere matters of curiosity but should be attentively studied with a view to enabling us to recognise the true nature of similar cases when they come again'. Dr Maunsell, accoucheur to the Wesley Female Institution and Magdalene Asylum, reviewed vaccination against smallpox and proved its efficacy. It must be remembered that Jenner's discovery was less than fifty years old at the time. In contrast to these two scholarly articles there was also one recommending the efficacy of applying oil of mustard to the skin in cholera as a rubefacient and vesicator. A more futile approach to a deadly disease is difficult to imagine.

The treatment of patients in hospital was a reflection of the state of medical knowledge. It must be emphasised that at this time hospitals catered for the poor and destitute. The upper classes, when they got ill, were cared for and operated on in their own houses. It was generally believed that hospitals were dangerous places. It has been calculated that a soldier on the field at Waterloo was safer than a patient in an early-Victorian hospital. The great enemy was infection. Hospital surgeons in spite of the lack of anaesthesia were able to perform operations with remarkable technical skill only to have their patient taken from them by post-operative infection. Even after the slightest operation the wound could become infected and the patient could die in a few days. Doolin has quoted Ericsen, a distinguished Victorian surgeon on the staff of University College Hospital London, who estimated the mortality in his cases of amputation as 25 per cent. According to Ericsen the mortality at the Edinburgh Royal Infirmary was 43 per cent and at the Glasgow Royal Infirmary 38 per cent. The mortality figure for amputation in the Crimea was up to 70 per cent.[9] Surgeons of the time produced many theories to explain the horror of sepsis. Their theories as regards its causation might have been wrong, but it is incorrect to suggest that they accepted the situation with equanimity. The most widely-held theory was that hospital infection was carried by noxious gas or miasma. The foul-smelling miasma originated as an emanation from cesspools and sewers. It entered the sick room and contaminated wounds. The contaminated wound in turn generated more miasma as evidenced by its evil smell and the miasma travelled on air currents to other wounds. Efforts were made to prevent the miasma from getting access to the wards. Clothing and bedding were soaked with chloride of lime and Condy's fluid. Sheets soaked in chloride of lime were hung over the walls. Chlorine gas was passed into the wards and huge fires were kept burning even in the heat of summer to draw off the miasma by way of the chimney.[10] Ventilation was also achieved by the ordinary means of doors and windows. Gratings were inserted in the floors or walls of passages, by louvres in the roof, and openings in the ceilings of both passages and wards. As regards toilet facilities water-closets were installed during the second half of the century. Baths were also installed around this time. Beds had curtains around them and from 1800 onwards hospitals were equipped with beds of iron frame with wire woven mattresses. In the first quarter of the century lighting was provided by candles. Subsequently gas lighting was introduced into the hospitals.[11] St Vincent's Hospital was nearly fifty years old before the great principles of antiseptic surgery were learned and put into practice. All these defects in Victorian hospitals must be admitted but there is an increasing tendency among medical historians to believe that the good points of the hospitals of the period have been forgotten. They concede that the hospitals gave some strength and support to patients who were neglected; and by good nursing care, and the provision of suitable meals, enabled patients to stimulate their natural immunities to combat disease. For the terminally ill they ensured that the patient could spend his or her last days in moderate comfort and dignity.

CHAPTER 4

EXPANSION

From the very beginning the need for a hospital such as St Vincent's was evident. So great was the demand for the service that the hospital had no choice but to expand almost immediately. Within a few months two additional female wards were opened and in 1836 a children's ward to care for fifteen infants from one year upwards was established. In the same year the stables and out-offices at the rear of the house were taken down. In the space thus provided a male ward was erected together with a bathroom, consulting room and post mortem room.

St Patrick's ward, with eighteen beds for male patients, was opened officially on 15 August 1836.[1] The main building was connected to St Patrick's and offices at the back by a long tunnel-like corridor. St Vincent's now had sixty beds and new staff had to be added to deal with the increase in the volume of work. At this point there was a standstill in building for five years. All the available ground was occupied and there seemed no possibility of further enlargement.

On the recommendation of Dr Murray, Dr O'Bryen Bellingham, although a Protestant, was appointed second medical officer in ordinary to the hospital. He was different in every way from his colleague O'Ferrall. He came of a family that could trace its lineage back to William the Conquerer. He was the son of Sir Alan Bellingham of Castlebellingham, Co. Louth, the second baronet. Born in 1805 he was educated at the Feinaiglian Institute (now Aldborough House). He became Licentiate of the College of Surgeons in 1828, proceeded M.D. Edinburgh in 1830 and Member of the College in 1833. He was appointed Professor of Botany and Librarian to the Royal College of Surgeons.

At first he resided at 63 Eccles Street. Although he lived at a great distance from the hospital (!), nine o'clock always found him at his post. He subsequently moved to 19 Kildare Street. E.D. Mapother wrote of him: 'He was towards all men courteous and generous, and if he entered into any controversy it was to elicit truth, never to gain a personal triumph. He had an intellectual and earnest appearance. He was a skilled practitioner and accurate observer. During the Famine years he found that scurvy was caused by a lack of potatoes.' Amongst Dr Bellingham's noteworthy operations was tapping the skull for hydrocephalus, the patient surviving three weeks. His fame rests on observations on aneurysms and their treatment by compression—a shabby paper-bound duodecimo published in January 1847. His book *Diseases of the Heart* was published a few days after his death on 11 October 1857.

> In him were combined the most gentle disposition, the most perfect freedom from envy or guile, with the utmost integrity of conduct and most accomplished manners. Few people have undergone greater annoyances, the offspring of professional jealousy in his inferiors, and few—few indeed—would have borne them with such a Christian spirit. It was in his painful and fatal illness that the noble mind of Dr Bellingham shone forth with such lustre—he met excruciating pain with resignation, death without fear.[2]

Mrs Aikenhead also appointed two consultants to the staff of the hospital. Sir Henry Marsh was appointed consultant physician and Sir Philip Crampton was appointed consultant surgeon. They were two of the most eminent practitioners in the Dublin of the period. Sir Henry was physician to Dr Steevens' Hospital. Sir Philip Crampton was the Surgeon General and was a very colourful figure in the professional and social life of the city. There is a famous story about a reception in Dublin Castle which Sir Philip attended dressed in the striking uniform of Surgeon General: a guest asked who he was and was informed that he was an officer in the 'Lancers'. For many years there was a memorial to Crampton at the junction of D'Olier Street, Pearse Street and College Street, which looked remarkably like a pineapple. Crampton and Marsh were probably called in for difficult or unusual cases but do not appear to have played an active part in the daily functioning of the hospital.

Mrs Aikenhead appointed Mother Francis Magdalene McCarthy first Rectress of St Vincent's Hospital. Helena Brigid McCarthy was born in London in 1798 and was the fourth daughter of Charles McCarthy and Mary Strange. She was cousin to Dr Wiseman, the future Cardinal Archbishop of Westminster and leader of the Catholic hierarchy in England. She was educated by the Benedictine nuns of Old Heath Hall in Yorkshire. A friend of hers, Mary Hennessy, had become a Sister of Charity and after her father's death she made a decision to join the same order herself. She left for Dublin in September 1829 and entered the congregation.

Sister Camillus Sallinave was appointed to organise nursing in the hospital, a position which would now be described as matron. It is interesting that Sister Camillus was the only one out of the three nuns sent to Paris to train who took an active part in the establishment and running of St Vincent's Hospital.

From 1 January 1838 to 1 January 1842, 500 patients a year were admitted to the hospital. A dispensary or out-patients' department was opened for the treatment of patients whose ailments did not necessitate admission to the hospital. The number of patients attending proved how necessary a dispensary was in the working of the hospital. For the year ending 1 January 1839, 5,093 patients attended; 8,411 in 1840; 14,498 in 1841; and 15,105 in 1842.[3]

For about ten years up to 1845 Mrs Aikenhead generally resided in the hospital. When her health permitted she would descend from her room on the top floor of the building and walk through the wards, speaking to and encouraging both the patients and the sisters. It is recorded that the first operation performed in the hospital was on a little boy named Daniel O'Connell who was suffering from an abscess on his leg. Tradition has it that Mrs Aikenhead took the young lad on her lap and consoled and comforted him while the surgeon incised the abscess. This of course was in the days before anaesthesia.

The following notice appeared in Pettigrew and Oulton's Directory for Dublin for 1837:

> This noble Institution was opened in 1835 by the religious Sisters of Charity with the concurrence of their Founder the Most Reverend Dr Murray, Catholic Archbishop of Dublin. The hospital contains sixty beds, constantly occupied by cases of great urgency and has attached to it a dispensary where great numbers of sick are relieved. Both are open to the afflicted without any regard to religious distinction. The plans and economy of the hospital are modelled on those of Notre Dame de la Pitiè, Enfans Malade etc. of Paris, for which purpose some of the Sisters have for some time resided in these establishments abroad. Its funds are derived from voluntary subscriptions, donations and bequests. It incurs no expense for superintendence as it is conducted exclusively by the Sisters of Charity who devote their whole time to its management and contribute liberally to its resources.

In 1841, 57 St Stephen's Green, the house next door to the hospital, belonging to the Earl of Westmeath, came up for sale. The house with its fine banqueting room had been built by Anthony Lee, a portrait painter, in 1760. It was subsequently sold to John Fitzgibbon, father of the future Lord Chancellor. Young Fitzgibbon passed his early days there until his father died in 1780.[4] This was a golden opportunity to expand the hospital which was already much too small for the demands made upon it. With a sum of money providentially supplied by Sister Lucy Clifford, a member of the congregation, the house was purchased.

The joining together of the two houses presented many difficulties as the landings were at different levels and the chimney stacks were insecure. The builders had only been at work for a short period when the main building of the new acquisition collapsed one Sunday morning. The banqueting hall and ballroom which were connected to the house by a vestibule survived. Mrs Aikenhead was in the convent at Sandymount at the time. She received the news of the collapse of the house more with relief than resignation. She is reported to have said, 'My dears, I am greatly obliged to the Lord for taking down that house. It was really the right thing to do; but I should have been considered deranged if I had done it. The connection of the two houses would have always been a botched affair. Now proper plans can be made and all done as it should be.' She had realised that the connection between the two houses would be unsatisfactory.

Now she was able to draw up new and more comprehensive plans for the joining together of the two buildings. This cost the sum of £8,000 which was raised by subscription. No. 57 was fully incorporated into no. 56 and the numbers of the remaining houses stretching towards Leeson Street were now changed accordingly. The large granite staircase winding past the chapel to the first floor of the hospital marked the boundary between no. 56 and the old no. 57.[5] In 1848 another male ward (St Laurence's) was provided. It was the first ward to be constructed as such in the hospital; all previous wards were originally rooms. St Laurence's contained twenty-eight beds and 2,000 cubic feet of space were allotted to each patient. It was described as 'one of the finest wards in the Empire'. By 1850 St Vincent's had ninety beds.

In the early hours of 25 June 1854 the hospital was visited by near catastrophe. A fire broke out in one of the rooms adjoining the community refectory. One of the night nurses smelled fire and raised the alarm. A sister prudently turned off the gas supply at the meter. The fire brigade was called, staff members were mobilised and they deluged the room and the fire with buckets of water so effectively that by the time the fire brigade arrived the fire had been extinguished. Neighbours of the hospital including the Chief Baron Pigot and the Lord Mayor also arrived to offer their help. If the fire had not been discovered so early the whole hospital might have been destroyed. Practical as always, Mrs Aikenhead arranged for the builders and representatives from the insurance company to be present in the hospital early the next morning. She discussed the problems arising from the fire in a letter to the Rectress of the Cork convent:

> I think the insurance of convents and establishments connected with them is universally sanctioned, if not directed or even ordered by the ecclesiastical authorities; and we have now before us a very painful instance to recommend the securing of this precaution . . . I am now about to acknowledge by note and stamped receipt the sum of twenty seven pounds, eighteen shillings sterling from the Sun Insurance Office to pay for the repairs and losses incurred by the late fire at St Vincent's Hospital. This statement will prove to you that any amount I may have mentioned to you as of the losses was pretty correct. Of

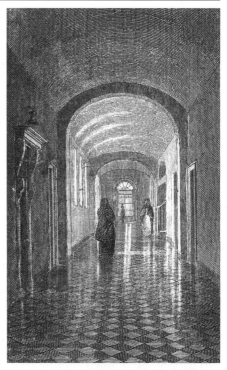

Corridor in the hospital, *c.* 1860

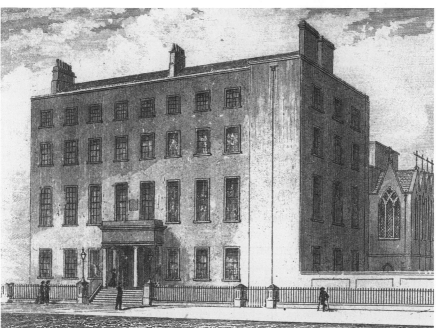

Drawing of the hospital, *c.* 1860

course we shall have to add some pounds more but this sum is the amount of the estimate of builder etc. etc. sent in and allowed.

Her letter also described the lighting in the hospital at night:

> You know the great staircase is all of stone, on it one lamp of gaslight burns, another in the long stone corridor, as you may remember upwards of 100 feet long; and at this time no candles are at all used in the house except the taper which a steady Sister who has charge of the gaslights carries in her own hand.[6]

In 1869 Francis Quinlan, physician to the hospital, at a meeting to inaugurate the thirty-sixth medical session of the hospital gave an interesting account of the structural development of the hospital over the previous fifteen to twenty years. The portico which was one of the distinguishing features of the hospital was an early addition to the building. It now stands in the grounds of Elm Park. In the hall of the hospital there were two busts: stationed on the right was one of Mrs Aikenhead, and on the left one of Dr Murray. A painting illustrating a gospel scene hung also in the hall between the two busts. These two busts now stand in the main hall of the new St Vincent's Hospital.

In 1856 it was decided to demolish the long passage connecting the front and back of the hospital and the old male ward which was now unsuitable. It was planned to connect the front and back of the establishment by a block of buildings containing cellars and an under-passage; then a first storey with a new corridor; a second storey containing a new children's ward and another male ward; and an upper tier with additional accommodation for the sisters. The construction was carried out in a year and a half. The house at the southern end was purchased about 1861 and removed 'to great improvement of ventilation'. A new chapel which Quinlan described as 'an exquisite chapel of the renaissance style' was constructed at the back. A little gothic mortuary chapel was also built at the back.

In 1864 a large residence in Stillorgan was purchased as a convalescent home through the munificence of Mr Francis Coppinger of Mounttown Castle. The approach to the house, the former seat of the Earls of Carysfort, was planted with rows of lime trees. Hence the name of the house. Linden was the first convalescent home established in Ireland. In 1878 the Mullins Convalescent Hospital was opened in the grounds. It was maintained by the bequest of Michael Bernard Mullins of Merrion Square who desired that it should be placed under the care of the Sisters of Charity. Books, newspapers and games were provided for the convalescent patients. According to Quinlan one third of the patients in St Vincent's passed through Linden. Stables were constructed at the back of the hospital to house vehicles taking patients to Linden. Between the hospital and the convalescent home 120 patients were accommodated daily. Quinlan stated that 800 patients were admitted each year to the hospital of whom about sixty died. Six thousand patients attended during each year at the out-patients' or dispensary. There was absolutely no religious discrimination and clergy of all denominations were admitted to see the patients of their own particular religion. Concluding his account, Francis Quinlan stated that it was the object of the hospital 'to teach the poor, to visit and heal the sick, to save from falling and to rescue the fallen'.[7]

It is hard to appreciate the intense interest that the establishment of St Vincent's generated amongst the Victorian public. Hospitals organised, founded and run by women were a complete novelty in the social, political and medical customs of the time. Mrs Aikenhead and community had no shortage of visitors who came to study this new phenomenon and to see how it was working. The visitors included many famous people well known in politics and in the public affairs of the nation. In 1839 Fr (later Cardinal) Wiseman visited his cousin Mother McCarthy in the hospital and also had a long interview with Mrs Aikenhead. He had come to Dublin to preach on the occasion of the consecration of St Andrew's Church, Westland Row.

Daniel O'Connell was very interested in St Vincent's. In July 1840 he attended a meeting in the hospital and made a speech in its support. Edmund Rice, the founder of the Christian Brothers, and Gerald Griffin, the poet and novelist, were frequent visitors. Gerald Griffin's sister, Sister Baptist, was a member of the congregation. Another famous poet of the time, James Clarence Mangan, was for a period in the hospital, not as a visitor but as a patient in St Patrick's ward. He was treated for over-indulgence in opium and he contrasted the luxury of the clean sheets of the hospital with the wretched garret in which he lived. Not surprisingly he was a rather troublesome patient. One of the sisters who was willing to excuse his peculiarities simply remarked, 'Those poets have nerves at every pore.' Thomas Moore also made a tour of the hospital.

The title of hospital poet must go to Richard Dalton Williams. He was born either in Tipperary or in Dublin in 1821. He was educated by the Jesuits in Tullabeg and in St Patrick's College, Carlow. He entered St Vincent's in 1843 as a medical student under the direction of Dr Bellingham. He was described as a shy young man who spoke but little and rarely lifted his eyes or even his spectacles in the presence of the Sisters of Charity but he had written some fiery war songs and was known as 'Shamrock' of the *Nation*. Together with Kevin Izod O'Doherty, a future surgeon to the hospital, he was one of the registered proprietors of the *Irish Tribune* newspaper.

When the nuns heard about his poetic gifts he was immediately pressed into service and he translated the *Stabat Mater*, the *Dies Irae* and the *Adoro Te Devote* which were inserted in the manual of the hospital. One of his poems was 'The Dying Girl', the inspiration of which he found in St Vincent's in 'an Ormond peasant daughter with blue eyes and golden hair', who died, presumably from consumption.

When I saw her first reclining,
Her lips were moved in pray'r,
And the setting sun was shining
On her loosened golden hair.
When our kindly glances met her,
Deadly brilliant was her eye,
And she said that she was better,
While we knew that she must die . . .

Some of his best-known lines are in his poem entitled 'Sister of Charity', in which he praises the work of the sisters:

Sister of Charity! gentle and dutiful
Loving as seraphim, tender and mild
In humbleness strong and in purity beautiful
In spirit heroic, in manner a child.

Williams fell foul of the authorities in the 1848 Rising and was accused of trying to depose and levy war against the Queen by publishing certain articles in the *Irish Tribune*. In his defence he read out in court 'The Sister of Charity'. The jury returned a verdict of not guilty. In 1849 he went to Edinburgh and took his diploma. In 1850 he was house officer in Dr Steevens' Hospital. He emigrated to America in 1851 and was appointed Professor of Belles Lettres in the Jesuit College at Mobile. In 1856 he practised medicine in New Orleans where he married Isobel Connolly, a girl of Irish descent. He died of the disease about which he had written so much, in Louisiana in July 1862.[8]

On a more academic note Dr Edward Pusey, co-founder with John Henry Newman of the Oxford Movement in the Church of England, climbed the stone stairs to the top storey of the hospital where Mrs Aikenhead's office was situated. He was looking for a rule for the Anglican sisterhood he was about to establish. When John Henry Newman was Rector of the Catholic University in the 1850s he lived in Harcourt Street and frequently said Mass in the hospital chapel.

In the summer of 1852 one of the most eminent Victorians of them all visited the hospital. At that period Florence Nightingale had decided that her aim in life was to nurse the sick or rescue the fallen. She was most anxious to train as a nurse. When on a visit to Rome in 1847 she became friendly with Henry Edward Manning, a distinguished Church of England clergyman. By 1852 Manning had become a Catholic and at this stage was a Catholic priest. He was subsequently to be Cardinal Archbishop of Westminster. Manning said of Florence, 'She was torn at one time between her vocation to God and to humanity, at another time between the Church of her home and the Church of Rome.'

Florence Nightingale appeared to be on the verge of joining the Catholic Church. In the Church she felt that she would better carry out her mission of nursing. In June 1852 she wrote to Manning:

> If you knew what a home the Catholic Church would be to me. All that I want I shall find in her . . . The Daughters of St Vincent's would open their arms to me this they have already done so . . . for what training is there compared to that of a Catholic nun . . . there is nothing like the training (in these days) which the Sacred Heart or the Order of St Vincent's gives to women.

She wrote in July 1852 to Manning:

> The question which you were kind enough to say you would ask for me is whether they would take me at the hospital of St Stephen on the Green in Dublin (which is served by the Sisters of Mercy) for three months as I am: I could not go for more at present and therefore it would not do for me to go into the noviceship. Novices are seldom, postulants never I believe, employed in the hospital. I want to be employed there at once, for it is not for the purposes of retreat that I go, which I could do elsewhere with less anxiety to my people, but to learn their trade. I have a particular reason for wishing to be under St Vincent; I have obligations to him. I do not wish to trouble you for information which I could get myself. But I do not think they would take me on these terms without a recommendation which you alone could do for me. I should not wish the patients to know I was not a Catholic nor anyone but the Reverend Mother and the priest . . . I really believe that it would give my dear people less pain for me to become a Roman Catholic and marry than it would be for me to become a Sister of Charity.

She wrote again:

> I really don't know what I am going to do but if I do not see you again, St Vincent's Hospital, St Stephen's Green is the place and the Reverend Mother's name is (or was) McCarthy. Eight years ago I tried to do this and failed.

She wrote again on 7 September 1852:

> I am leaving Ireland without having accomplished one object for which I came; I shall try once more at Dublin whether it is possible to do anything there. We shall be there tomorrow 'till Saturday and then I suppose we will return to England.

A comment can be made on this correspondence. Florence Nightingale got her orders mixed up; the hospital 'St Stephen on the Green' was of course under the direction of the Irish Sisters of Charity and not the Sisters of Mercy. The Sisters of Mercy Hospital, the Mater, was not to open until 1861.[9]

According to her biographer Cecil Woodham-Smith, Florence Nightingale was in Dublin in August 1852 and visited St Vincent's. Apparently the hospital had got a holiday as it was being repaired, so there was nothing to be seen. Also according to Woodham-Smith, Florence Nightingale had an unhappy experience in a Dublin hospital. In a 'memorandum of 1852' she wrote of a 'terrible lesson learned in Dublin' and her inclination to Roman Catholicism vanished.[10] It is quite reasonable to accept that construction work was being carried out, as the hospital was constantly under repair and expanding. However, the main reason for refusal to accept her for training was that only members of the congregation were being trained as nurses at this time. One can only wonder what would have happened if Florence Nightingale had started her nursing training in St Vincent's. It is one of the big 'ifs' of Irish medical history.

Perhaps the greatest tribute to the work of the young hospital came not from Ireland or England, but literally from the other side of the world. The hospital's fame had spread to Australia. In 1836, Archbishop Polding, Vicar Apostolic of New Holland and Van Diemen's Land, wrote to Mrs Aikenhead asking that a community of Irish Sisters of Charity would be sent to Sydney, New South Wales, at that time a penal colony. His Vicar General, Dr Ullathorne (afterwards Archbishop of Birmingham), visited Mrs Aikenhead on his trip to Ireland in 1837 and requested her to send out sisters to Australia. Mrs Aikenhead consented to his request.

Six sisters volunteered for the Australian mission, and five were selected including one who had already studied in France. They left Dublin for London on 12 August 1838 and set sail from Gravesend on 18 August. Dr Ullathorne was also on the voyage. They arrived in Sydney Harbour on the last day of 1838. St Vincent's Hospital Sydney was founded in 1857. This is not the place to describe the achievements of the Australian mission, but it is good to know that St Vincent's Hospital Sydney and St Vincent's Hospital on the Green in Dublin share common origins and ideals.

In the early 1840s Mrs Aikenhead's health was deteriorating and the hospital was an unsuitable residence for her. In addition to the spinal trouble, she was developing bronchitis. She found the climb up the stone stairs of the hospital to her room very difficult. There were to be no lifts in St Vincent's for many years.

In 1844 the congregation had purchased a large house belonging to the Society of Friends at Harold's Cross. It had become the novitiate and mother house. Harold's Cross was at this time well situated in the country and was ideal for Mrs Aikenhead. She took up residence there and it was her home until she died on 22 July 1858.

The working men of Dublin sent a deputation to beg the honour of carrying her coffin to the grave. This was conceded and—very fittingly—it was not the great of the land, but sons of toil, men such as those whom she had first known and loved at Eason's Hill, who were privileged to carry the remains of Mary Aikenhead to her final resting place.[11]

CHAPTER 5

A TEACHING HOSPITAL

A part from caring for the sick it was also the duty of the voluntary hospital to educate the doctors of the future. It was the good fortune of St Vincent's to open its doors during a most fertile period in the history of medical education. Up to approximately the end of the 1820s it was possible for medical students to qualify without ever examining a patient. They had little opportunity to examine patients at the bedside and their lectures were long, boring and didactic and in many cases written in bad Latin.

Robert Graves of the Meath Hospital introduced to Dublin a system of teaching that was unique to Ireland and Britain and had its origins in the German schools. The main emphasis was on bedside management and the examination of the patient in the ward. The student was encouraged to take a history directly from the patient, then to examine the patient, to make notes and finally to discuss the diagnosis, pathology and treatment. In its essentials this method of teaching students is still used throughout the medical world. Such sensible and practical methods of teaching obviously fell on fertile soil in St Vincent's. Teaching in the hospital was expertly organised by O'Ferrall no doubt with the active encouragement of Mrs Aikenhead who as ever realised the importance of adequate training.

By 1839 the hospital could announce that the clinical lectures delivered in St Vincent's and certificates of attendance and its practice were recognised by the Colleges of Surgeons in Dublin and London. Many of the students attending St Vincent's took the Licentiate of the Royal College of Surgeons. This was a four year course and three of the four years had to be passed in attendance at lectures in hospitals recognised by the Council. Some students sat for the Licentiate of the King and Queen's College of Physicians in Ireland. This course also lasted four years and again the student had to attend lectures in a recognised hospital. Tuition at a hospital like St Vincent's was eight to nine guineas per year and the total cost for a medical student in those years was approximately £400–£500.

The Medical Act of 1858 revolutionised medical education in the United

Kingdom. It instituted a General Medical Council which was empowered to keep a register of qualified medical men. The General Medical Council supervised professional study and examinations and reported defects to the Medical Council.

O'Ferrall has left an account of the methods of teaching in St Vincent's Hospital during the second half of the 1850s. It shows that the Irish medical schools of the period were well ahead in their methods of teaching students.

> The pupils to be arranged in pairs and to each pair be assigned the care and registry of two or more cases. The pairs to consist of one senior and one junior pupil; the latter to be employed by the former in writing and other duties directed by his more experienced colleague. The cases committed to their care for registry to consist of an equal amount of instances of external and internal pathology or of surgical and medical cases as they are commonly called. A registry of the private facts of each case to be kept at the head of the bed and the senior pupil whose duty it is to keep it shall be required to read the report at each visit. One morning in each week, after the visit the class shall be assembled in the theatre and the senior pupils shall be required to produce the finished cases or registries and to give an account of the grounds on which the diagnosis has been made. At the foot of every bed in the hospital and fixed to the iron rails there is a long metal tray; on this are placed every morning several glass vessels containing specimens of the renal secretion, expectoration, discharges from abscesses and from the vesications of blisters etc. as the case might be. The eye is thus trained to observe the different tints, degrees of transparency and deposits, which a walk through wards ninety feet long shall bring to his notice.

Apparatus for chemical analysis, such as litmus, acids and alkalines, test tubes, spirit lamps etc. were left on a table in every ward. Post-mortems were carried out in the pathology theatre, which was a separate building connected by a small courtyard with the lecture and operating theatres. The building was 24 feet square and 26 feet high with a lantern window at the top through which the 'lighter gases immediately escape'. Under the top light was a table with leaden cover with an aperture in the middle through which liquids escape to the sewers. The assembling of the class in the lecture theatre to discuss the diagnosis of cases is still very much in vogue today, and is called a clinical pathological conference.[1]

In May 1845 a Bill to establish the Queen's University of Ireland with constituent colleges at Belfast, Cork and either Galway or Limerick was introduced into the House of Commons by the government of Sir Robert Peel. The colleges were to be strictly non sectarian; there was to be no religious test for admission, nor religious instruction in the colleges. In 1847 the proposed establishment of the colleges was condemned by Pope Pius

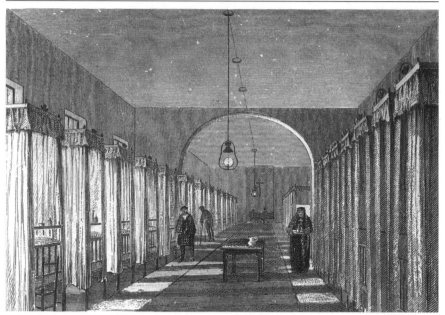

Male ward in the hospital, *c.* 1850–60

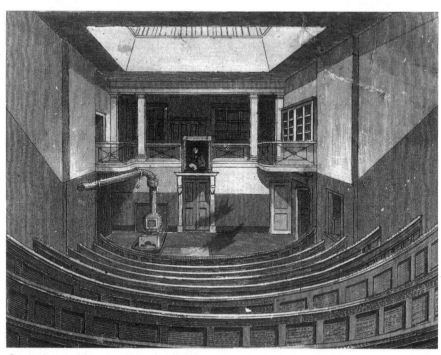

Operating and lecture theatre, *c.* 1865

IX. They were described as the 'Godless colleges' and were vehemently opposed by the Catholic hierarchy. A Synod of the Bishops was held in Thurles in August/September 1850 and the bishops of Ireland formally denounced the Queen's colleges as unsuitable for Catholics.

The hierarchy resolved to found a Catholic University modelled on the University of Louvain in Belgium. Dr (later Cardinal) John Henry Newman, an outstanding Catholic intellectual of his day, was formally invited by the Irish Catholic bishops to become Rector of the new Catholic University which was to be established at 86 St Stephen's Green. The new Rector gave ample proof that he realised the importance of establishing a medical faculty in the new university. In one of his famous discourses on university education he stated: 'Looking at medicine merely as an art, and that one of the most primary and necessary arts of life, the difference which results to a Catholic population is incalculable between the presence of a body of practitioners who recognise the principles and laws of its religion, or of a body of men who are ignorant or make light of them.' Newman quickly sized up the medical situation in Dublin, as can be seen from his report to the hierarchy for the session 1855–56 of the university:

> The medical establishments have been simply in the hands of the Protestants; and without going out of my way to complain of the fact, I may fairly record it as a reason for feeling satisfaction at the prospects which are now opening upon us of its alleviation. I understand that at this time out of all the Dublin hospitals, only three have any Catholic practitioner in them at all, and that even in these three, the Catholic officials do not exceed the number of Protestants. On the other hand out of sixty-two medical officers altogether in the various hospitals, the Catholics do not exceed the number of ten. Again out of five medical schools in Dublin (exclusive of our University) three have no Catholic lecturers at all, and the other two have only one each; so that on the whole, out of forty-nine lecturers only two are Catholics. Putting the two lists together, we find that out of one hundred and eleven medical practitioners in situations of trust and authority, twelve are Catholics and ninety-nine Protestants. And while the national religion is so inadequately represented in the existing schools of medicine, so on the other hand, in a Catholic population there is an imperative call for Catholic practitioners.

The school of the Apothecary's Hall which was situated in Cecilia Street, a short narrow street which runs between and parallel to Dame Street and Wellington Quay, was shutting down. Through an intermediary Newman purchased the building for the site of the new medical faculty of the Catholic University. The school was formally opened on 2 November 1855. In the 1850s Dublin possessed nine general teaching hospitals, most of them small, and rivalry between them was considerable. This feature of Dublin medicine has existed up to modern times. Each hospital had a traditional loyalty to a particular medical school. As Newman had observed, practically all the hospitals were Protestant in their philosophy of teaching. For Newman's medical school there was only one hospital to which he could turn for the clinical training of the students and this was St Vincent's. As Rector of the Catholic University Newman was a frequent visitor to the hospital. Negotiations between the hospital and the university for the admission of medical students to the hospital for teaching purposes commenced in the summer of 1856. Much of the negotiation is outlined in correspondence between Scratton, secretary to the university, R.S.D. Lyons, the first Professor of Medicine in the Medical School, and O'Ferrall. Lyons, the son of a Lord Mayor of Cork, was one of the leading physicians of the period. He was an expert on the microscope and had been pathologist to the British forces in the Crimea. Negotiations obviously were rather difficult at times.

In a letter from Lyons to Newman dated 18 June 1856, Lyons had reported on an interview with O'Ferrall. O'Ferrall thought St Vincent's would be giving more than receiving, but according to Lyons he was most friendly and did not view the proposed connection of the hospital with the Catholic University in an unfavourable light. Lyons felt that for the present Newman should be satisfied with having the hospital declared a 'clinique' of the university—'more advantageous arrangements could be subsequently effected'.

In a letter from Scratton to Newman on 19 June 1856, Scratton stated that O'Ferrall was willing that St Vincent's would be a 'clinique' and that the students should go to St Vincent's for instructions in clinical medicine. O'Ferrall was prepared to give Lyons all necessary apparatus for teaching pathology in the hospital. Scratton also said that the Archbishop, Dr Cullen, was very anxious that the school should have the great blessing of working side by side with religious—'and that the nuns would advance the glory of God by allowing students to be associated with them'. On 20 June O'Ferrall wrote to Scratton:

> In my interview with Dr Lyons I expressed my willingness to make the accumulated resources of my present position as Clinical Professor of St Vincent's Hospital available for the advantage of your pupils, but I frankly avowed a resolution (long since made) not to undertake any new responsibilities which must encroach on the time and attention required by the daily duties of private practice.

Another difficulty O'Ferrall had was outlined in a letter from Scratton to Newman dated 21 June; O'Ferrall would not undertake the professorship of clinical surgery and medicine unless the students were prohibited from attending any other hospital than St Vincent's. Scratton believed that Ellis (Professor of Surgery) would object to not being able to take students to

Jervis Street. Newman informed Lyons on 20 June that he proposed to offer O'Ferrall the chair of clinical instructions and Lyons that of the practice of medicine and pathology, but added: 'If I do not succeed in getting medical officers in St Vincent's Hospital I am at a loss what to do as regards this offer to you as I cannot offer you the practice of medicine unless you are able to get into a hospital without one.' Lyons, although proposed Professor of Medicine in the university, had no hospital appointment.

In August 1856 Lyons wrote to Newman concerning what he described as 'the all important subject of hospital'. He wanted also to discuss the succession to Dr Bellingham: 'This highly accomplished physician and excellent gentleman is attacked by cancer and his tenure of life is from the circumstances, I am informed, of the shortest. I am getting applications made for the succession to this post.' He asked Newman could he put any influence in motion in this matter. He observed: 'Mrs Aikenhead is, I believe, the final authority but Mrs McCarthy, the Superioress of the hospital is very influential. She is I am informed a cousin of the Lord Cardinal of Westminster.'

On 4 September, Lyons wrote to Newman that he had heard that 'It is of the very first importance that the Professors of Medicine and Surgery should have a recognised connection with some hospital.'

Certain facts can reasonably be deduced from this correspondence. The university authorities were anxious to use St Vincent's as a teaching hospital of the Catholic University and O'Ferrall did not appear to welcome this proposal completely. He wished to have the monopoly of teaching Cecilia Street students; it is possible also that he did not wish to have his private practice interfered with. Lyons had to wait another year for an appointment to a teaching hospital and in 1857 he was appointed physician to the Charitable Infirmary in Jervis Street. In any case St Vincent's was to have a long and fruitful collaboration with Newman's medical school in Cecilia Street in the teaching of generations of medical students.[2]

Admission ledgers of patients for the years 1853–57 give a picture of the type of cases admitted to the hospital during this period and of the clinical material for teaching medical students. The wards which admitted female patients were St Joseph's, St Anne's, St John's, St Camillus's and St Mary's. Admission to the hospital was usually achieved by sponsorship from members of the aristocracy or of the wealthy middle classes who were donors to the hospital. Subscribers to the hospital funds had obvious influence in getting poor people, in whose welfare they were interested, admitted to the hospital wards. Clergymen were also frequent sources of referral. In the case of acute admissions to the hospital the reason for admission was tersely given in the appropriate column in the ledgers as 'necessity'.

Many of the diseases from which the patients were suffering have disappeared but there are some which still haunt medical science today. Rheumatism and rheumatic arthritis in its various manifestations was a very common cause of admission to the hospital. Others recorded were phthisis erythema nodosum, bronchitis, epilepsy, anthrax, dropsy, eye conditions, chlorosis, varicose ulcers, hepatitis, erysipelas, haemorrhoids, diseases of the heart, tetanus, and many gynaecological conditions. Many of these diseases have now vanished but enough of them are left to challenge the medical skill of the late twentieth century. In the results column of the ledger the remarks are equally short. The patient either died or was relieved or improved or in some cases cured.

The majority of patients came from the inner city area but many of them came from the suburbs and around the country. Some came from Athlone, Longford, Clonmel, Kingstown, Co. Louth, Co. Kildare. One patient came from as far away as Anglesey, North Wales. The majority of patients were in the twenty to forty age group and their occupations reflect a social structure which has long disappeared. Over 90 per cent of the women admitted to the hospital were classified as servants. Other occupations were laundress, toymaker, waistcoat maker, dressmaker, egg-counter, book-folder, washerwoman, milliner, and the occasional factory girl, glovemaker, school mistress.

There were many admissions to the children's ward (which was apparently St John's) and the ledger entries make sad reading. Daniel aged four from Athlone died of tetanus following a laceration of the foot and toes. James aged six from Cross Kevin Street died with symptoms of tetanus inflammation of the brain and acute pneumonia. Andrew aged three of Cuffe Street was suffering from disease of the spine and was slightly improved. Luckier were Alfred aged five from Abbey Street whose scrofulous ophthalmia was much improved and Kate aged three from Great Brittian Street was relieved of her bronchitis.

The entries in the ledgers of the men's wards follow roughly the same pattern. There were more cases of injury and in general the men were of an older age group than the women patients. Conditions from which males suffered were rheumatism, rheumatic arthritis, diseases of the abdomen, emphysema, Bright's disease, phthisis, leg ulcers, dyspepsia. The wards in which they were treated were St Patrick's and St Laurence's. Far and away the most common occupation given in the charts was that of labourer. Other frequent occupations were butler, baker, cabinet-maker, carpenter, plasterer, coach-driver and game-keeper. In November 1855 forty-five men and seventy women were admitted to the hospital during the same period. In November 1865 thirty-four men and thirty-eight women were admitted to the wards. Sponsors for their admission to hospital were again friends of the congregation and many clergymen.

CHAPTER 6

NEW GENERATION

By the 1860s St Vincent's was ready for further expansion under the direction of a new generation. Many medical historians consider this decade to be particularly important in the history of medicine. It was at this time also that the language of medicine became modernised into terms which are used today. From the beginning of the nineteenth century, however, medicine was gradually illuminated with what we call the scientific outlook, whereby observations, experiments and inference were rated more highly as mental processes than untrammelled speculation. In the middle of the decade there emerged one of the most significant discoveries in the history of medicine: the concept of antiseptic surgery with all its implications was born.[1]

The Rectress of the hospital Mother Magdalene McCarthy was appointed Mother General in 1858 and she was succeeded at St Vincent's by Mrs Margison. The hospital now had one hundred beds. Like her predecessor, Mrs Margison had strong English connections. She came from Preston, Lancashire. When she came to Dublin in her twenty-third year to join the congregation she was accompanied by her brother, a Benedictine monk. He had heard that the novitiate was very austere and tried to persuade her to come back to Preston with him. She remained undaunted and was eventually to become Mother General.

O'Ferrall was beginning to age and his eyesight was failing. According to Edward Dillon Mapother, O'Ferrall always assumed the mixed title of medical advisor to St Vincent's, considering the words 'chief' or 'first' to be unnecessary, for there were only two—and Bellingham always used the title of 'surgeon'. Again according to Mapother, by 1851 O'Ferrall retained scarcely any vision.

> By concentrating his visual organs for a few seconds he had some sight and by means of a slit in a card could read line after line of print very slowly. He would find his way by aid of what I would term a tactile cane and with the assistance of anyone who would truly recount the

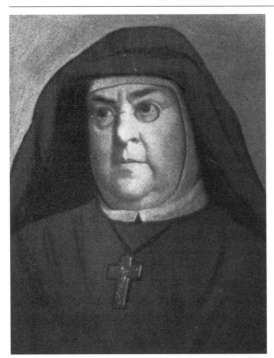

Mother Francis Magdalene
McCarthy, Rectress 1836–58

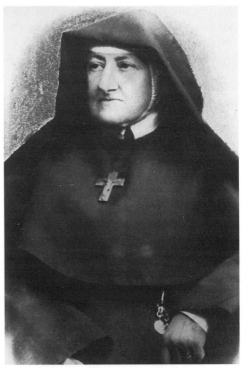

Sister M. Camillus Sallinave

phenomena of a case to him, would make a diagnosis and then promptly advise treatment which was never fallacious. Without such aid his mistakes were often ludicrous. His memory was well and fully stored and his judgement never erred.

His receipts from practice were not what he could have made them with a little more economy of time. His only relaxation was to make frequent trips to London, where he was the welcome guest of the famous surgeon Sir Benjamin Brodie. Although generous and outgoing in his youth, according to Mapother he became parsimonious in his old age. He died in 1866 and was interred in the vaults of St Teresa's Church, Clarendon Street.[2]

In 1857 Kevin Izod O'Doherty and Francis B. Quinlan were appointed assistant surgeons, William J. O'Doherty was appointed surgeon dentist and Mr Patrick Dwyer was appointed apothecary. In the next year O'Doherty and Quinlan were described in notices of the hospital as medical advisors in ordinary.

Kevin Izod O'Doherty, who was born in Gloucester Street, Dublin in 1823, had a stormy career. The son of a solicitor, he was educated in Dr Wall's School in Hume Street, in St Vincent's and in Cecilia Street. In 1848 before he had passed his examinations he became involved in the Young Ireland movement. He started a newspaper, the *Irish Tribune*, together with Richard Dalton Williams. Convicted of treason felony he was transported for a period of ten years. Most of this time was spent in Tasmania. He was pardoned in 1854. Having studied for two years in Paris he obtained the Fellowship of the College of Surgeons in 1857.

He did not stay long on the staff of St Vincent's. He emigrated with his family to Queensland, Australia where he practised medicine. He founded the Hibernian Queensland Society in 1871. He returned to Ireland in 1885. He became a Freeman of the City of Dublin and a Member of Parliament for North Meath. He emigrated to Brisbane in 1888. By this stage he had lost his practice and he died in poverty in 1905. His wife Mary Kelly (Eva of the *Nation*) was a well-known poet—noted for her patriotic poems. A volume of her poems was edited by Justine McCarthy in 1910.[3]

Francis Boxwell Quinlan was born in Mountjoy Square in 1834. His father was the proprietor of the *Dublin Evening Post*, a newspaper of liberal principles. He received his medical education in the College of Surgeons, Trinity College and the Catholic University and was a student of the Richmond, Whitworth and Hardwicke Hospitals. In May 1856 he became a Licentiate of the College of Physicians. He was Professor of Materia Medica in the Catholic University School of Medicine from 1859 to 1900. He gave many years of devoted service to the hospital and to the school, particularly in the realm of teaching.

Mapother was appointed medical officer in ordinary to the hospital in 1859. He was an extraordinary genius and a man of many talents. His portrait shows an intimidating personality with a large thick black beard and

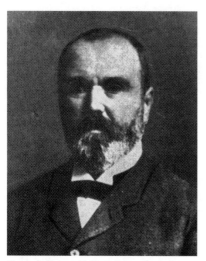

Francis Boxwell Quinlan, physician
1864–89

List of patients

a stern visage. He came from an old Roscommon family, his father being an officer of the Bank of Ireland. His mother Mary Lyons was also a member of one of the principal families of Roscommon. He was educated in the College of Surgeons and the Carmichael School and Queen's College Galway, Jervis Street and the Richmond. MacAlister, Professor of Anatomy at Cambridge, left a description of the young Mapother as a demonstrator:

> Mapother was about the only one of the demonstrators who really did his work. The chief work of the demonstrator was to give an impromptu lecture, on any dissected part he could find, to a mob of students who crowded around him. In this kind of work he excelled; he had a clear voice, a very rapid utterance, and a lucid method of description. I can, even after the lapse of half a century, remember some of his commonest phrases and turns of expression.

In 1857 he graduated M.D. in the Queen's College Galway and received the Letters Testimonial of the College of Physicians in 1862. In 1864 he was appointed to the chair of Hygiene in the College of Surgeons and in 1867 he was elected Professor of Anatomy and Physiology in the same school. According to Doolin, 'As a surgeon Mapother was painstaking but not brilliant.'[4] One of his literary ventures took place under peculiar circumstances. Carmichael, Mapother's old teacher, left £3,000 to the College of Surgeons, the interest of which was to be awarded every fourth year as a prize of £300 for the best essay on medical education. Mapother was himself a Professor and member of council, but entered under the pseudonym of 'United and Prosper'; apparently he felt some embarrassment receiving the prize, particularly as it was given in public session.

In addition to these duties and to his work in the hospital, Mapother took a very active part in the political, social and medical questions of the day. Some of his writings and solutions to contemporary medical problems in Dublin have even this day a particularly modern ring. In an article in the *Dublin Builder* Mapother gave his views on the organisation and running of hospitals.[5] He enumerated nine hospitals, the Adelaide, City of Dublin, Jervis Street, Mater, Meath, Mercer's, Richmond, Dr Steevens', St Vincent's. To these hospitals between 1 January and 31 December 1863, 11,991 patients had been admitted. Of these 552 died. Mapother made the point that mortality was proportionately greater than among cases treated in their own homes. He went on: 'I must acknowledge that till every effort is made to prevent by pure air and perfect sewage the occurrence of fever, the treating of it may be compared to the task of Sisyphus . . . I may here express my conviction that with full regard to the necessity of fresh air in these institutions the most contagious diseases may be mixed up with ordinary patients.'

Mapother also had definite views on the organisation and building of hospitals. He was an advocate of numerous windows in hospitals; the hospitals should be surrounded by gardens so that the patients could enjoy the scenery from their wards. Window spaces should be half the wall space. The walls and ceilings should be of light colour and the material should not be porous but hard and polished. He recommended 'pale green paper, not arsenical; varnished has been found the most suitable in the city. Whitewashing of walls to be effective for the removal of carbonic acid should be repeated every three to four weeks.' He stated that ordinary plaster became in a few years loaded with organic matter. The surface of floors should be polished and impervious to moisture. Stairs and landings should be made of stone. Latrines which were projecting out at the end of the pavilion should have their closets along their outer walls. Partitions should not reach the ceiling and the latrines should be kept aired by opposite windows kept open.

In an essay on the medical profession and the education and licensing bodies,[6] he pointed out that the number of beds per inhabitant in Dublin was 1 to 254, London 1 to 500, Edinburgh 1 to 375, Paris 1 to 167 and Glasgow 1 to 530. He said there were ten hospitals in Dublin and they were too small. He stated that hospitals are injudicious and old-fashioned institutions and that a well-organised system of home treatment was more calculated to aid the sick and at a lesser expense. He believed that the appointment of a whole-time pathologist could not be afforded without amalgamation of hospitals.

He noted that St Vincent's had one hundred beds, four clinical teachers and was directed by the Sisters of Charity. It received £300 from Dublin Corporation. It possessed a sanatorium with twenty beds at Stillorgan. There was a separate ward for children at St Vincent's. According to Mapother £90 paid for all the lectures in hospital needed for the Diploma of the Dublin College of Surgeons. Private instruction and books required £20 more. He was rather caustic about the system of examinations. He said that up to 1834 the exam for the Licence of the College of Physicians was in Latin and took thirty minutes. In 1834 two of the examiners in the London College of Physicians were respectively eighty-three and ninety-five years of age.

In June 1869 he addressed the Statistical and Social Inquiry Society of Ireland on the subject of the Dublin hospitals, their grants and governing bodies.[7] He drew attention to the fact that St Vincent's, with the exception of £300 obtained yearly from the Corporation, depended completely on subscriptions and charitable donations. It was wholly managed by the Sisters of Charity who appointed medical officers with the advice of their existing staff.

Apparently an article in *The Lancet* of 5 June 1869 had criticised the system of appointing medical officers or—as we now call them—consultants in Dublin hospitals. It was stated in this article that merit and ability did not have a fair chance and had no chance at all unless backed by the necessary purchase money. Mapother made the point that when some hospital places

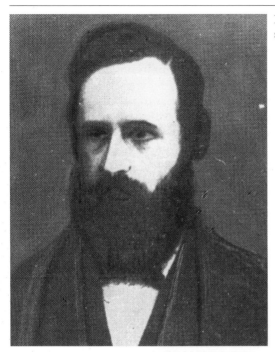

Edward Dillon Mapother,
surgeon 1859–89

Pathological theatre,
c. 1860

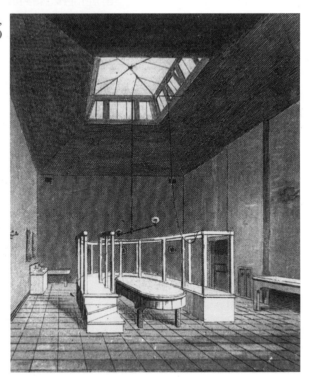

on the staff were bought an element of sectarian prejudice and nepotism also played a part. At the same meeting William Hegarty O'Leary stated that he had the honour of being one of Mapother's colleagues in St Vincent's and that he did not buy his position but worked up from the rank of student to that of assistant.

Mapother returned to the attack in an address to the Dublin branch of the British Medical Association in 1888.[8] Regarding his own hospital, he stated: 'I will only say that although it is large as regards occupied beds and paying pupils, the managers desire to acquiesce in any condition which may increase the usefulness to the sick poor and to the cause of the medical profession. Its distances from neighbouring hospitals are to Mercer's 74 yards and to the Meath 1,000 yards.'

He advocated for the southside the amalgamation of Sir Patrick Dun's Hospital and the City of Dublin Hospital which were only 700 yards apart. He was of the opinion that one hospital should be kept for surgical purposes and the other for medical purposes. For the northside, he agreed with the findings of a recent commission which recommended the amalgamation of Dr Steevens' and the Richmond Hospitals. He said there were too many clinical positions, i.e. twenty-five physicians and thirty-eight surgeons, and the beds in Dublin hospitals were relatively few.

Mapother married Ellen, daughter of John Tobin M.P., of Halifax, Nova Scotia, and had one son and six daughters. He emigrated to London in the 1890s and he became well known there as a skin specialist. He died in London in 1908. His son Edward became a distinguished psychiatrist on the staff of the famous Maudsley Clinic.

William Hegarty O'Leary was born in Dublin in 1836. His father was connected with the building trade and owned a slate quarry in the Vale of Avoca. He was the only surviving son of his parents and he later prefixed an O to his patronymic. He was educated in a small school in Peter Street and subsequently in the Catholic University School of Medicine. In 1862 he became a Licentiate and in 1871 a Fellow of the College of Surgeons.[9] He was appointed assistant surgeon in St Vincent's in 1866 and surgeon in 1869.

O'Leary came to prominence with his involvement in the famous case of The Queen v. Kelly. One evening in July 1871 ex-Head Constable Talbot was returning home to Dorset Street. As he walked up North Frederick Street from Cavendish Row a man ran out in front of him, raised his arm and fired a pistol in his face. Subsequently a man carrying a gun was arrested in Hardwicke Street and was identified by Talbot as his assailant. Talbot died five days later in hospital and his assailant Robert Kelly was tried for his murder before the Lord Chief Justice and the Lord Chief Baron accompanied by the Lord Mayor.

It was the Crown's case that Talbot had died as a result of bullet wounds from the pistol fired at him. The Defence claimed that Talbot had died from bad surgical management of his wounds. At the instigation of Isaac

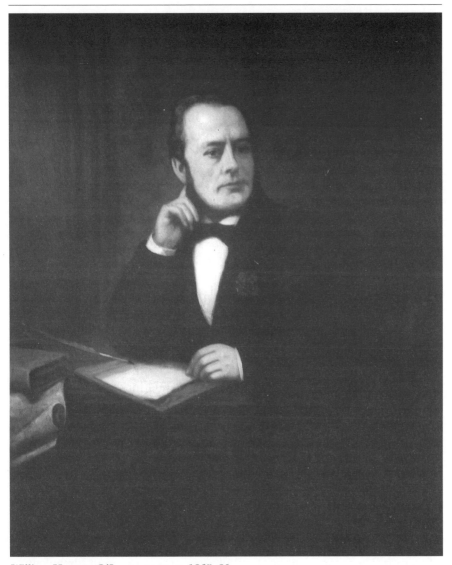

William Hegarty O'Leary, surgeon 1865–80

Butt, the veteran Home Ruler, O'Leary gave evidence for the Defence. Basically the result of the trial depended on the medical evidence and there were obviously political overtones to the case. The doctors from what might be described as the establishment hospitals insisted that Talbot died as a result of the bullet wounds; O'Leary criticised their treatment and maintained that Talbot had died as a result of bad surgical practice. The jury believed O'Leary and Kelly was found not guilty.[10] The trial was dramatised in the play *Trial at Green Street Courthouse* by Roger McHugh.

As a result of the Queen v. Kelly case O'Leary became involved in politics. As Doolin has percipiently stated: 'By saving one man's life O'Leary had to sacrifice his own some ten years later.' He was an example of the aphorism: 'Medicine and politics do not mix.' In 1874 he was elected M.P. for Drogheda, in the Home Rule interest. He had the reputation of being the smallest man in the House of Commons: he stood 4 feet 6 inches, and it was said that his ambitions were 6 feet 4 inches. According to Cameron he spoke very eloquently though rather floridly. He was a fervent admirer of Disraeli and pronounced him the greatest statesman since William Pitt.

An interesting story is told about O'Leary. In 1878 Isaac Butt was seriously ill. He was being attended by Dr Butcher, a well-known practitioner of the time who was also notable for bearing a striking resemblance to Disraeli. O'Leary asked Dublin journalist James Collins what treatment Butt was receiving. On being told, he stated that the treatment was a mistake and asked Collins to arrange for him to be let into Butt's house at 39 Great George's Street so that he could have a consultation with Butcher. The consultation was predictably stormy and Butcher observed, 'I did not come here to learn my profession and if I wanted to learn it I would go to someone else rather than to the member for Drogheda.' Three weeks later Butcher adopted the treatment recommended by O'Leary. O'Leary was informed of this. 'Too late James, too late,' answered O'Leary. Butt died a week later.[11]

Robert Cryan was born in Boyle, Co. Roscommon in 1826. He was educated in the Carmichael School and in the University of Glasgow. In 1847 he passed through the College of Surgeons and through the College of Physicians in 1849. In 1873 he was elected a Fellow of the College of Physicians. He became one of the Professors of Anatomy and Physiology in the Catholic University School of Medicine in 1855. He was appointed to the staff of St Vincent's in 1868 and was the first to practise as a pure physician in the hospital. According to Doolin, Cryan was wealthy and had an unassuming demeanour and this prevented him from making that 'figure before the public eye which a more pushy man would have done'.[12] Cryan may have been shy but he certainly had a distinguished career in Dublin medicine. According to his colleague Byrne, Cryan was a most highly-regarded lecturer in anatomy and physiology and as a clinical teacher in pathology and medicine he displayed remarkable powers. 'He had kindness of heart and simplicity and a thorough modesty in professional matters.' He was particularly interested in midwifery and gynaecology although he did not practise in these specialities. He was instrumental in the establishment of a special ward for gynaecology in the hospital. He died suddenly in 1881.[13]

Around the early 1870s the *Freeman's Journal* published an article on St Vincent's which illustrates the esteem in which the hospital was already held for its work in combating sickness and disease:

> If popularity be any advantage to a hospital St Vincent's may boast of a large share. One of the Sisters' greatest trials is having to refuse admittance to persons who have set their hearts on getting in and yet are not fit cases for the hospital. Sometimes in spite of rules and reasons the poor creatures contrive to have their wish gratified, as was the case on one occasion with a girl whose look of infinite distress and piteous appeal to be received 'until she made her peace with God' so won the Sisters that admission was granted and the afflicted soul restored to grace and happily prepared for death.
>
> People from all parts of the country are to be met with. Even from England will they sometimes come to look for healing. In Lancashire especially the establishment is held in high repute. Whenever there is a Frenchman in the hospital there is sure to be a constant succession of foreign visitors. The French are remarked for their kindness to their sick compatriots and on such occasions they bring in all kinds of dainties and the nicest little dishes imaginable to tempt the languid appetite. Italians too are found on the list from time to time and it is an affecting scene when one of the poor fellows dies and the rest come to mourn over him in the passionate southern manner and take him away for burial. On the return of the Irish brigade from Rome a great many of the brave Zouaves found their way to St Vincent's. I think there were at one time fifteen to sixteen of them, some with wounds and some with agues and chest infections caught in the campaign . . . If bodily strength be not restored the mind at least will be subjected to good influences. If death cannot be averted the passage from life to life through a brief darkness will be made a happy one.
>
> As might be expected the gratitude of the patients is evidenced in many touching ways. I have been shown all kinds of gifts from corkscrews and medicine mugs to ornamental productions for bazaars testifying to the anxiety of former patients to do something for the institution.
>
> One man who had emigrated to Australia used to send half a sovereign every year to the hospital in the old land. The faith and charity of the illustrious order of which it is the special work have found a response worthy of our people. Every class makes some

offering. The poor give their mite. The well-to-do their larger gift. Subscribers of course enjoy the privilege of recommending patients. Rich people who are charitable as well give considerable donations occasionally or have a bed in the hospital to which they can always send a patient. I noticed ten or twelve of these endowed beds which represent twenty pounds per annum each. I am surprised that there are not many more, that all the large manufactories and extensive establishments in the city do not have beds in this or other hospitals to which without strain of public charity the workmen who meet with accidents in their employment by falling from scaffolding, or having been badly scalded or injured by machinery could be sent at once as a matter of right.

Though it is hardly necessary to do so I may as well add that the religion of applicants makes no difference whatever in their reception or rejection. Seldom is the hospital without Protestant patients who are as accessible to the Minister as the Catholics are to the Priest. Amongst the subscribers are many Protestants and I have myself known members of that creed who are warm friends of the institution and constant visitors.

A few years ago the Superiors of the hospital made an application to the Corporation of Dublin stating the difficulty of keeping up the work from year to year and claiming such assistance as similar establishments were in receipt of. Promptly and considerately the claim was allowed and since then a yearly grant of £300 has been allowed to St Vincent's. This is honourable to the Corporation and a great help to the Sisterhood. However, lest it might be supposed that the grant goes further than it really does, it might be as well to mention that the meat bill alone mounts up to nearly £1000 per year.[14]

CHAPTER 7

THE MEDICAL BOARD

In October 1869 a Medical Board was established. It consisted of the physicians and surgeons of the hospital. Present at the first meeting were Dr Quinlan, Dr Mapother, Dr O'Leary and Dr Cryan. The functions of the Board were to organise the teaching of students in the hospital and to advise the Reverend Mother on appointments to the hospital and on matters of medical policy. The members also received fees from the students for teaching, and these were distributed amongst themselves. Rules for the administration of the business of the Board were drawn up. The ordinary time of meeting was to be 11 a.m. and the meeting was called by written notice left at the private residence of each member at least a day before the meeting setting forth the time and place of the meeting and the business to be transacted. The secretary was empowered to call a meeting whenever he thought fit or when he had received a personal or written requisition from a member of the Board to do so. Three members of the Board comprised a quorum for the conduct of business.

Dr Quinlan was appointed the first honorary secretary of the Medical Board. The secretary was instructed not to pay any dividend to any member of the Board who had not declared that he had returned all the names of the students and lodged all fees for the Medical Board of the hospital received by him. The secretary was personally liable to the other members of the Board for the fees due upon every certificate issued by him. It was stated that this liability 'must in every instance be discharged at the dividend meeting next succeeding the issue of such certificate and cannot under any circumstances whatever be held over beyond such meeting'. It was the duty of the secretary when a new student presented himself at the hospital to apply to him for a deposit of at least £1 for his fee. If the pupil declared himself to be an apprentice of any member of the Board then the secretary had to apply by letter to that member for the deposit or a memo of it. Should the secretary not receive that deposit or memo within a week he should again apply in the same manner, and should a second application not be complete then the pupil was treated as an ordinary non-apprenticed student.

In that period there were two types of students: students who were apprenticed in general to the hospital and students who were apprentices to one particular member of the hospital Board. In the second case the appropriate member of the Board had to make sure that the fees were paid to the Board.

In January 1870 the first accounts of the Medical Board were audited. The expenses of the Medical Board, which consisted of newspaper advertisements for the medical posts, stationery and printing, and residency rent, made up a total of £30.15s.4d. This sum deducted from the amount of £86.2s.0d received from the medical students left a balance of £55.6s.8d. Thus, a dividend of £13.16s.8d was ordered to be paid to each member of the Board. There were six clinical lectures given each week in the hospital: on Monday Dr Quinlan, on Tuesday Dr Mapother, on Wednesday Dr O'Leary, Thursday Dr Cryan, Friday Dr Quinlan and Saturday Dr O'Leary. Two resident medical students were also appointed, one for the winter and one for the summer session. Over the next twenty years the number of residents was gradually increased.

Appointments were made by competitive examination. The first resident students appointed to the hospital were Messrs. Ryan and Laffan; they were appointed for the winter session on 27 November 1869. Following these appointments a communication came to the Board from the Reverend Mother expressing a wish that in future the names of all candidates would be communicated to Mrs Margison previous to the holding of the examinations. In November 1869 the Board also booked a lodging house where the students could stay during their term of office. The most suitable lodging house was that of Mr Bolton at no. 1 Lower Leeson Street, who offered a sitting-room and a double bedded room. The terms demanded by the owner were £28 for eight months inclusive of attendance but exclusive of fire, light and washing of house linen.

In May 1869 a house surgeon was appointed. The first holder of the office was a Dr Hillary. The appointment was not made without some friction between the Medical Board and the Reverend Mother. Apparently the Reverend Mother was not too happy with the method of selection of a house officer. The duties of the house surgeon were to attend to all cases of accident and emergency, to superintend or perform post-mortem examinations and to be available daily at 5 p.m. to visit such cases as he might be called upon to visit either by the physician or surgeon in charge, or by the resident pupil or the ward sister. The appointment was for three years at a salary of £100 per annum. In 1889, a physician and a resident surgeon were appointed at a salary of £50 per annum each, instead of one resident medical officer.[1]

In December 1872 the Medical Board organised the construction of a pathological laboratory in the hospital, the first of its kind in Ireland. A sum of £30 was placed at the disposal of the secretary of the Medical Board to carry out the construction of benches and to provide gas apparatus. He was also instructed to devote the residue of this sum to the provision of equipment such as a coarse scales, a sand bath, water bath and an apparatus for drying precipitates. It was settled that each member of the Board should be at liberty to pursue in the laboratory such researches as he should see fit. Chemicals and apparatus would be at his own expense. Each member of the Board who wished it could have a part of the space privately allotted to him; and it was decided that all apparatus provided by the Board should be for the general use and that no part of it would be removed from the laboratory without the special order of a Board meeting entered in the minutes.

Strict rules were laid down for the use of the laboratory by the students. No student whose name did not appear upon the hospital register for the current session would be admitted into the laboratory to the demonstrations or otherwise. No students were to be permitted to remain in the laboratories unless one of the physicians or surgeons was present. The resident students were supplied with keys to enable them to enter the laboratory for the purpose of doing anything directed by the physicians or surgeons. They were not permitted however to lend their keys to any person or to bring any student in, in the absence of the physician or surgeon. No article belonging to the laboratory could be removed from it by any person without the special order of the Medical Board conveyed in writing by the secretary.[2] O'Leary must obviously have had difficulty in combining his medical work with his parliamentary duties at this time, and a plan was drawn up to supplement his duties.

The summer of 1876 witnessed the dawn of specialisation in St Vincent's. Dr John A. Byrne was appointed gynaecologist to the hospital. A special ward for the diseases of women was established and there were to be two gynaecological dispensaries held weekly. It was decided to allow the title Obstetric Physician to be superseded by that of Gynaecologist in accordance with the practice of continental schools. Dr Byrne was empowered to collect his own fees from teaching medical students.[3] John Augustine Byrne was born in 22 Wellington Quay, Dublin on 9 April 1827. His father was a wholesale hat-manufacturer. In 1847 he became a Licentiate of the College of Physicians. He graduated B.A. and M.B. in Trinity College Dublin in 1848. In 1858 he became assistant Master to the Rotunda Lying-In Hospital. He was appointed Professor of Midwifery in the Catholic University School of Medicine in 1859. Byrne died on 13 January 1891.[4] He strongly advocated the building in Dublin of a Catholic obstetric and maternity hospital.

The next specialist appointed to the hospital was Dr Denis Redmond who became ophthalmic and oral surgeon in March 1880.[5] Denis Redmond was the son of Denis Redmond of Belmont Lodge, Sandyford, Co. Dublin. He was educated in the Royal College of Science and the Catholic University School of Medicine. He became Professor of Ophthalmic Surgery in the Catholic University School of Medicine. Neither Redmond nor Byrne was given a seat on the Medical Board. Redmond was allotted the use of ten beds in the hospital so that it would be recognised as an ophthalmology teaching hospital. Redmond died suddenly in 1892.

In 1879 there were changes in the university education structure of the country which had a profound influence on a teaching hospital like St Vincent's. Up to this time practically all the medical students of the hospital took the Licentiates of the Royal College of Surgeons and of the Royal College of Physicians. In 1879 the Royal University with its headquarters in Earlsfort Terrace was established. The Royal was not a teaching but an examining body empowered to give degrees to all candidates on condition of their successfully passing the prescribed courses of the university. For the first time medical students in St Vincent's had access to university medical degrees. At this period Dublin University (Trinity College) was not considered suitable for Catholic students.

In the 1880s the medical course took at least four years to complete. Candidates for the M.B. of the Royal University had to pass the first university examination in arts before embarking on a medical career; they were then obliged to pass the first and second university examinations in medicine and the degree examination. Studies were divided into two periods of two years each. In the first period the student studied botany, zoology, chemistry, histology and materia medica. In the second he took anatomy, physiology, midwifery, medicine, surgery, mental disease and medical jurisprudence. During the first period he attended a teaching hospital for six months, and in the second period for eighteen months. It was also necessary to have six months attendance in midwifery. The medical courses in the Royal College of Surgeons and the Royal College of Physicians were similar; each student had to pass four professional examinations before qualifying.

The Medical Act of 1886 laid down that a person should not be registered under the Medical Acts unless he had passed a qualifying examination in surgery, medicine and midwifery. Shortly after the passing of this Act, the College of Physicians and the College of Surgeons set up the Irish Conjoint Board to conduct qualifying examinations in surgery, medicine and midwifery. From 1 January 1892 an extra year was added to the medical course by the General Medical Council, making it a five year course. From the time that a medical student entered the Royal University he or she could not present him or herself for the final examination until six years had elapsed. The financial burden of an extra year's study for the degrees of the Royal University meant that many Cecilia Street students were unable to avail of the opportunity of obtaining university degrees. During the lifetime of the Royal University, approximately 40 per cent of Cecilia Street students took its course, while 60 per cent sat for the Diploma of the Royal College of Physicians or the Royal College of Surgeons.[6]

In February 1880 O'Leary contracted pneumonia while crossing to England for the sitting of parliament. The pneumonia proved fatal and he died in London at the age of forty-four. Four days later the funeral cortège left his house in Merrion Square. It travelled via Clare Street, Nassau Street and Grafton Street to Glasnevin followed by a large number of mourners including many medical students. Many prominent people, among them the Lord Mayor and Lord Chancellor, attended the funeral or sent their carriages. O'Leary left nine young children to be provided for: a fund was organised among the medical fraternity to pay for their education. It is nice to record that among the first to contribute were some of those doctors whom O'Leary had contradicted in the murder trial some ten years previously. One of his children became a distinguished Jesuit and constructed the first seismograph in Ireland in the grounds of Rathfarnham Castle in 1915.

To fill the surgical vacancy caused by the death of Dr O'Leary, Matthew J. Kehoe was appointed surgeon to the hospital in 1880. In the same year the Medical Board proposed: that St Laurence's should be the medical ward, and St Patrick's the surgical ward; that the children's ward should be turned into an addition to St Patrick's; and that a reasonable number of beds for children should be reserved in the female wards.[7]

In February 1890, the Board discussed the desirability of re-opening the children's wards so that medical students would not have to go elsewhere for lectures on diseases of children. The secretary of the Board was instructed to impress on the Reverend Mother the need to open such a ward. It is interesting to note that over the years since the foundation, the children's ward had been run down and finally closed. In the early advertisements the fact that St Vincent's had a children's ward was specifically emphasised. A possible reason for the change of policy is that in 1876, the Sisters of Charity were invited to take over the administration of the Children's Hospital in Lower Buckingham Street (subsequently in Temple Street). Perhaps the congregation felt that their work for sick children should be concentrated in the Children's Hospital.

In 1882 the Board decided that candidates appointed to any position should undertake, while connected with the hospital, to maintain a permanent residence in Dublin and within a reasonable distance. In 1883 the Board decided that as far as possible the physicians and surgeons should confine themselves to their own speciality.

In January 1883, Dr Quinlan moved that the hospital be placed on the telephone exchange for a period of one year at a cost not exceeding £10, it being clearly understood that no further grant should be sought from the Medical Board for this purpose. The matter was held over for consideration.[8]

On the death of Cryan, Michael Francis Cox was appointed physician. Born in Roscommon in 1851, he was educated at St Mel's College, Longford and the Catholic University School of Medicine and qualified L.R.C.P.I. in 1875. His boyhood was spent in the depressing years following the famine and he was deeply affected by the sufferings of the people. There was considerable criticism over his appointment as physician, it being thought by many that Cox was too young and inexperienced for the position. He was the choice of the Reverend Mother, Mrs Seagrave. Time proved her correct. Cox was to become one of the most eminent physicians of his time. It is interesting that another candidate for the position was Dr George Sigerson who was also destined to play a major role in the professional and social life of the country.

In 1882, there was another significant and important appointment to St Vincent's. John Stephen McArdle replaced Matthew Kehoe. McArdle was to have a glittering career in Irish medicine and in the social and political history of the country. Born in Dundalk in 1859, he was educated at St Mary's College, Dundalk and the Catholic University School of Medicine.

In 1885, new types of appointments were made to the hospital. Michael McHugh was made assistant physician and Richard F. Tobin assistant surgeon. McHugh was born in Dublin in 1855. Before taking up medicine he studied chemistry in Berlin for three years. He graduated in medicine in 1882 after studying in the Catholic University School of Medicine and Trinity College. He also took an M.A. in Modern Literature. Richard Francis Tobin was born in Waterford in 1843 and was educated at the Catholic University School of Medicine. He became L.R.C.S.I. and L.R.C.P.I. in 1864. After qualification he joined the Army Medical Service and was Assistant Professor of Surgery at the Royal Victoria College, Netley. In 1885 he was a field surgeon during military operations in the Sudan. At one stage during the campaign he had 129 wounded men under his care. Of these 124 recovered. This was a considerable surgical feat given the conditions under which he worked.[9]

It was indicative of the importance of the dispensaries in the hospital that the main duties allotted to McHugh and Tobin were to take charge of the medical and surgical dispensaries. McHugh's duties were to attend the hospital at 10 a.m. every day to conduct the dispensary if required. He was also to conduct post-mortem examinations and render such general assistance to the physicians and surgeons in the discharge of their duties as might from time to time be required. In the absence of any physician or surgeon from illness or other causes, the assistant physician was to discharge his duties if called upon to do so. The assistant physician should also discharge the vacation duties of the physicians or surgeons. The assistant physician would not be a member of the Medical Board and would not receive any share of the fees except one fifth of the fees paid by him for his own pupils. The duties of the assistant surgeon were laid down on lines identical with those of the assistant physicians.

Subsequently the Income Tax Commissioners wrote to the hospital to find out the remunerations of the assistant surgeon and physician. Some things never change. It was pointed out to the Commissioners that the assistant physician and surgeon as well as all members of the visiting staff of the hospital gave their services freely and without charge to all patients in

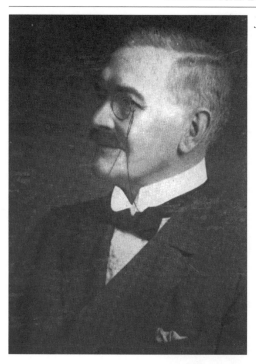

John S. McArdle, surgeon
1882–1928

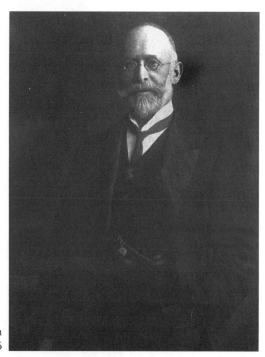

Michael F. Cox, physician
1881–1925

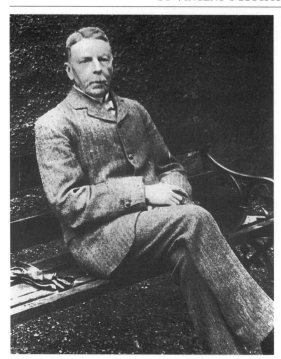

Richard F. Tobin, surgeon
1885–1917

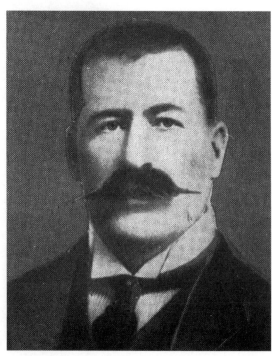

Michael McHugh, physician
1885–1915

the hospital. This system was to last well into the second half of the twentieth century.

Assistant physicians and surgeons had no right to official beds in the hospital, but according to the goodwill of the ward sister were given the occasional bed when the necessity arose. While many of them were subsequently elected as full consultants to the hospital, with beds and a seat on the Medical Board, they had no automatic right to such positions. Again this was a system that lasted until recent years.[10]

CHAPTER 8

THE END OF THE CENTURY

1884 was Golden Jubilee Year for St Vincent's. The *Dublin Journal of Medical Science* for January 1884, like the edition of fifty years previously, contained a mixture of scientific and possibly less scientific articles. An article by Dr Walter Smith of the Adelaide Hospital has a rather modern ring. He pointed out that when two drugs are given one can counteract the effects of the other. He defined an antagonist as 'a substance which operates in a manner physiologically opposed to that of another substance and annuls its action i.e. counteracts not the drug itself directly but its effect'. Another article by an Irish medical graduate on the effects of the climate in the Indian hills on young soldiers is perhaps a reminder that at that time Ireland was a part of a far-flung empire. On a slightly lighter note there was a review of a book entitled *The Law of Sex*; the author's theory was that the father with a Roman nose was more likely to have daughters than sons. The reviewer did not seem to think much of this theory.

In 1884, 15,000 patients attended the various dispensaries in the hospital. There was a statement in the report for that year which sounds familiar to many of us today: 'It may surprise many but it is nevertheless a lamentable fact that unless renewed help be forthcoming from time to time some of the wards may have to be closed as has happened to some of the London hospitals.' Receipts for the year September 1883 to September 1884 amounted to £4,490.15s.10d. This included a recently-increased grant from the Corporation of £400. The other monies came from charity sermons, sales of work, concerts, penny collections and bequests. Expenditure was £5,185.15s.7d leaving a deficit of £694.19s.9d.

In January 1884, seventy-six women patients were admitted to the hospital. Most of them came from Dublin and district, but some came from Roscommon, Longford, Louth, Kildare, Limerick, Kilkenny and Westmeath. A very large proportion of the patients' occupations was given as 'none', but the most common occupation was that of 'servant'. Other common occupations were shop assistant and dressmaker. Emergency admissions were still described as 'of necessity'. Five died. Margaret aged sixty-five died of debility. O.N. aged twenty from cardiac disease. Mary aged forty from pulmonary phthisis. Julia aged fifty from gangrene of the foot. Laura aged twelve from cerebral arachnitis. Mary a dressmaker aged twenty-three suffering from paralysis was deemed incurable. Three young women suffering from pulmonary phthisis were also considered incurable as was Maura aged fourteen with paralysis of the eye and Mary aged forty with facial cancer. Some of the most common problems which are still with us appear to have been adequately treated and cured. They were such conditions as eczema of the legs, haemorrhoids, tonsillitis, enlarged glands, sprained ankles and alcoholism. A rough calculation shows that the average stay in the hospital of the first twenty women admitted in January 1884 was approximately thirty-seven days.

Teaching in the hospital continued to be of very high quality and attracted many medical students—as can be gauged from this table published in the 1891–92 report.

Table
Average Annual attendance during the ten years ending 30 June, 1870: 30
Average Annual attendance during the ten years ending 30 June, 1880: 46
Attendance during session 1880–81: 44
Attendance during session 1881–82: 35
Attendance during session 1882–83: 39
Attendance during session 1883–84: 54
Attendance during session 1884–85: 84
Attendance during session 1885–86: 112
Attendance during session 1886–87: 119
Attendance during session 1887–88: 80
Attendance during session 1888–89: 102
Attendance during session 1889–90: 101
Attendance during session 1890–91: 110

The Golden Jubilee celebrations took place on 23 January 1884. In the morning High Mass was sung by the auxiliary bishop in the presence of Cardinal McCabe, the Archbishop of Dublin, attended by the Chapter of the Cathedral. The music for the occasion was extremely well rendered by the blind choir from the asylum for the blind at Merrion, one of the many noble institutions carried on by the Sisters of Charity. The sermon was preached by Fr Edward Kelly S.J., Rector of Clongowes, who eloquently pointed out the immense good effected for the poor by the holy alliance of charity and science.

In the afternoon a *conversazione* was held in the hospital. According to a contemporary account, all the great rooms, corridors and staircases of the beautiful old house, formerly the residence of the Earl of Meath, were thrown open to the guests. They had been decorated with flowers and plants from the gardens of the blind asylum, and with wonderful scrolls and

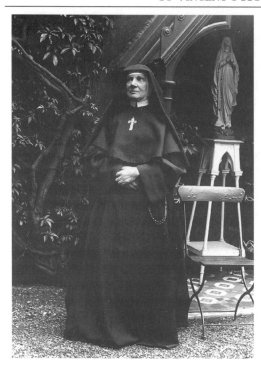

Mother Canisius Cullen, Rectress
1882–1905

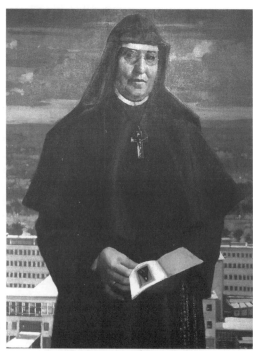

Mother Bernard Carew, Rectress
1905–18, 1924–30 and 1931–35

emblems (religious and national) artistically wrought in flowers and colours on the walls. In the fabrication and mounting of the scrolls the patients of the hospital had assisted, a convalescent carpenter having been found exceedingly useful for the occasion. Lord Meath's former reception rooms, with their richly-decorated ceilings, brown polished floors and conventional simplicity of arrangements, had put on a festive air which for the moment pushed thoughts of pain and sickness into the background, and recalled the old days when brilliant gatherings assembled within these walls at the bidding of a noble host. In the old dining-room of Westmeath House (as it was called in former days), refreshments were served, and the staircases and corridors were alive with visitors hurrying to the drawing-room where a concert was taking place, or to one or other of the apartments where various amusements were provided. Here a phonograph was talking and singing, there the microscope was transforming a cobweb of lace into a fishing net stout enough to gladden the heart of a Claddagh fisherman; while in another room marvels of electricity delighted the astonished audience. From a retired room at the end of the corridor the benevolent Sisters of Charity enjoyed the festivities in their own way, peeping out occasionally like children at a show, receiving a few friends who had discerned them in their retreat, or coming forth when requested to assist and direct, or to conduct visitors to the cheerful homelike hospital wards. One present remarked, looking around the assembly, 'Curious to think that fifty years ago, so many respectable Catholics—even Catholics fit to be seen—could hardly have been found in Dublin'!

That evening at a brilliant concert given in honour of this occasion at Dr Mapother's house in Merrion Square, a fine poem of considerable length was read. With many skilled varieties of metre it told the story of St Vincent's. Few among the fashionable audience appreciated the subtle device of the poet who, when the connection between Richard Dalton Williams and the hospital came to be alluded to, suddenly adopted the measure of Williams's 'Adieu to Innisfail':

> And you great Saints! one first divinely fired
> To give your life for Him who died for man;
> And one whom equal charity inspired
> A code of living martyrdom to plan;
> Stephen and Vincent! join with Charity,
> And fitting laureates of St Vincent's be.[1]

To answer the ever increasing demand on its services, the hospital had to expand. In 1879, no. 55 St Stephen's Green had been purchased at a cost of £1,300 to provide accommodation for the resident medical and surgical officers and for the resident pupils. In 1888, nos. 58 and 59 were bought. No. 58 subsequently became a private nursing home. Another *conversazione* was held in the hospital on 27 February 1889. The purpose of this party was

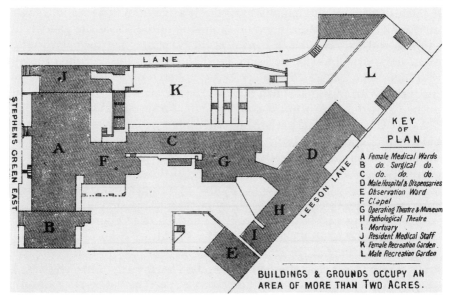

Plan of the hospital, *c.* 1890

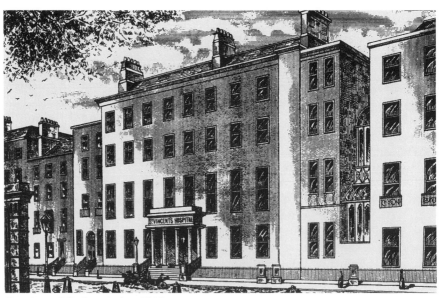

Drawing of the hospital, *c.* 1890

to inaugurate the inclusion of 58 St Stephen's Green in the main hospital. Again the corridors and wards were artistically decorated with garlands, emblems and rare exotics. Over every arch was written a suitable motto of welcome. The party started at 4 p.m. and there were approximately one hundred and fifty guests. They included all the well-known residents of Dublin.

> On arrival they were conducted to the various wards by the medical students of the hospital. The courtesy and conduct of the students was apparently a subject of universal remark. The weather was not too fine on that day but the wards were warm, well ventilated and scrupulously clean; neither did they lose that air of home comfort for which St Vincent's was justifiably famous. After visiting the wards the guests entered the various reception rooms in which entertainments were in progress. In one, amongst the marvels of science, the phonograph was still holding forth, in another a series of microscopes revealed things hidden to the naked eye; while in a third room vocalists of rare merit demonstrated that in the human voice, man has a gift greater than science or gold can ever buy. Excellent refreshments were served all round during the afternoon and the party was over at approximately 7.30 p.m. Again one lady was heard to remark as she left the party, 'The Sisters of Charity do nothing by halves.'[2]

A feature of medicine in the 1890s was the demand for private nursing homes from people who could afford to pay for their medical and surgical care. Up to this time the hospitals were exclusively for the poor, and the more well-to-do people were treated in their own homes. With the rapid development of medicine and surgery and the increasing complexities of treatment, to be cared for in one's own home was becoming impracticable, except for relatively minor ailments.

St Vincent's now expanded into Lower Leeson Street. In 1897, nos. 96 and 97 Lower Leeson Street were purchased and fitted up as a private nursing home. They proved so successful that two years later the adjoining houses in Leeson Street were rented. Communication with the hospital was provided by means of a bridge crossing Leeson Lane and leading directly to the rear of no. 97 Leeson Street.

Over the next ten years the block 93–99 Lower Leeson Street became part of the hospital. In 1908 the charges for rooms in no. 96 (always known simply as 96) varied from three to five guineas per week including dietary as ordered and ordinary nursing. Special nursing, stimulants and medicines were charged as extras. Patients had to make their own arrangements for medical and surgical attendants; no mental or infectious cases were received into the private rooms and nurses were not allowed to receive any gratuity. In 1911, no. 93 was rented by the Sisters of St John of God as a temporary convent during their period of training in the hospital. In 1912, no. 94

Lower Leeson Street which was originally used as a home for the staff nurses was converted into a semi-private nursing home with two to three beds to a room. No. 94 was known as St Winifred's. In 1917, no. 60 St Stephen's Green also became a semi-private nursing home. Nos. 58 and 96 St Stephen's Green were fully private nursing homes with single rooms. In 1911 a small operating theatre was added to no. 58. Up to 1908 operations were conducted in the patient's room in no. 96. Then a bathroom at the top of 96 was fitted up as an operating room and functioned as a theatre for many years. In 1914 a completely new and well-equipped theatre was constructed at the back of 96. The nursing homes were extremely successful and there was always a long waiting list for the rooms. It must be emphasised that all the profits from the private nursing homes went to the general hospital, and were its main financial support.

Over the next fifty years other private nursing homes sprang up near the hospital—in Upper Leeson Street, Mount Street and Herbert Street. Many of them were staffed by former Vincent's nurses and many of the consultants in the hospital attended patients in them. Most of them closed after the end of the Second World War when with the rapid increase in medical technology medical services tended to be concentrated on or around the hospitals.

Lasting until the 1970s, 96 was the most famous private nursing home in the country. Standing tall and imposing in Lower Leeson Street, it was the most regal of homes. Going in through the handsome Georgian door, one was immediately cut off from the noise and bustle of Dublin's traffic, and entered a domain of peace and tranquillity. On the left was the office where sister-in-charge wrestled with the daily task of finding out who was going home today and wondering how on earth she could fit in another dozen emergencies. As usual she could fill her thirty-five rooms ten times over. On the right there was the small elegant parlour where families could wait anxiously for news of their sick relatives.

On the ground floor were several large handsome rooms with exquisitely plastered ceilings and impressive fireplaces. On the first and second floor were similar rooms although slightly smaller. At the return on the first floor was the suitably named room 'Bella Vista' looking out on the back garden and approached by a polished staircase. One could take the lift to the third floor where there were smaller but still elegant rooms, and the ascent by short steep stairs to small rooms on the top storey. On each floor senior and junior staff nurses were constantly going up and down the carpeted corridors, in and out to patients, smoothing their pillows, organising and encouraging them for that awesome trip to the theatre, or preparing them for the all-important visit of their surgeon or physician.

Michael McHugh was appointed to the senior staff in 1889, when Quinlan became honorary physician. Subsequently McHugh became Professor of Materia Medica and Therapeutics in the Royal College of Surgeons. He took a particular interest in the education and training of

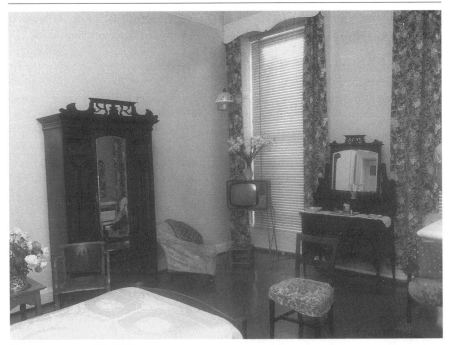

Bedroom at no. 96, 1960s

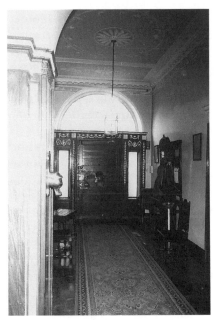

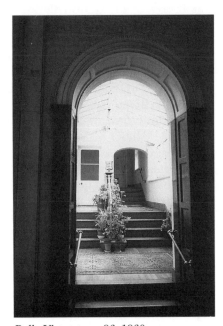

Hall at no. 96, 1960s

Bella Vista at no. 96, 1960s

nurses in the hospital and was also involved in medical politics. At the inaugural meeting of the teaching session 1904–05 in the hospital, he launched an attack on the government in the Castle. He stated that the doctors who administered the Poor Law or dispensary medical system were over-worked and under-paid.

There were several other important appointments made to the hospital during this period. In 1897 William Dargan was appointed physician to the out-patients' department. He was also in charge of the pathology department. Dargan who was a member of a distinguished family qualified M.B.R.U.I. in 1894. His uncle was William Dargan the pioneer of Irish railways and the founder of the National Gallery. He won a scholarship in pathology from the Royal University. He was essentially a bedside physician and was a skilled clinician.

Richard Shaw became anaesthetist and pharmacist to the hospital in 1895. He was described as 'a gentleman of the old school'. Although he had a flourishing general practice, he attended the hospital every day, dressed in a frock coat, tie and a tall hat. On entering the pharmacy department he discarded the hat and the frock coat and donned a small brown apron.

Ferdinand Odevaine was appointed ophthalmic surgeon in succession to Redmond in 1892. Patrick J. Fagan became assistant surgeon in 1895 and full surgeon in 1905. He was born in Co. Meath in 1863 and educated at Castleknock College and the Catholic University School of Medicine. He was Professor of Natural Philosophy in the school from 1901-1904. An interesting appointment in the early 1890s was that of Marcus Bloom, dentist, who lived and practised in Clare Street. This will be of interest to Joycean scholars as it is thought that one of the reasons that James Joyce gave the name of Leopold Bloom to his hero was because Joyce had known of the family of Blooms living in Clare Street.[3]

John A. Byrne was succeeded by Alfred Smith. Smith was born in Cavan in 1861 and educated in St Patrick's College, Cavan and the Catholic University School of Medicine. In his profession he was outstanding as a teacher and as a surgeon. He was appointed Professor of Midwifery and Gynaecology in Cecilia Street in 1891. His scientific mind enabled him to embrace new techniques in surgery.

At the turn of the century the hospital had 160 beds. Life in Dublin during the last decade of the nineteenth century was pleasant for the successful professional man. To be appointed to the staff of St Vincent's Hospital was an indication of great professional success. During this period there was no elaborate system of senior resident medical officers who looked after emergencies in the hospital at night and members of the staff were frequently called out for acute cases; therefore they had to live reasonably near the hospital. The Georgian squares, Merrion Square and Fitzwilliam Square, and their surrounding streets were ideal for the medical consultants of St Vincent's and the other voluntary hospitals. The medical consultants lived in and practised from the large Georgian houses.[4]

In 1908 there were forty-eight doctors living in Merrion Square and twelve in Fitzwilliam Square. The daily routine of the consultants was to visit the hospital in the morning and do ward rounds and examine the patients in their beds. If they were surgeons they would have one or two operating sessions per week in the morning. After seeing their hospital patients they would go down to the back of the garden, across Leeson Lane and into 96 to see their private patients, and if they had time would visit any patient that they might have under their care in the outlying private nursing homes. In the afternoon they would see their private patients in the house. Their consulting room or study would probably be the small front room on the ground floor, and behind it the large dining-room would serve as a waiting room during the day.

There was no such thing in those days as a highly-trained medical secretary answering the door, organising appointments and writing reports. Many of the consultants—particularly the surgeons—would have a butler or 'man' opening the door and letting the patients in and out. In Victorian times he probably acted as coachman also and lived in the mews at the back of the houses. When the internal combustion engine supplanted the horse he would frequently act as chauffeur. After seeing his quota of patients in his study the consultant, if he was busy, would usually go out to see the patients that he had not time to see in the morning, and would re-visit 96 or the private nursing homes. Usually he would dine with his family at approximately seven o'clock in the evening.

If the consultant was well known and at the top of the professional tree he might occasionally be summoned down the country to consult on some wealthy farmer or businessman who could afford the fees. If necessary a special train might be organised to speed him to the sick bed. Medical consultant work was a profitable occupation, during the nineteenth century. A large wealthy Catholic middle class had emerged who demanded the best medical treatment. Compared to modern times there were relatively few consultants and they were located exclusively in the cities.

There was considerable social life during the nineties. Dinner parties, musical soirées and dances during the season were common. A busy consultant in Vincent's had little time for politics; most of them could be regarded as supporters of Home Rule but in no sense could they be deemed radicals or separatists. Michael Cox had an association with Parnell, who spoke from the balcony of his house in Sligo. He was also a friend and associate of John Redmond. Johnnie McArdle with his fiery outbursts would appear to have been an active supporter of the campaign for Home Rule. Richard Tobin with his military background and education would have been an upholder of the status quo. The young members who came on the staff during the first part of the twentieth century were more open in their support of Home Rule than their predecessors, but again were not very actively involved in politics.

In April 1900 Queen Victoria and members of her family paid a visit to

Dublin. This visit came as a great surprise as she had not set foot in that part of her realm for almost forty years. The official reason given for the visit was that it was for the benefit of her health. A slightly uncharitable suggestion was that the real purpose of her visit was to recruit Irish soldiers for the British army—at this time engaged not too successfully in the Boer War. The Queen and her daughter visited many of the Dublin hospitals.

The Irish Times reported:

Yesterday Princess Henry of Battenberg (daughter of Queen Victoria), attended by Miss Minnie Cochrane and Lord William Cecil, visited St Vincent's Hospital, Stephen's Green. Her Royal Highness was received by Mrs Cullen, Superioress of the Hospital, and by the following members of the medical staff. Dr M.F. Cox, Surgeon M'Ardle, Surgeon Tobin, Dr M'Hugh, Dr Alfred Smith, Dr Odevaine, Dr Dargan, Dr Fagan, Mr O'Duffy and the members of the resident medical staff.

Amongst those present were: Most Rev Dr Donnelly, Bishop of Canea, Monsignor Molloy, Sir Gerald and Lady Dease, Madame O'Connor, Mrs Cox, Mrs Tobin, Mrs Shaw, Very Rev Fr Byrne, S.M., Miss M'Ardle, Mrs O'Duffy, Mrs Quinlan, Miss Wogan Browne, Master Cox &c.

In anticipation of the Royal visit a number of people had assembled outside the hospital, who, on arrival of the Princess, cheered Her Royal Highness. Mrs Kelly presented the Princess with a fine bunch of flowers, which the Princess graciously accepted.

The institution was opened in 1834 by the Sisters of Charity. In its external appearance it is not very tempting—there is nothing, in fact, to suggest its extent and magnitude such as would be realised by a walk through its various and spacious wards. The hospital contains 160 beds, which are at present all occupied. The Princess was first conducted to St Joseph's medical ward for females, under the charge of Dr M'Hugh. Her Royal Highness spoke to several of the patients and made inquiries respecting them, as she did in reference to the patients in the various wards which she subsequently visited. St Elizabeth's and St Camillus', medical wards in charge of Dr Cox; St Anne's, in charge of Dr Alfred Smith; St Vincent's female ward, in charge of Dr Tobin; St Patrick's surgical ward; St Laurence's, medical ward; St Bridget's female surgical ward, in charge of Surgeon M'Ardle.

A young soldier named Alfred Carroll Browne, who belonged to one of the Irish regiments, and who was severely wounded on 15 December at Colenso, lay in bed. The Princess heard with marked attention the character of the wound by which the young Irish soldier was put hors de combat. The bullet entered his leg just below the knee and took a somewhat extraordinary course, passing between the bones into the flesh just above the ankle. A few days ago by means of the

Roentgen rays the exact position of the bullet was located, and yesterday that accomplished operator, Surgeon M'Ardle, extracted the bullet, which he now exhibited to the Princess.

In the course of Her Royal Highness's tour through the hospital she was conducted to the handsome chapel of the institution, and viewed it with interest. Before leaving the hospital the Princess inscribed her name and date of her visit in the visitors' book, and Miss Cochrane, Lord William Cecil and Sir Gerald Dease also inscribed their names. Her Royal Highness was throughout her promenade most gracious in conversation with the Superioress, Madame O'Connor and other ladies, who were presented. On leaving she shook hands with the Superioress and Madame O'Connor, and with the principal members of the medical and surgical staff. It may be mentioned that all the decorations in front of the hospital on the occasion of the entry of Her Majesty the Queen to Dublin are still displayed. A crimson cloth was laid down for the visit of the Princess, who, on departing from the institution, was loudly cheered by all assembled.

Queen Victoria left Ireland at the end of April 1900 and within a year she was dead. Her visit to Ireland marked the end of an era. There were to be more Royal visits and the social structures were to continue for another few years but the imperial sun was setting and the sky was darkening.[5]

CHAPTER 9

NEW SPIRIT

The arrival of the twentieth century brought an increased period of social and political turbulence to the country. Inevitably the hospital and its workers were influenced by these sentiments. There was a new sense of nationalism abroad, particularly amongst the younger generation who were flocking to the universities in increasing numbers. Home Rule which had been the ambition of most nationalists was no longer the goal of the young; they were looking for radical solutions and complete independence from England.

They were no longer as respectful as they used to be to their elders and betters. A letter in *St Stephen's*, the University College magazine, 1 March 1904, illustrated this point. Although anonymous it complained that in St Vincent's Hospital 'there was no waiting room provided for the students when they arrived for their clinic at 9 a.m., and they had to wait in cold and draughty corridors. The Professor ambled in between 9.15 and 9.30 a.m. wrapped in sumptuous mantles of fur and frieze.' The writer also complained that there was not a second morning clinic and the morning dispensary did not start on time.

James N. Meenan was appointed physician to the out-patients' in 1906. He was born in Co. Tyrone in 1879 and educated at St Macartan's, Monaghan, Clongowes Wood College and the Catholic University School of Medicine. He became Professor of Hygiene and Medical Jurisprudence in the Catholic University Medical School in 1909. At the same time Robert McDonnell was appointed assistant surgeon to the hospital.

Medicine was rapidly developing into a science and this required more facilities in hospitals, trained staff, increased specialisation and more modern techniques and equipment. One of the most exciting discoveries in the last decade of the nineteenth century had been the discovery of Roentgen or X-rays. They transformed the diagnosis of most medical and surgical conditions. McArdle was quick to realise the importance of this new technique. It will be remembered that he demonstrated Roentgen-rays to the Royal visitor in April 1900. In 1895 with the help of an electrical engineer he installed an X-ray tube in a small workshop near Dublin Castle. He was anxious to get in on the ground floor of this new idea which promised so much in the diagnosis of fractures.[1]

Plans were drawn up in 1904 for an X-ray department in the hospital which was equipped with some primitive apparatus. The duty of supervising the X-ray department fell to the junior members of the hospital staff. J.N. Meenan was persuaded to take up the position of radiologist in 1905 but he soon discovered that his increasing practice would not allow him to continue in this work. He was succeeded by Gerald Tierney the gynaecologist; and Harry Meade was appointed to run the department in 1912. It was several years before a full-time radiologist was appointed in the person of Michael O'Hea.

O'Hea qualified in 1910 and had been assistant physician to the Children's Hospital, Temple Street as well as to St Vincent's. Always immaculately clad in formal attire, he had a fresh flower in his buttonhole every day. He presided over the affairs of the X-ray department with great skill and decorum. Patients were naturally overcome by the awesome X-ray machines and it was O'Hea's first care to put them at their ease. In the hospital he was considered the *arbiter elegantiarum*. The organisation of the annual staff dinner usually fell to the lot of the most junior staff member. He was a prudent man if he consulted Dr O'Hea about the menu. In 1916 a new X-ray apparatus was installed in the disused operating theatre of the hospital which was converted into an up-to-date radiological department.

Michael Curran was appointed laryngologist in 1903–04 and William L. Murphy, a member of the famous Martin Murphy family, was laryngologist from 1908–19. William Dargan became a full physician to the hospital in 1906. Pathology was becoming increasingly important. In 1906 a whole-time pathologist was appointed in the person of Thomas T. O'Farrell. O'Farrell was born in the Punjab, the son of Surgeon General O'Farrell. He qualified L.R.C.P.I. and L.R.C.S.I. in 1906 and subsequently F.R.C.S.I. O'Farrell had to wait until 1924 for a properly-equipped laboratory. Denis Kennedy was appointed assistant surgeon in 1908. He was a native of Tipperary with a formidable personality. He was held in high regard by his colleagues and was considered to be a first class operator in an emergency. He was a pioneer in many of the advances of surgery in the hospital.

In 1909 a new operating theatre was opened in the hospital. It was an octagonal building, well lighted and constructed in every detail with a view to having operations conducted in the conditions the most favourable to antiseptic surgery. The theatre was reached from the anaesthetic room and had a separate entrance from the outside for students. Sliding slabs of white marble were used instead of doors connecting the different rooms. This theatre was to serve as the main operating theatre of the hospital up to 1970.[2]

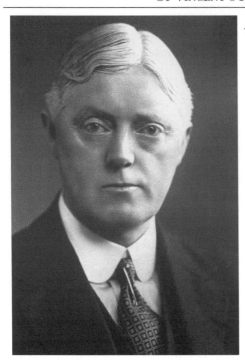

James N. Meenan, physician
1906–50

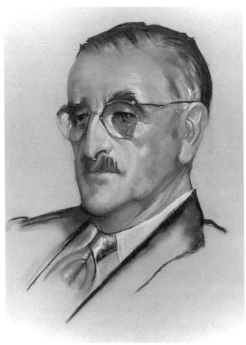

Harry S. Meade, surgeon
1910–52

P.J. Fagan gave an address at the opening of the new operating theatre entitled 'The Vice Regal Microbe'. The background to this was that Lady Aberdeen, the wife of the Viceroy of the period, was conducting a crusade to eradicate tuberculosis which was very prevalent in Ireland at the time. It would appear that Fagan felt that Ireland was unfairly singled out as a country in which tuberculosis was rife and that other countries, just as badly affected as Ireland, were not mentioned. Fagan might have been rather caustic in his speech. In any case Sir William Thompson, physician to the Vice-Regal Lodge, walked out in the middle of Fagan's address.[3]

On the sudden death of Patrick Fagan in 1910, Denis Kennedy became full surgeon to the hospital. Henry Meade was appointed surgeon to the out-patients' department in succession to Kennedy. Meade was born at Amoy, South China in 1884 and qualified L.R.C.S.I. in 1909 and F.R.C.S.I. in 1910. Mother Bernard Carew was appointed Mother Rectress of the hospital in succession to Mrs Cullen in 1905. She was to play a dominant part in the evolution and expansion of the hospital in the new century. It would be fair to say that the hospital was dominated by three members of the staff during this period: McArdle, Cox and Tobin.

In 1889 McArdle visited the famous J.B. Murphy of Murphy's button fame in the United States and studied his methods. In spite of many offers to stay on in the United States he returned to Ireland and to Vincent's. He succeeded P.J. Hayes as Professor of Surgery in the Catholic University School of Medicine in 1904 and was also surgeon to St Patrick's College, Maynooth. A special ward for Maynooth students was established in a large room off the bridge which crossed Leeson Lane at the back of the hospital. He was the most prominent surgeon in the country and his generosity to patients, students and colleagues was legendary.

McArdle was a man of enormous energy and also took a very active part in the social life of the city. In politics he was an avowed nationalist although on one occasion he got into trouble with the students when he stated that the British army had the best medical service in the world. It is said that on the occasion of Queen Victoria's visit to Dublin in 1900 he flew a black flag from his house in Upper Merrion Street. He later moved to Merrion Square South where he put in marble steps up to his front door and was subsequently known amongst Dubliners as Johnnie McMarble. The marble steps still shine outside 72 Merrion Square, one of the last symbols of an era when Merrion Square was the centre of Irish medicine. It is worthy of mention that McArdle was also an international lacrosse player. His father thought he was playing far too much lacrosse when a student and neglecting his studies; consequently he paid a visit to Dublin and confiscated his son's equipment. McArdle had a younger brother Joseph, who was equally brilliant. After qualification he joined the Army Medical Service and died at Khartum in 1903.[4]

Michael Cox, a tall distinguished patriarchal figure, was probably one of the best-known physicians in the country. He had the reputation of being an excellent clinician. He was also an expert on horse breeding and archaeology and wrote several authoritative books on these subjects. As has been noted, he was a great friend and supporter of John Redmond, the leader of the Irish Parliamentary Party, and Parnell had spoken from the balcony of his house. In 1911 Cox was made a Privy Counsellor for Ireland, a singular honour. In this period titles were given out freely to consultants in the Dublin hospitals but not one member of the staff of St Vincent's received such recognition. In Edwardian times Dublin was known as 'The City of Dreadful Knights'. A privy counsellorship must have compensated St Vincent's for the lack of titled members among its staff as it was a unique award. According to T.J. Morrissey, Michael Cox was the first choice of the government for the position of president of University College Dublin on the establishment of the National University of Ireland in 1908, but he refused the post.[5] He was the first chairman of convocation of the National University. He resigned his privy counsellorship in 1920 as a protest against the behaviour of the British forces in Ireland.

Richard Francis Tobin, known as Daddy Tobin, was a complete contrast to Cox and McArdle. He had been a Brigade Surgeon in the Army Medical Service and subsequently Assistant Professor of Surgery in the Military Hospital at Netley, England. He had an austere personality and was a strict disciplinarian. He had the highest standards of ethics and behaviour and required them also from his students. At one of the prize-giving ceremonies in St Vincent's he told a story about an examination in the military college, when one of the porters offered to give a young Irish candidate the details of the specimens which would be placed before him on the day of the examination. Apparently the porter was also an Irishman, was fiercely patriotic and wanted the Irish candidates to do better in their examinations than the English, Scots and Welsh. The Irish candidate refused to accept the information about the specimens and subsequently told Tobin about the episode. Bringing the example of this young man to the attention of the students and praising him for his rigorous honesty, he concluded by saying that it was only what could be expected of a Vincent's student.[6]

One Vincent's student of the nineties would have pleased Tobin. Thomas Joseph Crean was born on Northbrook Road on 19 April 1874. His father Michael was a barrister. His mother was Emma Dunne. He was educated at Clongowes Wood College. He played rugby for Ireland from 1894–96. He is credited with bringing a new dimension to scrummaging by developing the wheel. He joined the British army and was assigned to the first Imperial Light Horse (Natal). His rank was that of Surgeon Captain. He gained the Victoria Cross on 18 December 1901 at Tyger Kloof, South Africa. The citation stated that although hurt, he continued to attend the wounded under heavy fire, at only 150 yards range from the enemy. He did not desist until he was injured a second time himself. For good measure he also held the Royal Humane Society's Testimonial for saving life at sea. Crean died in London on 25 March 1923.[7]

Tobin was particularly interested in the training of nurses and especially theatre nurses in antiseptic technique. He was also a recognised expert on treatment of fractures of the femur.

Francis J. Morrin, who was to be a distinguished surgeon in St Vincent's Hospital, had vivid memories of Tobin:

> The surgeon in charge at the time was Mr Tobin, a retired army colonel who had gained distinction on the battle fields of Adowa and Omdurman. Instead of a sabre, he carried an enormous brass ear trumpet which he wielded like a Field Marshal's baton. I remember stuffing it with cotton wool while he was addressing himself to a trembling student in the class. He came to a recently admitted patient who was dressed up for the occasion in a new linen shirt taken fresh out of the manufacturer's pack. It was a strong linen or twill affair which hung on his frame in geometrical lines, like a problem picture out of Euclid. The sight of it exasperated the old man and he called out 'Sister'. 'Yes, Mr Tobin' was the demure reply. 'Was this shirt washed?' 'No, Mr Tobin, it is a new shirt'. 'Sister, do you, or do you not, wash new shirts?' 'No, Mr Tobin, I mean yes Mr Tobin' replied the now thoroughly frightened new Sister. 'What is it that you are saying Sister?' he roared. I broke in 'Say the Angelus, Sister, tell the old codger anything, he can't hear.' He turned like a flash. 'What are you saying? What did you say? What did you call me? Stand to attention when I am speaking to you'. For the first time in my life I received a good old British Army dressing down, in a voice loud enough to send the startled birds on Stephen's Green quaking wildly over the roof tops. Poor old Tobin. I became his house surgeon, may he rest in peace. He was a martinet and if he had a bark, he had a very gentle bite.[8]

In 1908 a new chapter was opened in the tortuous history of university education in Ireland. The Irish Universities Act of 1908 abolished the Royal University and in its place was instituted the National University of Ireland with constituent colleges in Dublin, Cork and Galway; also affiliated to the new university was St Patrick's College, Maynooth. The Catholic University School of Medicine in Cecilia Street became the Medical School of University College Dublin. The medical faculty of Cecilia Street transferred to the University College Dublin. From now on the vast majority of medical students from St Vincent's took the M.B. B.Ch. of the National University of Ireland.

Medical clinics were held in the wards between 9 a.m. and 11 a.m. daily. There were also special clinics for junior students held on Tuesdays, Thursdays and Saturdays. Surgical clinics were also held daily as well as a junior class three times each week. In the out-patients' department, medical dispensaries were held three times each week at which the students were given clinical instruction; similar instruction was given in the surgical dispensaries three times each week. The students also received instruction in the special departments: pathology, gynaecology, ophthalmology and otology, dentistry, pharmacy, diseases of children and diseases of the skin. There were courses in the application of X-rays to the diagnosis and treatment of injury and disease, and special arrangements were made to instruct the Vincent's students in fevers in Cork Street Hospital. Postgraduate courses were held during the summer and autumn months.

Two resident physicians and two resident surgeons were appointed half-yearly; each held office for six months and received a salary of £50 per annum with furnished apartments, attendance, light and fuel. Sixteen resident pupils were appointed annually, four at the beginning of each quarter. Clinical clerks and dressers were appointed in compliance with the requirements of the licensing bodies; a special certificate was given for this course. Examinations for medals and prizes were also held during the year. The Bellingham Gold Medal in Medicine was competed for in memory of O'Bryen Bellingham. A gold medal for excellence in surgery known as the O'Ferrall Medal was also competed for—this medal was in memory of the first medical director of the hospital.

P.T. O'Farrell (Patsy O'Farrell), a student in Vincent's during the first decade of the century, has left vivid memories of the hospital during that period:

> Even as he approached the hospital a row of handsome carriages would greet his eye, affording no small matter for discussion among connoisseurs of horse-flesh. On entering the portals of the hospital he would be directed by the dignified hall-porter, Kelly, to the students' room where he would be expected to enter his name in a large attendance book—a rule more honoured in the breach than the observance. This book like many other fancies has now passed into the limbo of forgotten things.
>
> Clinical lectures then, as now, were timed to start at 9 a.m., but the customary five minutes' grace allowed by the Hospital statutes was fully exercised by the Staff for the disposal of their top-hats and adjustment of their frock coats before meeting the class.
>
> Students were expected to be punctual in their attendance at clinical lectures. Woe betide the latecomer to Mr Tobin's class. More likely than not he would be summoned forward to the bedside to display his knowledge; many a defaulter will recollect the penalty paid: he might have been encased in splints as a 'practical demonstration', or put up in plaster of Paris, and subjected to even worse indignities to the unholy joy of his fellow students . . . At this time and for some years to follow clinical lectures were almost purely a matter of observation, for such trappings as blood-chemistry were only in the process of evolution, and the diagnostic instruments of precision of later days

were practically unknown or unused. Nearly all students carried a binaural stethoscope in their pockets . . .

Each physician and surgeon at the time had a distinctive personality of his own. 'Johnny Mac' who startled us with his spectacular operations, his diagnostic acumen, and inspired us with the fond hope that some day or other we might be able to emulate his manual dexterity, and afford his expensive cigars! The cynical McHugh, always referred to out of his hearing as 'Mickey', taught us many a good lesson in therapeutics and many a time enlivened his class with literary bon mots, accompanied by a self-satisfied chuckle.

Michael Cox, distinguished among Dublin physicians in both personal appearance and scholarly attainments, whose gentleness of character endeared him to his patients, and who was to our youthful eyes the living embodiment of the 'bed-side manner'. Or 'Paddy', Mr Fagan, of striding step and deep sonorous voice, anatomist to his finger tips and surgeon of no mean merit . . .

'Billy' Dargan, the youngest and most active member of the staff of those days, forms a vital and worthy link between the great men of the past and those of our own day.

Passing down the hospital corridor, the junior student might be amazed to hear a certain locality referred to as the 'dog-house'. In an unguarded moment he might be inveigled by an apparently kind-hearted resident to visit the locality. There he would be promptly pressed into the service of dressing septic wounds and varicose ulcers for hours on end. The 'dog-house' of course was the accident and casualty department.

The old operating theatre occupied the position of what was subsequently the X-ray department. It consisted, as was the prevailing custom, of a large hall with plenty of seating accommodation arranged in tiers. The students' entrance was situated on the landing close to St Laurence's ward. With increasing courage the student would gradually find himself appropriating the front seat directly overlooking the operating table. Rubber gloves were not worn in those days, and face masks had not come into vogue. Great care was expended on the disinfection of the hands, and on the preparation of the operation site. Iodine, as a skin and wound disinfectant, did not come into use until later years when Mr Tobin introduced this method for the first time in any Dublin hospital.

The sponges used during operation were picked up from the operation sheets with a long forceps, they were transferred to a series of basins which were hand-washed by relays of nurses before being deposited in boiling water. After boiling for some minutes the sponges were then wrung dry and used over again during the operation. Denis Kennedy, on his appointment in 1908 as assistant surgeon, introduced a system of 'dry-wipes' into the operating theatre.

The out-patients' department, or extern department, as it was then known, was situated under St Laurence's ward. The surgical and medical dispensaries were held in the one room, the assistant surgeon and assistant physician attending on alternate days. The arrangements for the examination of patients were simple. One end of the room was divided by a wooden partition and two rather dilapidated curtains closed over these primitive cubicles. Overcrowding was the rule, for the attendances at the extern department in those days exceeded eighteen thousand cases each year. The old pharmacy was situated close by and alongside the pharmacy was a special extern department for diseases of women.

O'Farrell recalled that the teaching of pathology was coming very much to the forefront in the hospital. In 1906 a full-time pathologist was appointed. The existing pathology laboratory occupied a small room on St Joseph's corridor. In 1909 O'Farrell was appointed a resident pupil and again has vivid memories of the therapeutics of the period:

The application of half-a-dozen leeches to a congested liver sounds a simple matter enough, but, even *hirudines medicinales* could be sluggards, and force or persuasion was sometimes necessary to make them 'tap the claret'. A piece of apple peel made a fine compelling agent, or else a drop of milk acted as a palatable inducement . . . During his term of residency the student had his first opportunity of becoming closely acquainted with the sisters in charge of the various wards. At that time these nuns wore the conventional black habit of the order with white sleeves and aprons; a full white habit has been an innovation of later years.

O'Farrell wrote that the new graduate had a better chance of being appointed a resident medical officer than previous newly-qualified doctors. In 1904–05 only two resident medical officers were appointed for a period of twelve months. After 1905 the practice was established of appointing four, holding office for six months.

In 1910 Tobin instituted a practical course in anaesthetics for senior students. It was mooted that the students should be charged a special additional fee for the course. Tobin strenuously opposed this suggestion, maintaining that it was the duty of Vincent's to turn out our students complete and proficient in every department of medicine without any addition to the standard teaching fees. Needless to say 'he had his way for he was always a mighty and successful fighter where students' rights were at stake'.[9]

CHAPTER 10

THE WAR YEARS

In the years leading up to the outbreak of war in 1914, the political situation in Ireland was explosive. There was threat of civil war between north and south, over the introduction of the Home Rule Bill in the British parliament. The students in Cecilia Street had the reputation of being very radical in their politics. A political club, known as the Dungannon Club, was started in the school in or around 1905. Its politics were Sinn Féin and even separatist. No doubt many of the students from Vincent's who attended Cecilia Street shared these sentiments.

In July 1914, McArdle addressed a parade of the National Volunteers at his home in Ballyteigue, Co. Wicklow. He was quite bellicose in his approach: if it became necessary for them to leave the paths of peace to which they were so much attached, and if the necessity arose of defending their wives and children he would not be there as their doctor. He would not be there as their friend merely but he hoped he would be there as one of the rank and file of the army that they had started for the defence of their country. Surgeon Boyd-Barrett from Temple Street Hospital who was also on the platform said that 'as McArdle has disembowelled many members of the aristocracy he should be made Minister of the Interior'.[1]

With the outbreak of hostilities the dangers of civil war in the country receded but provoked further divided loyalties. On one side many believed that Irishmen should rally to the defence of small nations and join the British army; while some nationalists believed that England's difficulty was Ireland's opportunity. This tension was illustrated at the inaugural meeting of the UCD Medical Society in November 1914, when Professor McArdle expressed himself dissatisfied with the evidence offered to prove that the German army in Belgium had been guilty of atrocities. When the name of Lord Kitchener, Secretary of State for War, was mentioned there was an outburst of hissing and booing.[2]

In the hospital there were several important changes on the staff. Michael McHugh died suddenly in 1915, and J.N. Meenan was appointed to the senior staff. On the elevation of Meenan, J.B. Magennis, the son of a well-known Dublin general practitioner, was appointed to the out-patients' department. William Doolin was born in Dublin in 1888, the son of Walter Doolin, an architect. He qualified in 1910. He was one of the first honours medical graduates to sign the roll of the National University of Ireland. In 1914 he had been appointed surgical chief in the Anglo-German hospital in Buenos Aires. The outbreak of war prevented him taking up the post. He was appointed assistant surgeon to St Vincent's.

Several present and future members of the staff saw war service. Harry Meade joined the French army, serving in France and in Greece; he was demobilised in 1918. J.B. Magennis also joined the French army. He was appointed Medicine Major in 1917. He worked in the Verdun sector and on one occasion had a very narrow escape from death. He had gone to lunch with the staff of a neighbouring hospital. After lunch he was going back to his own hospital when an intensive bombardment commenced. He took refuge in a nearby wood and discovered that he had lost his bearings. He finally made his way back to the hospital where he had lunched, to find that it had suffered a direct hit and all the officers had been killed. Another future surgeon to the hospital, Francis J. Morrin, joined the British army and was appointed bacteriologist on a hospital ship in the Mediterranean. P.T. O'Farrell, subsequently a member of the staff, served in the Royal Flying Corps and saw service in the Far East. The war was also to bring tragedy to two senior members of the hospital staff. Tobin's only son was killed at Gallipoli in 1915 and one of Michael Cox's sons who also joined the British army was seriously injured.

During the early years of the Great War Sean O'Casey the famous playwright became patient number 23 in St Laurence's ward of St Vincent's Hospital, 'under a Sister named Gonzaga, a delightful woman most popular with the patients, never lax, always lenient, always cheerful with a gay greeting for everyone'. O'Casey had developed tuberculous glands and was sent first of all by his Union to the Adelaide Hospital. There was no bed available for him in the Adelaide and his Union then requested his admission to St Vincent's. His experience there is recalled in *Drums Under the Windows*:

> But now he innocently passed in by the heavy wide double-folding door, glancing at the great brass gong in the vestibule—looking like the languishing shield of Oscar, now dedicated to God—giving different numbers of strokes for the different sisters, with a long solemn one for the Reverend Mother. He turned left down the long tiled corridor, with high French windows along its way, on one side, giving on to a lawn on which, in brief moments of leisure, sisters paraded determinedly up and down, decidedly reading some pious manual, so that not a moment should be allotted to the unthinking world. He passed by the gaudy image of St Michael shoving a tough spear throughout the twisted body of a spitting dragon; perhaps a

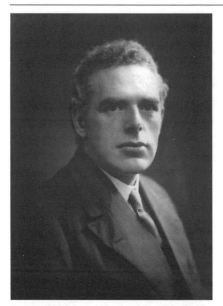

James B. Magennis, physician 1915–40

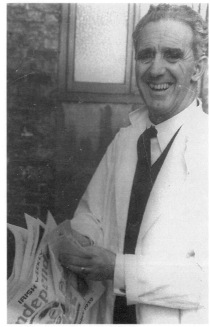

William Doolin, surgeon 1914–57

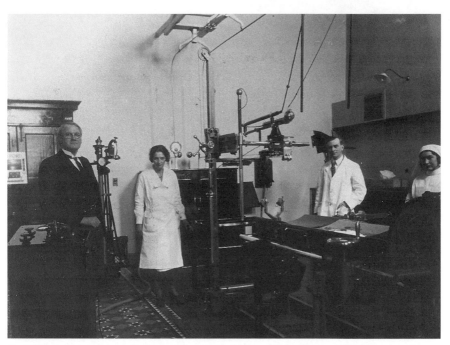

Radiology department. (Left to right) M.F. O'Hea, Molly Gunn, Billy Murphy, nurse

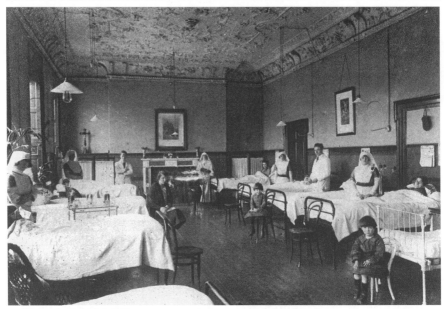

St Joseph's ward, *c.* 1920

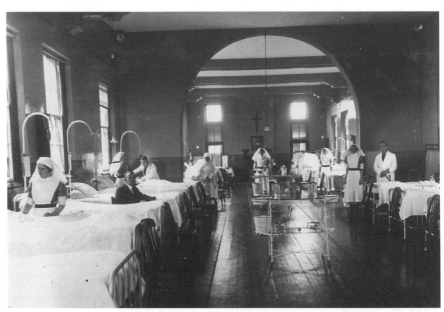

St Laurence's ward, *c.* 1920

white-coated surgeon flitted by, giving importance to a quick walk or a decorous trot, on his way to, or coming from, doing damage to some poor body. Silent nuns, on duty, soft-slippered, glided to and fro . . .

Then up a few steps at the corridor's end if he remembered right to St Laurence's ward, the saint himself frocked, cowled and tonsured, at the entrance, standing deep in stony meditation . . . The ward was a big one long and lofty with rows of beds on each side. At the far end was a huge fireplace with a bright fire blazing, for though it was a warm day the hot-water system had gone agley, and big black kettles simmered on the hob ready with healing or cleansing heat should a patient need it . . .

Many wounded soldiers were treated in St Vincent's at this time also:

. . . The whole city was sadly coloured now with the blue of the wounded soldier. They were flowing into St Vincent's as room could be made for them . . . Mr Tobin the head surgeon had lost an only son in Flanders, and it seemed he couldn't see enough of forms similar to what his son last looked like. Every free moment he plunged into the middle of those well enough to talk, and would stand there silent, for he was almost stone deaf, and could hear only a shout given into a circular disk with a delicate connection to a rod stuck into his ear. 'Where did you get your blighty son,' he'd say to a wounded man, sticking the rod into an ear, and inclining the disk towards the soldier's mouth. When he heard the faint echo of the place's name, he'd murmur, 'Ah! my son spent his last moment a long way off; but yours was near enough, son, near enough.' He seemed to think when he was close to them, he was closer to his son. When on the roof of the operating theatre, a group of them sang 'Tipperary', Tobin was in the middle of them, trumpet in ear, his old slender wavery hand trying to keep time, trying to conjure up the ghost of his son from the songs and stories of the wounded men.

Sean O'Casey had some slight difference of opinion with Sister Paul over the provision of chairs to celebrate a jubilee that was being held in the hospital, but he referred also to her kindness:

Sister Paul was still cold but she was kind on the morning of the operation. Under the warm blankets on the operating table she had stroked his arm and smiled down reassuringly . . . But when he was coming out of his sleep he sang 'Alliliu na Gamhna' and 'The Palatine's Daughter' at the top of his good baritone voice, the nurses in the ward standing round to listen to him, and when the songs had ended the theatre nurse bent over him to whisper coaxingly: 'Sing us another, 23, another in Irish, please do.' The doctor had said the wound was healing remarkably well and the beds were in great demand. St Vincent's was being pestered with petitions for help. A few days more at the most and he'd have to quit this clean airy place, the pleasant bed, the fine food and the peace and quietude surrounding the sick.

Before he left he had an interview with Sister Paul.

'Well 23', she said calmly, 'your wound's healing splendidly, and there is little more that we can do for you here. What you want now are good food and plenty of fresh air and sun. I've just got word that you are to go for a fortnight to our convalescent home; but it will be two weeks or so before there's a vacancy, so you'll have to remain with us here till they're ready for you.

Apparently Sean O'Casey did not take up the offer of the bed in the convalescent home.

He wrapped his razor, soap, brush and face flannel in an old ragged handkerchief, and thrust the little bundle into a pocket, and went over to Nurse Kelly making bandages in the centre of the ward. 'I am going,' he said, 'you can give my bed to someone else,' and he went from the ward, barely glancing at the tonsured head of the stony St Laurence, deeper in thought than ever; down the corridor, past the armoured Michael still thrusting a spear through a twisting dragon; past the great gong, just as the porter was giving it three strokes; out by the broad doorway into the Green opposite, and over the bridge, by the pond, under the trees, he took his first few steps homewards.[3]

Easter Week 1916 brought war to the steps of the hospital. On Easter Monday a detachment of the Citizen Army under the command of Commandant Michael Mallin and the Countess Markievicz occupied St Stephen's Green and the College of Surgeons on the far side of the Green opposite the hospital. They proceeded to dig trenches and put up barricades in the Green. The forces of the Crown were established in the Shelbourne Hotel and the University Club. Bullets swept from one side of the Green to the other. It was obviously a dangerous place to walk. Dr A.D. Courtney of Nenagh, Co. Tipperary, was house surgeon in St Vincent's Hospital during the Easter Rising and has left a vivid account of the events of that exciting week. On the morning of Easter Monday, he was having a cup of tea in the residency with some students when they heard a rifle shot. It was followed by a few others and Courtney said, 'This seems very peculiar.' One of the students commented, 'There are probably some manoeuvres on today.' Courtney replied, 'Manoeuvres around St Stephen's Green seem a bit improbable.'

However, they were summoned to the emergency room. Courtney and the students went over and found that a man had been brought in by ambulance. He was about forty-five years of age, well dressed and he was dead. It was evident that he had been shot through or in the region of the heart. Courtney asked the ambulance men what happened, and was told that the Sinn Féiners had broken out and were shooting everyone on the street. While he was talking to them a second body was brought in. He also was a middle-aged man, well dressed, and dead, having a single wound in his chest. The two men were taken to the mortuary; one of them, who was a buyer at Clery's, was on his way through the Green when he was shot. At this stage another wounded man came in. It was found that he had a bullet wound in his shoulder which was bleeding fairly freely. This man had just come out of a Masonic meeting in St Stephen's Green when he was apparently shot.

At this point Courtney and his colleagues realised that something major was afoot and they went immediately to Jim Ryan's room. Ryan was a resident medical student in the hospital. They found that his bed had not been slept in and he had not been seen anywhere in the hospital. His absence was obviously significant and it was clear to Courtney and his friends that Ryan was certainly associated with the events going on in the city. His exact whereabouts did not transpire until some days later when it was established that he was in the GPO. Although only a medical student, James Ryan was chief medical officer in the GPO. He was appointed to that key post because the doctor who was scheduled to look after the medical arrangements had not reported for duty. Dr James Ryan later had a very distinguished political career and was a Minister in many Fianna Fáil governments. He was Minister for Health at a particularly important time in the development of the medical services of the country.

On the Tuesday morning of Easter Week, at about five o'clock in the morning Courtney heard a fairly large chorus singing 'The Soldier's Song'.

> It was certainly very moving in the early hours of the morning to hear it echoing across the Green. It continued for about half an hour and came from either the Liberty Hall Group in the Green or the Garrison in the College of Surgeons. Later on, messages came in from people who were wounded or even ill in nearby parts of the city.

Later on Easter Tuesday the Reverend Mother of the hospital, Mrs Carew, sent for Courtney. She told him that someone would have to take charge of the hospital, as some of the visiting staff were away and some of them could not get to the hospital. She made what was to Courtney the astounding suggestion that he should take charge, direct what was to be done with the patients and summon the staff either by phone if possible or by messenger when necessary. Courtney objected very strongly to this on account of his lack of experience and he made the mistake of saying to

Reverend Mother that perhaps she had been reading too much of Macaulay's *Lays of Ancient Rome*, where in times of great peril it was well that one should hold sway. When he saw her reaction to this observation he just said, 'I will do whatever I can.'

Some members of the staff did come in to the hospital, like Surgeon Tobin, who lived just a few doors away. Tobin was fearless according to Courtney and felt in his element, but he was completely mystified and wondered what the rebels—as he called them—thought could be achieved by their action. He considered that St Stephen's Green was an absolute trap and that if and when the military took some of the surrounding houses nobody would escape alive from it. He was, of course, obviously and totally out of sympathy with the ideals of the Rising.

When he went down to Grafton Street Tobin found large crowds looting the shops. He immediately set to with his blackthorn stick beating them left and right and shouting, 'Looting in time of war is punishable with death.' The looters ran from him in all directions and he pursued this line from shop to shop throughout the city. One remarkable incident was described to Courtney when a young fellow who had been looting was to be seen in Baggot Street complete with bowler hat, binoculars and golf club, teeing up a ball in the middle of the street, belting it as far as he could and then following its progress with the binoculars. Tobin came back to the hospital and commented that although he could not understand the situation and did not approve of it, he would take off his hat to any man who took his gun in one hand and his life in the other to stand up for his principles.

Tobin was subsequently called to attend James Connolly in the Dublin Castle hospital and formed a very intimate friendship with him. Courtney reports that their first meeting was rather stormy, when in true military fashion Tobin upbraided Connolly and asked him if he realised he would be executed. Connolly answered that he did, and from then on Tobin's admiration for him increased. According to Courtney he was literally amazed at the books which Connolly asked him to bring in, when he offered to get him some reading matter. He saw him every day and Courtney had the privilege of going with Tobin to the Castle to see the wounded leader, but very little was said on that occasion. Tobin was also present at Connolly's execution on 12 May and came afterwards to the hospital rather downcast. But still he said (almost with sadness) that that was the punishment for rebellion in time of war, that Connolly understood this from the word go, and had no idea or hope or belief that anything else could occur.

On Easter Tuesday there was no ambulance attached to the hospital, so Courtney asked Mrs Carew if it would be possible to get one to deal effectively with the situation. They succeeded in getting one that day which remained at the disposal of the hospital until after the Rising had ceased. The ambulance was able to move around the area and pick up quite a number of wounded Volunteers—some of whom were reluctant or refused to go to hospital, because they feared that they would be subsequently picked up by the military. They also took a few overflow cases from Sir Patrick Dun's Hospital, which at that time was very overcrowded, with patients lying on mattresses in the corridors.

Amongst those cared for in the hospital was Canon Watters, the Parish Priest of Haddington Road.* He had received a bullet wound in the abdomen while going on a sick call. He was taken to St Vincent's but died five or six days later. Another patient was Michael Lennon, afterwards a District Justice in Dublin and very well known as a writer. Courtney recalls accompanying Dr Cox on his rounds. Lennon said to him, 'I don't suppose you would wish to attend me, seeing you are a Privy Counsellor,' or words to that effect. Cox replied very calmly and with an emphasis, 'I am first an Irishman, secondly a member of the medical profession and other matters only follow those.' As far as Courtney could remember, Lennon apologised.

On the Sunday Courtney went with the hospital ambulance to the Mount Street area and at approximately 3 p.m. learned that the occupants of Boland's Mills were surrendering. The ambulance stopped opposite what was then known as the Elpis Hospital and they watched while the garrison marched down in military order with their rifles, and dropped them as they passed the hospital. They looked exhausted, bedraggled and as Courtney said somewhat disappointed but under perfect control. He remembered seeing Eamon de Valera marching at their head. He was pale, tired, thinner and more gaunt than when Courtney had seen him previously, but as usual he carried himself erect and had the appearance of one still in command of his men, though then obviously handing over control to the British military. As a final observation Courtney adds that his account is very disjointed. Nevertheless, even if he was speaking from memory and without any notes, he gives a fascinating description of what was one of the most important weeks in the history of the country and of the hospital.[4]

Between the end of April and the middle of May 1916, eighteen women were admitted to the hospital suffering from either gunshot or bullet wounds. The youngest patient was aged twelve; two died. During the conflict the authorities of the hospital like the other voluntary hospitals in the city ignored a demand by the British forces to report cases of gunshot wounds and other suspicious injuries admitted to the wards.

The following letter stirred memories when it was published in *The Irish Times* on 13 April 1966:

> Sir,
> In Friday of Easter Week, 1916, I travelled to London by mail steamer from Kingstown to Holyhead and thence by the Irish

*Courtney said that Canon Watters the Parish Priest of Haddington Road was taken to the hospital with a bullet wound. This I feel is incorrect. Fr Watters was a Marist Priest from the Catholic University School, Lower Leeson Street. He had been on a call to Haddington Road. On his way home he was shot near St Mary's Road, presumably by a sniper. He was taken to the Royal City of Dublin Hospital and subsequently transferred to St Vincent's.

Mail to Euston. The train was packed with excited passengers and naturally the sole topic of conversation was 'The Rising'. Everyone had stories to tell of their experiences during that fateful week. A British tar in full uniform related how, completely unaware of what was happening, he was walking along St Stephen's Green on Easter Monday, when a man rushed out of a nearby hospital and dragged him into a hallway. The man, who was a doctor, told him, dressed as he was in naval uniform, it would be suicide for him to proceed further into the city, and the sailor added, 'he disguised me by giving me an old tall silk hat to wear, which I did.' I have often wondered what the people in Dublin, on that historic day, thought of the apparition he must have presented to their astonished gaze, clad as he was in a British tar's shore-going uniform, complete with bell bottomed trousers and surmounted by an ancient top hat. However the 'disguise' had been successful and he was on his way to rejoin his ship, safe and sound. About ten years later I was again a passenger on the Irish Mail proceeding from Euston to Holyhead and, as sometimes happens after the lapse of a decade, conversation turned again to 'The Rising'. I related the story of the sailor and the top hat as my contribution and when the laughter had subsided, one of my hearers said, 'that was a rather tall story'. 'Not so tall', retorted a man, who up to now had not joined in the conversation, although I had noticed that he was listening intently. 'I am the doctor who gave him the tall hat.'

Yours etc.,
'Dubliner', Co. Dublin.

At the height of the Civil War in 1922 the hospital also had to play a sad role. In early August the President of the Executive Council of the new Irish Free State, Arthur Griffith, was admitted to the private nursing home, at 96 Lower Leeson Street, to recuperate from an attack of tonsillitis. He was under the care of Dr Oliver St John Gogarty who thought he had suffered a slight stroke. On 12 August he was leaving his hospital room to go down to his offices in nearby Government Buildings when he collapsed in the corridor outside his room from another stroke. He was brought back to his bedroom but despite the best efforts of Dr Gogarty, Harry Meade and J.B. Magennis, who were rapidly on the scene, he died.

Ten days later on 22 August 1922 General Michael Collins was shot dead at Béal na Bláth, Co. Cork. His body was brought back to Dublin by sea and arrived at the North Wall in the early hours of 24 August. The body was brought to the mortuary chapel in St Vincent's Hospital for embalming.[5] After the embalming the remains were removed to the hospital chapel. The coffin was placed on a catafalque in front of the altar where it remained until the evening when the remains were brought to the City Hall for lying-in-state.

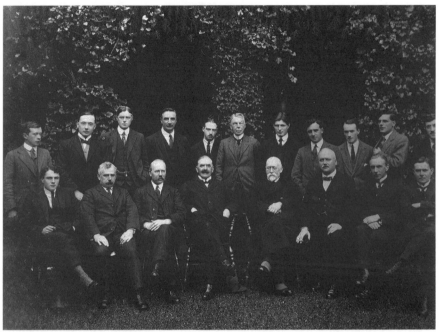

Visiting and resident staff, 1916. (Back row, left to right) W. Donnellan, Dr Courtney, Dr J.N. Meenan, Surgeon Kennedy, Mr McNamara, Surgeon Tobin, Mr J. O'Meara, Surgeon Doolin, Mr M. Smyth B.Sc., Dr Magennis, Mr Joyce; (front row, left to right) Mr Purcell, Dr Dargan, Dr Shaw, Surgeon McArdle, Rt Hon. Dr Cox P.C., Dr A. Smith, Dr H. Mooney, Dr T.T. O'Farrell

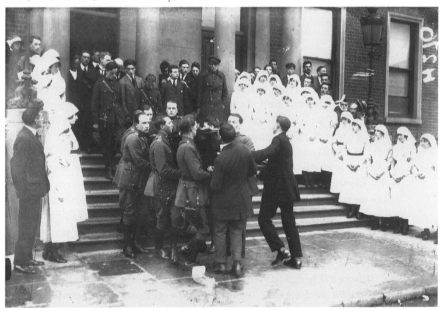

Removal of the remains of Michael Collins from St Vincent's Hospital, August 1922

Dillie Fallon (*née* Corcoran), who was night matron in the early 1920s, gives an interesting personal account:

> As night matron in the early twenties I had many exciting moments and heavy responsibility. The Black and Tans were constantly sniped at from the roof top of the hospital. One night they came ringing and pounding on no. 60, looking for 'Shinners'. On answering the door the guns were pointed at Sister Paula (R.I.P.) and myself. As the 'Shinners' appeared, who happened to be the lady medicals in night attire, there was silence as the British officer ordered them up to bed. Next day they were called to Mother Rectress's office and no. 60 was closed as a hostel.
>
> Curfew was on and the British used to surround a different section of the city each night to search people for arms. One night we had to give shelter to big numbers of people as they were unable to go home. That night we gave beds to clergy, (including Fr Byrne, later Archbishop of Dublin), in the nurses' infirmary. During this time Mr Meade worked very hard. I remember him coming back to operate at night after ambushes which took place during the day. We had seventeen operations on one occasion.
>
> I remember Joe McDonagh as a patient; Harry Boland with Michael Collins called each night to see him. Later I answered the hospital door to find Harry Boland being carried in on a stretcher. He put out his hand and said, 'It is nice to meet a friend.' Surgeon Kennedy was called, and operated on him at once. He died a day or two later. He told me he overpowered the soldier who came into his room in Skerries and would have got away but for a soldier in the back garden who shot him.
>
> Mr Griffith was also a patient in the top landing in 96. Going my rounds one night, his two guards said to me, 'Nurse, the Banshee is crying all night.' I had to cross the garden but I did not see or hear anything, so I mentioned it might be the cats from the Eastwood next door. I went back to the garden with the detective and I asked him to point out where the crying came from. He pointed to a spot. I passed it off. We nurses were off duty next morning when Mr Griffith collapsed and died. It was then I remembered the spot was exactly under his window.
>
> My next experience was receiving Michael Collins's remains. It was the most beautiful night I ever remember—full moon shining on the Green and silence everywhere, except for the slow step of the soldiers and the odd sob. His horse led the funeral, then his remains on the guncarriage followed by Mr W.T. Cosgrave, Mr P. Hogan, Mr Duffy and the remainder of the government. A few women followed weeping. We washed the clotted blood from his temple and round the

wound. His hands were soiled with clay, and afterwards members of the army changed his uniform.[6]

Dillie Fallon recounts another experience which had occurred a few years previously. After the death on hunger strike of Terence MacSwiney many other hunger strikers were released or transferred to hospital. One was J.R. O'Driscoll from Skibbereen who was taken into St Patrick's ward for artificial feeding. During curfew one night Dillie Fallon got word that 'a Priest' was at the main door seeking admittance. Josephine the night portress would not take the chain from the door without authorisation. When Dillie Fallon got to the hall 'the Priest' said that he had received a phone call to come and hear O'Driscoll's confession. He had a slight English accent which made her suspicious and she remembered the old ballad story of the 'Croppy Boy' and 'Father Green'. She managed to get rid of him. Next night when she was on duty O'Driscoll told her one of Michael Collins's intelligence men had told him that 'the Priest' was a soldier who had made a £5 bet that he would shoot O'Driscoll in his bed. This story might sound slightly amusing seventy years later but it shows the responsibility that the staff of St Vincent's and indeed other hospitals carried in those dangerous times.

As if war was not enough, in the last quarter of 1918 Western Europe was visited with a particularly virulent type of influenza. It was known as the Spanish flu as it was believed that it originated in Spain. It caused more deaths than the Great War. One of its features was that it was the young and healthy who succumbed to it. The epidemic first appeared in Britain and, judging by the admission book of the hospital, quickly spread to this country. The women's admission book of the last three months of the year illustrated the severity of the epidemic. In October the total number of cases admitted to the female ward was 102: fifty-one were suffering from influenza of whom five died. In November seventy-five were admitted: thirty-four with influenza of whom three died. In December thirty-two were admitted: nine with influenza of whom one died. In February there were eighty-six admissions: eleven with influenza of whom one died. In March there were seventy-seven admissions: twenty-seven with influenza of whom one died.

CHAPTER 11

THE TWENTIES

During the 1920s there was a continuous demand for expansion of the hospital. At the same time old buildings were crumbling and required renovation; the Great War had stimulated the swift growth of medical science; new techniques and specialities were rapidly evolving and young physicians and surgeons equally at home in the laboratories as at the bedside were seeking hospital appointments. All this was happening at a time when due to the ravages of the Great War bequests and subscriptions to the hospital were falling off and prices were soaring. The major building project of the decade was the new out-patients' department on Leeson Lane.

Over the years the out-patients' department had played an increasingly important role in the work of the hospital and attendances at the various clinics in the out-patients' department were rising rapidly every year. The old out-patients' at the back of the main building was becoming more and more unsatisfactory. Albert Fagan has left a description of it.[1] It consisted of a small room with a corner fireplace, table and one chair, and to the right a door to examining couches, separated by a partition with a green curtain covering the entrance. The waiting public stood in a cold draughty corridor leading on to the lane. One large ledger on the table was used to write in the names and addresses and no other records were kept. It was on the site of what became St Charles's ward. It was smoky and badly ventilated. It might also be added that there was a piggery next to the out-patients'—which certainly did not help the atmosphere.[2]

The building of the out-patients' took many years to accomplish. The money for the project came from the estate of Charles Lalor, former owner of the Imperial Hotel, O'Connell Street, Dublin, who left £15,000 in his will dated 1914 for such a purpose. His assets proved greater than his legacy and the sum was doubled, but the war in Europe halted building, with the result that the foundations were not laid until 1916. The building was further held up by a shortage of materials and the disturbances of the Civil War.

The new out-patients' department was finally opened in November 1924 by Dr Byrne, the then Archbishop of Dublin. Speakers at the opening ceremony were Sir Edward Coey Bigger, Chief Medical Officer, Sir William Thompson, President of the Royal College of Physicians (a Vincent's student), and Mr Justice O'Shaughnessy. The building which was of red brick and stone had its entrance on Leeson Lane. The building basically consisted of a large waiting hall, 103 feet long by 27 feet wide and provided with seating for 200 patients. Arranged around the hall were eight separate clinics or dispensaries, so organised as to be capable of working either as independent or as connecting units. In each dispensary unit the doctor had a large consulting room and several small examination rooms.

There were two operating theatres in the building. At the back of the hall the hospital pharmacy was situated. The pathology department was changed from its small area off St Joseph's ward and was re-located in a two storey building at the back of the out-patients' department. The department consisted of a large laboratory, preparation rooms, library and small laboratory. In the large laboratory there were pathological specimens and pathological lectures and demonstrations were held in this room. To staff the new department many fresh appointments were made to the junior staff. Many of those appointed were already working in the hospital, but their official appointments appear to date from 1924.

Patrick T. O'Farrell and H. Quinlan were appointed assistant physicians. P.T. O'Farrell was a brother of T.T. O'Farrell, the pathologist. Harold Quinlan was born in Limerick. He carried out postgraduate studies in Germany and his stories of the financial and economic crises in post-war Berlin were always most interesting.

Doolin, already assistant surgeon, and F.J. Morrin were the surgeons. Morrin after service in the Great War had joined the medical corps of the Free State army. He was surgeon to the military hospital in the Curragh with the rank of colonel. He was subsequently appointed director of medical services of the army. He used to say that he learned his surgery at the military hospital in the Curragh.

J.B. McArevey joined Herbert Mooney in the ophthalmological department. He was a Newry man who gained the Military Cross for gallantry in the war. He spoke with typical Northern candour and was a pioneer in corneal grafting. He was deeply religious and very charitable. Together with McArdle, McArevey was active in trying to obtain a reprieve from the British government for Kevin Barry after he had been condemned to death in 1920.

P.J. Keogh and Albert Fagan were the ear, nose and throat specialists to the hospital. Keogh was a skilled operator with a forceful personality. He was a prominent sportsman and captain of the Irish clay pigeon shooting team. Albert Fagan was the son of P.J. Fagan, former surgeon to the hospital. He had a sound practical approach to his speciality and had a large practice.

Reginald White was appointed gynaecologist in 1924 on the retirement of Alfred Smith. He had the reputation of being a skilled operator and a man

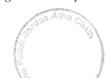

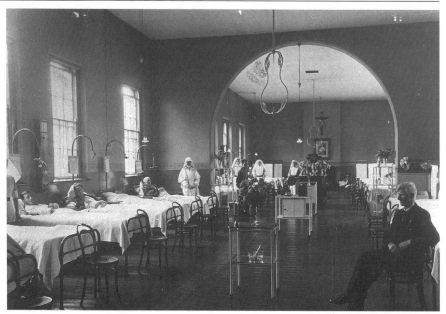

St Patrick's ward, *c.* 1920

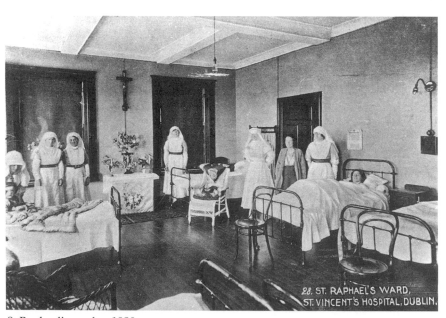

St Raphael's ward, *c.* 1920

of few words. The junior gynaecologist was John F. Cunningham. Cunningham carried out postgraduate studies in Vienna. He left the hospital in September 1931 to become Master of the National Maternity Hospital. He was replaced by Gerald Tierney. Tierney apart from his professional accomplishments was noted for his charitable work amongst the poor. He was an active member of the Society of St Vincent de Paul. He died in 1937, having lost his wife in a tragic car accident a few years previously.

The dentists were J.J. Murphy and Leo Smyth. Over the years the dental department had assumed an increasingly important role in the work of the hospital. Other dentists who worked in the hospital were Edward Corbett and Marcus Bloom—already referred to in connection with James Joyce. He was dentist from 1890–98. Kevin O'Duffy who was dentist from 1898–1903 was also dentist to the Lord Lieutenant. He played a prominent part in putting dentistry on a sound professional basis. His son Eimear was active in the Rising of 1916 and also gained fame as a writer—his major work was *The Wasted Island*. John I. Potter was in charge of dentistry from 1903–06. He subsequently became Professor in the dental school of University College Dublin.

Dr John Shiel was appointed pharmacist in 1926. He was also a barrister. Always dressed formally, he had the highest standards of social and professional etiquette. In a day before the dawn of the pharmaceutical industry he compounded most effective mixtures. He was most supportive of the junior members of the staff and helped them in many ways to build up their private practices. He frequently invited his colleagues to pleasant lunches in the Stephen's Green Club.

There were also several appointments at senior level. In 1924, as Michael Cox was ill, J.B. Magennis was appointed physician to the hospital. Magennis was one of the brightest stars in the medical constellation of the twenties and thirties. He was a pioneer in the treatment of pulmonary tuberculosis and was one of the first to use gold in its treatment. He was interested in theatricals and was an accomplished amateur actor. He could use a dramatic approach to his patients with great effect. He was especially devoted to the colour blue. He owned a blue Alfa Romeo car and smoked Du Maurier cigarettes, packaged in blue. He was also a successful horse-owner. He never married and in his day was one of Dublin's most eligible bachelors. There is a story that a wealthy Dublin industrialist offered his daughter in marriage to Magennis. Magennis understandably refused the offer, stating that if he wanted to get married he would make his own choice.

John (Jock) McGrath was appointed assistant pathologist to the hospital in 1927. He developed a particular interest in forensic medicine and was appointed State Pathologist. He was also assistant editor of the *Irish Journal of Medical Science*. In the same period Oswald J. Murphy returned from the post of Colonial Surgeon on the island of St Helena. His main interest was anaesthesia and he dealt with difficult anaesthetic problems. Subsequently

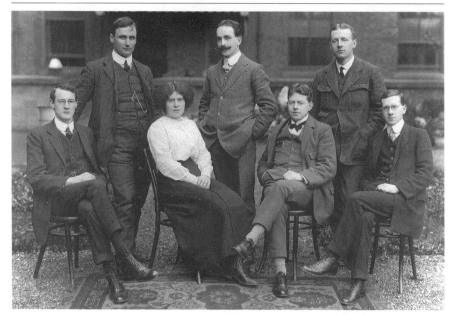

Resident medical staff, Easter 1911. (Back row, left to right) J.E. O'Sullivan, V.J. White, R.A.W. Ford; (front row, left to right) Dr M.F. O'Hea, Dr B. Griffin (house surgeon), Dr D. Murnaghan (house physician), Dr P.T.J. O'Farrell

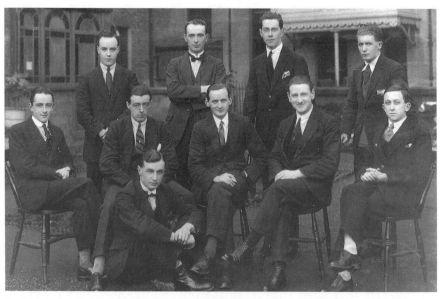

Resident medical staff, 1924–28. (Back row, left to right) E.J. Gallagher, M. O'Leary, A.J. Kirby, C.M. Saunders; (front row, left to right) J.J. Silke, J.S. O'Donovan, P.J. Kerley M.B., T.J. Prendergast M.B., A.J. Mooney B.A.; (seated) R.J. Cullen

Michael Mullen who was in general practice became anaesthetist to the out-patients' department.

McArdle died in April 1928 and his death was the cause of widespread grief. The Free State government sent a plane to circle the cemetery while his remains were being interred.[3] He had won a special place for himself in the heart of Irish society and medicine. He was one of the best-known men in Dublin. His routine would be that having finished his hospital work he would go to lunch, probably to the Dolphin Hotel, where for forty years he was a familiar figure; frequently he would be accompanied by a country doctor or two, and usually by his resident student. The 'surgeon's table' was a centre of joviality for the next hour. His progress through the city was one continuous salutation—a wave of his hand—everyone knew 'the surgeon'. After lunch he enjoyed a large cigar and a brief rest. Then he was off to lecture at the Catholic University School of Medicine, where he was Professor of Surgery—an honour bestowed on him in 1904—or home to Merrion Square, where his patients were being marshalled by 'Mustoe', his man-servant. From his long association with the household Mustoe considered himself an essential part of the surgeon's establishment, and it was no unusual thing for a patient to be told: 'We cannot see you today,' or 'We are going to the country.' The surgeon's home hours were from 2 p.m. to 4 p.m. but he was rarely out of his consulting rooms before 6 p.m. One of his students wrote a poem in his memory:

> The High Gods smiled on him, His youth they clothed
> With genius, and by them was he betrothed
> To Surgery—as yet a child—and they
> Grew up together.

The opportunity was taken by the President of University College Dublin to consolidate the professorial structure in the medical school. The chair of medicine was split into two professorships, the professorship of medicine in the Mater Hospital and the professorship of systemic medicine in St Vincent's. Both chairs were of equal prestige and importance. A similar system was applied to surgery.

James Nahor Meenan was appointed Professor of Systemic Medicine. He had been appointed Professor of Hygiene and Medical Jurisprudence in the Cecilia Street School of Medicine and subsequently in the School of Medicine of University College Dublin. He was consultant physician to St Patrick's College, Maynooth. His was the last professorial appointment in Cecilia Street before its closure. Tall and dignified, with a shock of white wavy hair, he possessed considerable diplomatic skills, with which he frequently used to solve the most difficult human problems. He had won a reputation as a fine clinical teacher and kept himself fully up-to-date with the rapid advances in medicine. His bedside clinics were very popular.

He took a keen interest in the welfare of his students, possibly slightly more in those who spoke with a Northern accent. He used to attend Mass in Catholic University School oratory on Sundays. On two Sundays during the year before the beginning of the final medical examinations the church would be crowded with devout students who were sitting for their finals. He was immensely loyal to his hospital and to his university. He showed a particular skill in picking out promising young men and women who would be suitable for appointment to the hospital. As one of his colleagues said, 'He was always looking for likely lads for his beloved Vincent's.' He was a great man for Vincent's.

Harry Meade had established himself as one of the leading surgeons in the country, and many patients owed their lives to his dexterity and skill. He was technically brilliant and spent much of his free time visiting European hospitals. He was President of the Royal College of Surgeons from 1948 to 1950 and President of the Association of Surgeons of Great Britain and Ireland in 1949. Like many surgeons he had a dogmatic approach to most problems, which thinly concealed a friendly and generous personality. He was always ready to help students down on their luck. His clinics were extremely practical and his aphorisms concerning the physical examination of patients were appreciated by generations of Vincent's students.

At the same time Thomas T. O'Farrell was appointed Professor of Pathology in University College Dublin. He was a pioneer in many departments of pathology. An expert histologist, his opinion was very much sought after in the diagnosis of difficult cases. He took a great interest in the affairs of the hospital and its welfare. He was to play a leading role in the purchase of the Elm Park site.

The death of McArdle left a vacant place on the surgical staff. This was filled by William Doolin who had spent a long period in the out-patients' department. Doolin was a man of many gifts and his surgical prowess tends to be forgotten in the light of his other accomplishments. He was a pioneer and achieved remarkable results in the treatment of cleft palate. He is most remembered for his literary pursuits. He was editor of the *Irish Journal of Medical Science* and in later years editor of the *Journal of the Irish Medical Association*. He made many contributions to medical history but recognition of his achievements came rather late in his career; when it did come, however, it was impressive. He was given a personal chair in the History of Medicine at University College Dublin. He gave many lectures to various distinguished bodies in Great Britain and Ireland. He was President of the Royal College of Surgeons in Ireland from 1938 to 1940. He was also interested in sport, particularly lawn tennis, and acted as umpire in the Davis Cup matches which took place in the Fitzwilliam Lawn Tennis Club.

Extensive alterations and building were carried out during this period in other parts of the hospital. In 1926 the old dispensary premises at the back of the hospital were completely renovated and two wards, St Charles's and St Teresa's, were established. In the same year an extra floor was added to the nurses' home. In 1926 an electric lift was installed in the private nursing home. Alterations were made in the houses so that direct communication extended from 93 to 97 Lower Leeson Street. At this time also the brick-work on the south side of the chapel was replaced with cement. In 1921 the back wall of 56 St Stephen's Green, the original home of the hospital, had to be repaired. A donation from the executors of the late Thomas Leonard paid for these alterations. In 1924 a special appeal in the form of a Violet Day gained £14,000 for the hospital. In 1928 an annalist for the hospital commented wryly:

> Future generations born in the age when electric power is transmitted by wireless may yet read these annals and doubtlessly be surprised to learn that only in 1928 a lift was erected in St Vincent's Hospital. Will they realise that previous to that everything, coal, food, milk, linen as well as patients had to be carried up those long winding stairs? Surely they will say they were giants on earth in those days.[4]

In 1929 extensive reconstruction had to be carried out on the private nursing home in Leeson Street and it was closed down until July 1931, with consequent great loss of income to the hospital. A bill from the period shows some of the costs faced by the hospital:

Repair Chapel Wall and Balcony £230.
St Anne's Theatre £350.
Quartz Mercury Lamp £90.
Electro Cardiograph £250.
Lift £1,250.
Kitchen £1,000.
Girls' Dining Room, Laundry and Drying Room £320.
Central Heating £950.

It is proper at this stage to pay tribute to the various voluntary bodies and private individuals who raised funds for the expenses of the hospital. Flag days, violet days and charity sermons played their part in raising significant amounts. Various ladies' committees organised sales of work, bazaars and other schemes to help with purchasing equipment for the various departments in the hospital. The committee consisted of wives of members of the staff, members of the community, nursing staff and other friends and supporters of the hospital.

About the end of the 1920s St Vincent's, like all the other Dublin voluntary hospitals, was in dire straits financially. The main source of income now was that from paying patients. According to Barrington the income from paying patients in six voluntary hospitals averaged £2,000 a year before the First World War. In the 1920s it rose to an average of £24,000 per year.[5] In the 1920s two of the Dublin hospitals had run sweepstakes sporadically on major horse races to raise money. This was strictly illegal but the government turned a blind eye towards the venture. Apparently Kevin O'Higgins the Minister for Justice was against the running of sweepstakes as he did not think it was possible to run them without fraud. It was also rumoured at the time that a well-known Jesuit theologian came out strongly in favour of the morality of sweepstakes.

The Public Charitable Hospitals Temporary Provision Act of 1930 was the Act under which the Hospitals Sweepstakes were first started. By the terms of this Act public charitable voluntary hospitals and similar institutions were empowered to raise funds by means of sweepstakes on condition that 25 per cent of their bed accommodation was provided for patients unable to pay for treatment or paying a sum not exceeding ten shillings per week. The Sweeps were held on major English races which would excite the interest of more people than local ones.

The first Sweep was held on the Manchester November Handicap in 1930. The first three Sweepstakes raised £1.25 million for the voluntary hospitals. Six hospitals took part in the first Sweep; seventeen more in the second Sweep and thirty-four in the third Sweep. After the first Sweep there was rather unseemly competition between the participant hospitals for their share of the proceeds and the government passed another Act in 1931 laying down that proceeds should be divided as two thirds to voluntary hospitals, one third to local authority hospitals; and a committee of reference was set up to administer grants to the voluntary hospitals.

In 1933 the new Fianna Fáil government passed a much more draconian Act. By the terms of the Public Hospitals Act of 1933, legal authority for the Irish Hospitals Sweepstakes was established and the Hospitals Commission was set up. The function of the Hospitals Commission was to advise the Minister on administration of Hospital Trust funds and to survey the hospital facilities in the country and submit ideas for improvement and co-ordination of medical facilities. The Sweep on the 1931 Derby was the first one in which St Vincent's participated and it received the sum of £20,950.19s.7d. This sum was put to modernising the X-ray department. From the first four Sweeps in which the hospital participated it received a total of £94,443.13s.4d. St Vincent's was the object of a certain amount of criticism for joining in the Sweepstakes only when their success was established.[6] Up to 1969 St Vincent's St Stephen's Green received a total of £2,092,011.5s.7d and St Vincent's Hospital, Elm Park received £3,073,368.3s.11d.[7]

The Irish Hospitals Sweepstakes were a tremendous success and were the brain child of Richard Duggan, a bookmaker, Joe McGrath, a former minister in the Free State government, and Spencer Freeman, an engineer. Sixty years later, it is hard to appreciate what a dominant part the Irish Hospitals Sweepstakes played in the social and economic life of the country, particularly in the 1930s. Ireland became internationally known for its Sweepstakes and the draws received overwhelming press coverage from all

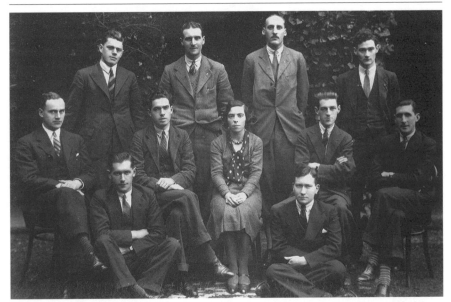

Resident staff, 1931. (Back row, left to right), D. Deasy, T.D. Phelan, S.B. Potter, J. McCormack; (middle row, left to right) Dr F.P. Ryan, Dr E.J. Prendiville, Miss T.A. O'Donnell, Dr T.J. Conlon, Dr J.W. Roche; (front row, left to right) J. Walsh, E.L. Murphy

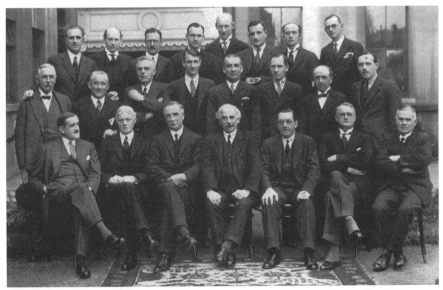

Consultant medical staff, 1933–34. (Back row, left to right) Mr Doolin, Dr Shiel, Dr Tierney, Dr McGrath, Mr Morrin, Dr Mullin, Mr Fagan, Dr W.P. Murphy; (middle row, left to right) Mr Mooney, Mr Keogh, Dr Magennis, Dr Quinlan, Mr Smyth, Dr O.J. Murphy, Mr J.J. Murphy, Mr Shortall; (front row, left to right) Mr Meade, Dr J.N. Meenan, Mr Kennedy, Dr Dargan, Dr White, Dr O'Hea, Dr T.T. O'Farrell

parts of the globe. The Sweep was declared illegal in the United States and in Britain. In Ireland itself the Sweep was an enormous source of employment, especially in the women's section of the working population.

Farmar,[8] in his account of the impact of the Hospitals Sweepstakes on the Dublin of the 1930s, states that the whole working of the Sweepstakes was a triumph for Irish organisation. Three to four times a year Dublin was treated to a colourful spectacle, a parade of 200 girls from the Hospitals Sweepstakes escorting the counterfoils of the tickets from the Sweepstakes Headquarters in Earlsfort Terrace down to the old Plaza Ballroom in Middle Abbey Street where they were mixed in a large drum. For each Sweep the girls were dressed in bright costumes illustrating one particular theme. For the 1932 Derby Sweep they were described as 'vividly garbed jockey girls'. In the Plaza Ballroom itself, nurses, six at a time from the different hospitals which participated in the Sweepstake, immaculately uniformed and starched, sat sideways to the drum which contained the tickets. The feature writer of the *Irish Independent* rhapsodised that one could see their profiles and realise that being a patient in hospital would have its compensations. Another nurse sat facing the audience behind a little glass container which held the names of the horses in the race. The ceremony was organised by General Eoin O'Duffy, Commissioner of the Garda Síochána. The writer continued:

> 'One' snaps General O'Duffy, like the crack of a whip. Six bare left arms open the six portholes as the drum comes to a standstill and six bare right arms are held aloft with open palms. 'Two' comes the sharp military command, and six right hands are inserted through the porthole to emerge a moment later with six tiny slips of paper which are held aloft for all to see. 'Three', the nurses slam the portholes simultaneously with their left hands while General O'Duffy walks across the stage and takes the counterfoils from their right hands. Meanwhile the name of a horse is drawn from a glass container after innumerable hefty spins and its name announced.

The final philosophical reflection of the reporter was, 'What would happen if some day a left handed nurse was assigned to the job at the porthole?'[9]

CHAPTER 12

ANNUS MIRABILIS

The year 1934 was a significant point in the history of the hospital. During that year St Vincent's celebrated its centenary and was entitled to look back with pride on a century of service to the sick and poor people of Dublin and of the country. The city itself had changed; it was no longer the declining second city of an empire but was the capital of a small new independent State. It had experienced years of famine, fighting in the streets and possibly worst of all, civil war. However, the scenes of poverty and disease described by the travellers of 100 years ago were no longer witnessed and for that St Vincent's on the Green could take a fair share of the credit. Nevertheless much remained to be accomplished. There were still vast areas of slums. Political tensions were high and, due to world-wide depression and the economic war, the times were not prosperous. Furthermore the new Nazi Germany was beginning to cast its shadow over Europe.

It was also a year in which the hospital took a decision to ensure that its service would continue for many years to come. The *Irish* (formerly *Dublin*) *Journal of Medical Science* in its edition of January 1934 illustrated the enormous changes in medicine over the previous 100 years. An authoritative review article on recent advances in medicine and therapeutics illustrated the rapid progress in medicine and surgery.[1] 'A critical survey of the medicine of recent years reveals not only a number of concrete gains, it enumerates the triumphs of medicine in the twentieth century.' The advent of biochemistry caused a complete change in outlook and investigation. The discovery of insulin, the liver treatment of pernicious anaemia, the delineation of coronary thrombosis and sub-acute bacterial endocarditis were some of the major advances of the period. The techniques of radiology were developing rapidly. The progress in medicine was matched by similar progress in surgery. The reviewer also made the point that the archaic hospital system in Dublin militated against advances in medicine and surgery. The hospitals were too small; he pleaded that an effort should be made, that hospitals should be amalgamated and that Sweepstakes money should be used to accomplish this.

The centenary celebrations began on 23 January 1934 with the Archbishop of Dublin Dr Byrne presiding at a High Mass of thanksgiving in the hospital.[2] Over the previous months the hospital chapel had been extensively decorated. A new tabernacle had been designed and on 17 December the Blessed Sacrament had been placed in it. The tabernacle was decorated with precious stones presented by members of the congregation, the community and the staff of the hospital. The Archbishop was attended by Dr Wall, Bishop of Thásos. The High Mass was sung by the chaplain Rev. F. Kenny; Rev. M. Allen C.C. and Rev. J. Robinson C.C., former chaplains in the hospital, were the Deacon and Sub-Deacon. Other former chaplains were in the choir with the Canons and some of the regular clergy. The following telegram was read during Mass:

> On the auspicious occasion of the centenary of the foundation of Ireland's first Catholic hospital the Holy Father, highly appreciating the laudable work done by the good Sisters of Charity, most lovingly bestows his Apostolic Blessing upon Mary Aikenhead's devoted children of St Vincent's Hospital, the medical staff, nurses, attendants, friends, benefactors, praying continuation of divine assistance in the future.
> Cardinal Pacelli.
> (Cardinal Pacelli was the Cardinal Secretary of State, later Pope Pius XII.)

The chapel was filled to capacity by members of the staff, their wives and a few special visitors. After Mass the visitors made an extensive tour of the hospital and the wards which had been decorated for the occasion. On 24 January 1934 the *Irish Press* wrote:

> The celebration of the centenary of St Vincent's Hospital, Dublin is one in which the whole nation joins. Not only is the order under whose charge this famous centre of healing is conducted, venerated by the Irish people for its innumerable works of charity but the institution itself has won the gratitude of every class in the capital, and outside it, the city's poor most of all. Some five per cent of the patients whom it has relieved and restored to health have been treated without charge.
>
> St Vincent's was established a hundred years ago by the founder of the Irish Sisters of Charity, Mother Mary Aikenhead. It was then a small building with one ward of twelve beds. Ever since, it has been increasing in size as well as in prestige and service and today it has more than two hundred beds. It was the first hospital in Ireland to have a children's ward and the first to open a nursing home. In its hundred years some of Ireland's greatest men have been associated with it. When a full record of their work has been written, the Irish

Sineaó
(H ní at)
CDN 8|15 1950 22 CITTADELVATICANO ETAT

REV MOTHER SUPERIOR ST VINCENTS HOSPITAL
ST STEPHENS GREEN DUBLIN

AUSPICIOUS OCCASION CENTENARY FOUNDATION IRELANDS

FIRST CATHOLIC HOSPITAL HOLY FATHER HIGHLY

APPRECIATING LAUDABLE WORK DONE BY GOOD SISTERS OF

APOSTOLIC
CHARITY MOST LOVINGLY BESTOWS ~~~~~~~ BLESSING

UPON MARY AIKENHEADS DEVOTED CHILDREN ON ST VINCENTS

HOSPITAL ITS MEDICAL STAFF NURSES ATTENDANTS FRIENDS

BENEFACTORS PRAYING CONTINUANCE DIVINE ASSISTANCE

IN FUTURE

CARDINAL PACELLI

Telegram from His Holiness the Pope on the occasion of the Centenary of St Vincent's Hospital, 1934. Cardinal Pacelli subsequently became Pope Pius XII.

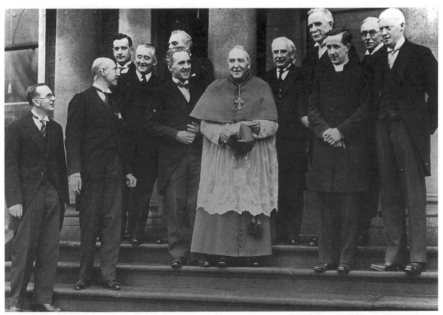

Medical staff with Archbishop Byrne on the occasion of the Centenary. (Left to right) W. Murphy, F.J. Morrin, M. Mullen, P.J. Keogh, J.B. Magennis, W. Doolin, Archbishop Byrne, W. Dargan, Denis Kennedy, Fr Kenny, Herbert Mooney, J.N. Meenan

Sisters of Charity in their hospital and in the many others which they have instituted, will be found to have made a contribution to the science of healing which few other organisations in any country can equal.

In the afternoon of 24 January, 1,400 guests attended a reception in the hospital. They were received by Mother Rectress, Mother M. Bernard Carew, on the grand staircase of the hospital leading up to St Joseph's ward. Mother A. Joseph Smith also received guests on St Brigid's ward and Mother F. Angela on St Laurence's. Many people prominent in the social and political life of the community attended the reception. President de Valera (then President of the Executive Council of the Irish Free State), and the Lord Mayor Alderman Alfred Byrne were conducted around the hospital by members of the staff and had tea in the nuns' refectory.

According to contemporary accounts, the President had announced his intention of remaining half an hour in the hospital but after one hour and a half he was still engaged in inspecting the many items of interest. Alderman Byrne who was one of the most famous Lord Mayors of Dublin and well known for his penchant for shaking hands also toured the hospital extensively. In St Charles's ward a little boy grasping the ever-extended hand of the Lord Mayor volunteered the remark, 'My father knows you.' 'Then I must know your father,' was the reply, 'and so I will make you the new Lord Mayor.' Then the Lord Mayor lifted the chain of office from his shoulders and placed it on the small boy. Another visitor prominent in the political life of the country at that time was General Eoin O'Duffy, former head of the Garda Síochána.

Visitors from the various houses were entertained on Thursday 25 January; and on Friday 26 January a large number of working-class people were entertained to tea in the out-patients' department. Sunday 28 January was also a memorable day. One hundred poor families from the district had a conducted tour of the hospital with its decorations of fairylights, gigantic palms and silver hanging; they were also entertained to a meal in the out-patients' department. The menu included beef, ham, mashed potato, greens and celery. Music was provided by the Irish Transport Union's Reed and Drum Band.

Monday 29 January witnessed the reunion of past nurses of the hospital. Two former matrons were present, Miss Campbell and Miss Sutton. Miss Campbell, although nearly eighty years of age, came from Scotland. Lunch after Mass was served in St Mary's nurses' home. That evening to conclude the centenary celebrations the medical staff were hosts at a banquet in the Council Chamber of University College Dublin which had been kindly lent to them by the President Dr Coffey. Dr Dargan the senior physician to the hospital presided and amongst the distinguished guests were President de Valera, Mr Sean T. O'Kelly, Minister for Local Government and Public Health, and the Lord Mayor. One of the toasts, that of 'the ladies', was

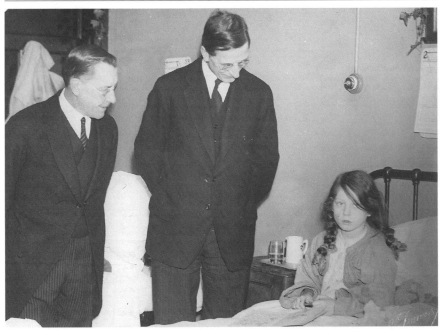

Centenary Year—President de Valera visiting the hospital accompanied by Dr Reggie White

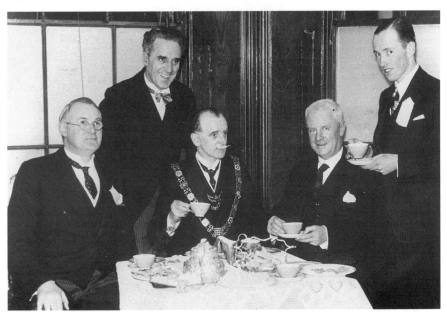

Centenary Year—Lord Mayor Alfred Byrne visiting the hospital accompanied by (from left) M.F. O'Hea, W. Doolin and (far right) P.A. FitzGerald

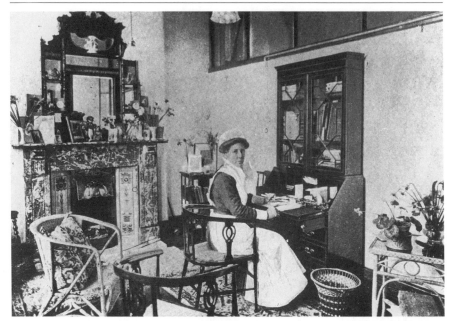

Miss Sutton, Matron, 1906–18

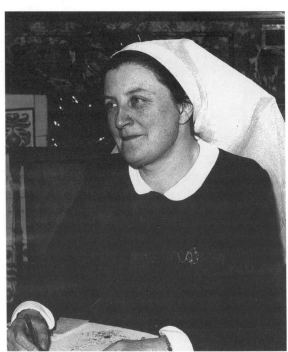

Miss Annie Kelly, Matron,
1946–68

responded to by Miss Alice Curtayne, the well-known historian. Miss Curtayne with William Doolin edited a book entitled *A Century of Service*. It was, and still is, a most valuable record of the work and achievements of the hospital during the first hundred years.

Following the centenary celebrations the Gardaí, as a token of appreciation to Sister Louis Gonzaga Butler who had had charge of St Brigid's ward—the Guards' ward—contributed to the purchase of a new monstrance for the hospital chapel. The medical staff wishing to commemorate the occasion in a lasting memorial presented a new crucifix for the high altar. The crucifix was designed by Oswald Reeves of the School of Art, Kildare Street.

It is surely no coincidence that in the Centenary Year appointments were made to the hospital of two brilliant young graduates who were to play a major role in its evolution over the next fifty years. T.C.J. (Bob) O'Connell who was born in Dublin spent three years in postgraduate study in Berlin. He was appointed assistant surgeon and also to give assistance in the X-ray department on the resignation of Dr William Murphy.

Denis Kenry O'Donovan was born in Limerick in 1909. He had an outstanding academic career and obtained first class honours in all his examinations. He was appointed junior physician to the hospital immediately after qualification. In 1935 he did postgraduate studies in McGill University in Montreal. It was here that he took up the study of the endocrine glands which was to be his main interest in medicine. In recognition of his service in helping to organise the centenary celebrations, T.T. O'Farrell was appointed to the Medical Board. He was the first specialist to be appointed.

Approximately six months after the ceremonies of the Centenary Year a most important event in the history of the hospital took place. Over the years, the old hospital—which was basically a terrace of Georgian buildings —had been renovated, expanded and transformed. Still the accommodation was never sufficient and the patchwork methods necessarily employed made the institution an awkward and uneven place in which to work. Modern medicine was rapidly expanding and the old buildings on the Green could not keep pace with these developments. It was a problem constantly worrying the hospital authorities. It was no mean feat and a credit to all who worked in the hospital that, in spite of its physical disadvantages, St Vincent's was able to maintain a dominant role in Irish medicine. But if St Vincent's was to retain its position as a leading hospital it had to seek new horizons.

In the summer of 1934 due to the good offices of T.T. O'Farrell it was brought to the attention of the Sisters of Charity that the lands of Elm Park at Merrion were for sale. The property consisted of a large mansion, Nutley House, standing in its own grounds of fifty acres with almost infinite space for extensions. It was approximately eight miles from the centre of Dublin.

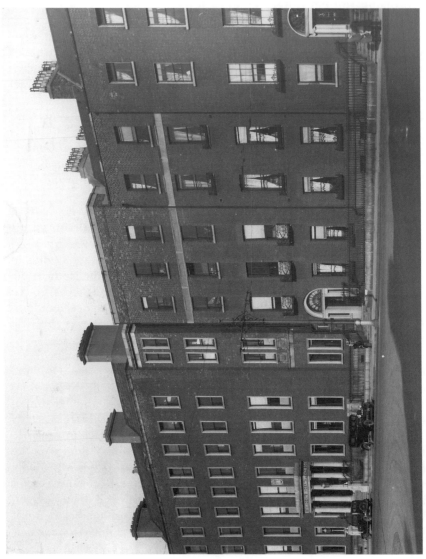

St Vincent's Hospital, St Stephen's Green, c. 1930

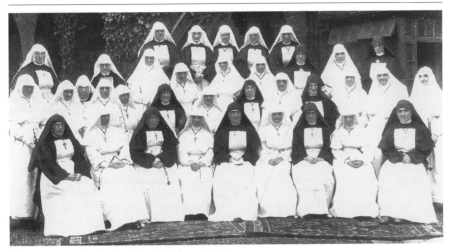

The community, St Stephen's Green, 1934

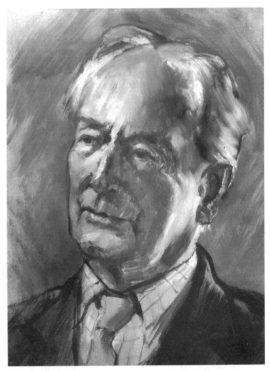

Denis K. O'Donovan, physician 1934–76

It bordered on the main roads to Bray and to Dun Laoghaire which were served by buses and trams. It was an ideal site for a general hospital.

On 7 June 1934 the Archbishop of Dublin gave permission for the Sisters to bid for Elm Park. On 5 July 1934 the congregation of the Irish Sisters of Charity purchased the lands at Elm Park for £24,000 (plus £1,700 auctioneer's fees). The *Irish Press* carried the story on 7 July under the heading:

BIG NEW HOSPITAL FOR DUBLIN
St Vincent's Plans: Site at Merrion Chosen.

The *Irish Press* understands that the purchasers of Elm Park, a mansion which stands in its own grounds of 50 acres, at Merrion Road, Dublin, are the Board of St Vincent's Hospital. It was learned last night that St Vincent's Hospital has planned to erect a huge new hospital on the site at Merrion and is at present negotiating with the Hospitals Commission for an allocation of the Sweepstake proceeds. A member of the Board said to an *Irish Press* representative last night, that they hoped to erect at Elm Park, the largest hospital in Dublin. The Board hoped to make it the administrative headquarters of St Vincent's, he added.

T.C.J. O'Connell told a (doubtless apocryphal) tale about the purchase of the Elm Park lands. In 1934 he was a junior member of the hospital staff. Like so many other people in the summer of 1934 he went on a visit to Germany to see the new Nazi state in action. During his holiday he received a telegram from the Reverend Mother asking him to come home to advise her on providing equipment for the new hospital. He broke off his holiday and came home immediately, feeling that he might be too late to help in the organisation. He could have completed his holiday—it was to be another thirty-six years before St Vincent's Hospital Elm Park opened its doors.

St Vincent's Hospital on the Green was built on ground that was an integral part of the history and development of the city of Dublin. The new Vincent's was built on no less historic ground, and the land surrounding it had also played a particular part in the history of Co. Dublin during medieval times.[3] As is well known, the grounds belonged to the Fitzwilliams of Meryon and subsequently passed through intermarriage to the Earls of Pembroke. The historic castle of the Fitzwilliams was sited just beside the chapel of St Mary's School. It was the main home of the Fitzwilliams for many years; there is now no trace of it. In medieval times there was a route via Donnybrook which the citizens of Dublin took when they wanted to travel to Blackrock. There was an old field path and double ditch that started at Seaview Terrace and went across the lands at Nutley emerging on Rock Road at the old Merrion churchyard. This route was especially important because it marked one of the limits of the franchise of the municipality of Dublin. Old maps of Dublin particularly Taylor's Map of 1816 and Duncan's Map of 1821 show very clearly this double ditch and path running just exactly behind Elm Park grounds and then behind St Mary's where it entered on to the Rock Road.

In medieval times there took place yearly the ceremony of 'riding the franchise'. The Lord Mayor, Aldermen and Councillors of the city of Dublin processed in state from out the Dame Gate riding past the Priory of All Saints, now Trinity College, to Ringsend. Then they advanced to near the present Poolbeg where they sent a yeoman to fling a dart into the sea to mark the admiralty jurisdiction of the Corporation. From this point they rode to Blackrock where the city sheriffs of the day held a court. From Blackrock the procession proceeded along the line of the present Rock Road until it came to the old Merrion chapel and churchyard. They then turned up into the fields and made their way to Simmonscourt along the ancient route. Approximately halfway along the route on the right hand side when facing the city of Dublin, there was an old well, the well of the Blessed Virgin.

In December 1892, Dr G.T. Stokes, accompanied by a distinguished antiquarian Mr James Mills, proceeded to investigate the lines of the route taken by the Lord Mayor and the Councillors and to see how much of it still existed. At Merrion churchyard they turned up the lane which was then known as Churchyard Lane and entered the grounds of Nutley just at St Mary's School. The grounds of Nutley were then owned by Mr Justice Madden who resided at Nutley House, which is now Elm Park Golf Club. They were able to trace the route behind the grounds of St Mary's across the field until they reached the grounds which are now on the Dublin side of Nutley Lane, behind Ailesbury Road. There was no trace of the well of the Blessed Virgin, but Dr Stokes was able to locate it at the back of the garden of the house which is now St Michael's College. From this area there was still a double ditch which ran parallel to Ailesbury Road, entered Seaview Terrace and then on to Simmonscourt.

However, the lands on which the hospital is built might have had an even earlier historic association. Antiquarians have stated, and made a good case for it, that this line of the franchise of the city of Dublin was based on a pre-historic road. Dr Petrie (the famous historian) has been quoted as saying that one principal road led from Tara through Dublin to Wicklow, and that this road went through the fields of what is now Nutley and Elm Park. Possibly, King Laoghaire himself, in the days of St Patrick, when he wished to inspect his fleets or to take the fresh air and salt water, drove straight from Tara through Dublin and through these lands to Dun Laoghaire and beyond to Wicklow. It is believed that St Patrick, when he came to bring Christianity to Ireland, landed on the shores of Wicklow. There is good reason to believe that at some stage he must have travelled along this road.

CHAPTER 13

THE EMERGENCY YEARS

I t became clear to the members of the staff in the late thirties that there was no glittering new hospital over the rainbow. Any faint hopes that it would be feasible to start working at Elm Park in the near future were removed by the outbreak of war in September 1939. The question now was not expansion but survival. For the foreseeable future the staff would have to continue working in and making the best of a relatively small hospital.

On 2 September 1939 a special meeting of the Medical Board was held to consider a letter which had been received from Dr Kerry Reddin, medical officer ARP Public Health Department, Dublin Corporation. Dr Reddin was anxious to know whether the hospital would reserve 100 beds for the treatment of casualties arising out of potential air raids upon the city. The Board was willing to co-operate but wanted further details about the scheme.[1]

A meeting of the Medical Boards of the various Dublin hospitals was held on 12 September 1939 to discuss an emergency scheme. The principal feature of the scheme was that a hospital of 400 beds (an evacuation hospital) a short distance out of Dublin would receive civilians as patients from those city hospitals which were being turned into casualty clearing stations. Along with the other Dublin hospitals, St Vincent's would be turned into a casualty clearing hospital with fifty beds. As far as possible the hospital would also carry on in its normal work. When the call came the top floors of the hospital were to be vacated, and the out-patients' department was to be a receiving station. Minor casualties would be treated and immediately discharged, but more serious cases would be accommodated in the wards adjacent to Leeson Lane. Other cases would receive first aid treatment and would be sent to the parlours at the front of the hospital for transfer to the base hospitals.

Air raid shelters were prepared in the underground passages and cellars of the hospital. Windows were covered on the inside with steel wire to protect from flying splinters of glass. Nurses and porters were given instructions on air raid precautions. Several sisters from the hospital attended the special classes for nuns at Portobello Barracks. Here the sisters were initiated into the mysteries of gas precaution and learned to adjust the gas masks—which involved the removal of all headgear. Later they went to an actual demonstration out on the hills where they had to put on masks and run through clouds of various gases. All sisters received certificates after examination.[2]

Over the next few months all was quiet on the Western Front. The war entered the phase known as the 'phoney war'. The hospital settled down into its normal peaceful routine again. In June 1940, however, there was a real threat that Ireland would be involved in the fighting. The plans for turning the hospital into a casualty clearing station were hurriedly revived. T.C.J. O'Connell organised a national blood transfusion scheme. In an article on the scheme he ended with the prophetic words, 'The establishment of a national blood transfusion service now under emergency conditions has in it the nucleus of a national peace time service which will be a boon alike to our patients and ourselves.'[3]

During this period the relationship between the Dublin voluntary hospitals and the Department of Local Government and Public Health was not particularly peaceful. The voluntary hospitals were worried that the Hospitals Commission, which had the power of allocating monies from the Sweepstakes, would have too much influence in the running of the hospitals and gradually take over their control. The situation was not improved when the Commission established a bed bureau in 1940. The function of the bed bureau was to control the admission of patients to the voluntary hospital wards, thus effectively depriving the hospital authorities of control over their own admissions.

The war years were a time of deprivation and shortage, frustration and denial. In many ways the hospital was thrown back on its own resources. There were shortages of essential fuels, gas, electricity, petrol and surgical gases. Medical personnel did not escape the effect of petrol rationing. Many distinguished consultants from St Vincent's and other hospitals were seen cycling in the streets of Dublin. They discovered the rather bumpy pleasure of travelling by train and bus and frequently found to their cost that the last tram actually did leave Nelson's Pillar at 9 p.m. They also learned to cope with that demon of the emergency years, 'the glimmer man'.

Doctors received a meagre allowance of petrol which had to be reserved for hospital work and for emergency duties. The shortage of dressings and of surgical equipment was frustrating. Nothing was sacrosanct—even nurses' uniforms were affected. The snowy white veils of the junior nurses which flowed gracefully down their backs were ruthlessly chopped off at the neck. The glowing coal fires which used to make the wards more cheerful were things of the past and while turf fires helped they were no substitute for coal, particularly in the making of toast. Members of the staff were envious when they heard of the miraculous properties of the new wonder drug penicillin now available in Great Britain and the United States. Thanks to the ingenuity of our chemists small doses of penicillin were made in Ireland, but the war was practically over before penicillin could be made generally available in the wards of the Dublin hospitals. The wartime shortages did not completely halt progress in the hospital. In the mid-1940s two new surgical theatres were built at a cost of £1,200 and the X-ray department on the site of the old disused operating theatre was expanded as a new X-ray theatre. New dietetic and physiotherapy schools were established.[4]

James Benedict Magennis died in the autumn of 1940. His death initiated many staff changes. P.T. O'Farrell and Harold Quinlan were promoted to senior physicians in the hospital and Francis J. Morrin to senior surgeon. O'Farrell was a pioneer in cardiology and organised the first cardiological service in the department. His slightly brusque manner was basically due to a rather shy and modest personality. When one got to know him better one realised that he had a distinct twinkle in his eye. He had a most distinguished career. He was Joint President of the Irish Medical Association and the British Medical Association for their meeting in Dublin in 1953 and was subsequently elected President of the Royal College of Physicians of Ireland.

Harold Quinlan was tall and elegant with a distinctive soothing bedside approach. He enjoyed the social round and was a very keen rider to hounds. He was a first class physician and possessed an acute brain. Even as a junior physician he built up a very large practice. He specialised in chest diseases and his opinion was sought all over the country. According to D.K. O'Donovan, 'Quinlan was before his time in his emphasis on the value of a dietary history and stressed the importance of malnutrition as a cause of poor resistance to infection. His emphasis on the background of the ultimate disease revealed to us the earliest faltering footsteps of social medicine as we know it today.'[5]

Francis J. Morrin was tall and spare with a military bearing. He spoke in short staccato phrases and was intolerant of any kind of verbiage or cant. He was a first class surgeon with a reputation as a decisive and speedy operator. He was so quick in his surgical manoeuvres that frequently, by the time one of his student assistants had scrubbed up, the operation was practically over. According to Bob O'Connell, 'Morrin had a reputation for attacking hopeless cases in ruthless fashion. Disease was an enemy to be destroyed relentlessly. Many a story might be told of his "marathon" operations in an attempt to remove the last vestige of malignant growth.'[6]

Fortunately there was no shortage of candidates to take up the vacancies created on the junior staff by the elevation of O'Farrell, Quinlan and Morrin to the Board. There was a galaxy of youthful stars waiting to take their place. O'Donovan and O'Connell were the first in a stream of brilliant young Vincent's graduates who had returned to their hospital.

Kevin Feeney had been appointed assistant gynaecologist to White in 1937 following the death of Gerald Tierney. Sylvester Boland, who had been a captain in the Irish army, and Denis O'Farrell, son of T.T O'Farrell, had been working in the X-ray department. They were appointed assistant radiologists in the department in 1938 and subsequently full radiologists. O'Connell states that 'Denis O'Farrell's principal hobby was shortwave radio and electronics. He was appointed by the Irish Government as head of monitoring services in 1939 and he was known to Ham Radio enthusiasts throughout the world. When he was on his honeymoon in the West in 1939 plans for weather stations along the coast were unwittingly revealed to him by an English Ham. The weather stations were picked up shortly after the outbreak of war.'[7]

Oliver FitzGerald and Patrick FitzGerald were appointed assistant physician and assistant surgeon respectively to the hospital in 1940. Both were destined to have distinguished careers in the hospital and in the academic and professional life of the country. Born in Waterford, they gained many prizes as students and vied with each other for first and second places in all their professional examinations. Oliver FitzGerald had just returned from Switzerland where he had been doing basic research.

Edward L. Murphy was appointed as junior physician in 1941. He had returned from the Johns Hopkins Hospital in Baltimore where he made neurology his special interest. As a neurologist he also served on the staff of several other Dublin hospitals. He was considerably influenced by American culture and habits. He was a first class clinician and wrote widely on various topics in medicine and allied sciences. His out-patient clinics in the hospital were legendary. He attracted large numbers of elderly patients for whom he was extremely caring and to whom he gave support and confidence.

Frank Duff, after a first class student career, was appointed assistant surgeon. Brian H. O'Brien was appointed ear, nose and throat specialist in 1941. He had been working in an unofficial capacity in the out-patients' department for several years. In his early days he also worked in London and regularly took the Night Mail from Euston on Friday to do his clinic in the hospital on the Saturday morning. As soon as the war ended he went to the United States to study the fenestration operation for the restoration of hearing. He became a recognised expert in this particular procedure.

William Dargan retired in 1943 after many years service to the hospital. He died a year later.

Denis Kennedy also retired in 1945, but was to lead an active life for another ten years. The retirements of Dargan and Kennedy brought O'Donovan and O'Connell to the Medical Board.

Philip Brennan, who had an outstanding student career, was appointed assistant physician in 1944. He was a first class clinician with a thorough knowledge of all branches of medicine. He was especially interested and expert in chest diseases.

During and soon after the war two important appointments were made in the medical faculty of University College Dublin—those of John F. Cunningham and D.K. O'Donovan. John F. Cunningham completed his period of Master—with extension—of the National Maternity Hospital.

Shortly afterwards Reginald White died and Cunningham was re-appointed gynaecologist to Vincent's, a position he had vacated on his appointment to the National Maternity Hospital. In 1943 he was appointed Professor of Obstetrics and Gynaecology in UCD. To his many patients he was known as 'Divine John'—he had a most soothing and courteous manner and was always immaculately groomed even if called out in the middle of the night to a case. Such attributes were the signs of complete attention and care for all his patients. Despite the demands of a busy professional life he also found the time to write a text book on obstetrics and gynaecology which achieved much popularity among students from many medical schools. In 1947 D.K. O'Donovan received academic recognition when he was appointed lecturer in medicine in the medical faculty of UCD.

Like all wars the Second World War had caused an upsurge in science. Torrents of new discoveries and concepts in medicine were pouring from centres of medical research all over the world. New specialities were constantly evolving, and the more senior ones expanding rapidly. These features were to lead to a rapid expansion in the medical staff of the hospital.

New techniques and horizons in surgery required more expert and skilled anaesthesia. G.R. Davys, who had service with the Royal Air Force during the war, was appointed anaesthetist in 1945 and joined the staff in 1946. Michael Nash, a late vocation to medicine, had postgraduate training in anaesthesia in England. Well versed in the classics he would soothe his patients with suitable quotations. Denis O'Leary, who subsequently joined the department in 1953, had also done postgraduate training in England.

One of the medical lessons of the war was the importance of the mind in the causation of disease. The then Professor of Medicine (the late James N. Meenan), anticipating the growth of the subject, decided to open a department of clinical psychiatry at St Vincent's and convinced Mother Carew (the Mother General) of the wisdom of this decision.[8] Psychiatry became a major part in medical treatment. Francis McLaughlin, a Donegal man, who served as a psychiatrist to the British army in the war, was appointed as the first psychiatrist to the hospital in 1945.

In 1949 Kevin Feeney was appointed Master of the Coombe Lying-In Hospital and his position in Vincent's was taken by Charles Coyle. After postgraduate work in the United States Francis Duff returned to the hospital and took up the position as specialist in genito-urinary surgery. F.O.C. Meenan, who had carried out postgraduate studies in London and Leeds, was appointed first whole-time dermatologist in 1949. Oliver McCullen joined Fagan and O'Brien in the department of otorhinolaryngology in 1951. He also had studied in London and Leeds. Philomena Guinan was appointed assistant ophthalmologist. She was the first woman consultant on the staff of the hospital. Nicholas Martin with the double qualification of dental surgeon and medical doctor was appointed dentist in 1949. James Maher came from Tipperary and joined the staff as assistant surgeon in

1948. A first class surgeon, he was to become one of the most popular and respected members of the staff of the hospital. After qualification he had been appointed house officer to Morrin. On one occasion Morrin was going away and instructed Maher about the management of a patient who was seriously ill at the time and who required constant supervision. Maher, who was an outstanding rugby player, had been selected to play in an important match and it was believed that if he performed well in this match there was a possibility of an international cap. With Maher, however, his patient came first; he did not tell Morrin about the match but rang his team captain to state that he would not be able to play. The principle that the patient always comes first was firmly held by 'Jamsie', as he was affectionately known during his professional life. Before taking up surgery Maher had practised as a gynaecologist; consequently he had no senior degree in surgery. In the 1950s the rule was instituted that hospital specialists must have a senior degree in the speciality in which they practised. At a mature age Maher had to settle down and study for the appropriate degree in surgery. This he accomplished successfully without any problem or fuss.

This chapter has recalled many of the appointments made in St Vincent's during the 1940s. It is well to recall also another important development at the beginning of this period when a rather rigid hierarchical system still prevailed in the hospital. The Medical Board consisted of the senior physicians and surgeons who were also in possession of the beds in the hospital and shared students' fees. The junior physicians and surgeons had to serve out their time at the out-patients' department relying on the good-will of the admissions sister for the use of an occasional bed. They had to wait until such times as a senior physician or surgeon retired and a vacancy occurred on the Board. It was usually the most senior of the junior physicians or surgeons who was elevated. Depending on the longevity of the senior members of the staff the juniors had to put in a varying degree of service in the out-patients' department.

Most assistants were eventually appointed to the senior staff, but this was by no means a universal rule. There were several examples in the history of the hospital of young physicians and surgeons resigning before the opportunity came for them to be appointed to the senior staff. Some decided to resign because there was no foreseeable vacancy on the senior staff. Others wished to further their careers in medicine outside the hospital. Such men as C. Burke Gaffney, assistant surgeon 1896–99, Glasgow Patterson, assistant surgeon 1889–93, Matthew B. Savage, assistant physician 1890–92 and Christopher Shortall 1927–35 gave outstanding service to the hospital.

Students' fees were divided by the members of the Board. Obviously such a situation was fraught with the possibility of friction between the senior and junior members of the staff. Juniors would be asked at times to give lectures. In 1940 the junior staff approached the Board and asked that they should be paid for giving these lectures to the students. This request rather upset the senior medical members and for a period the relationship between senior and junior staff was slightly cool. However, a solution was found through the good offices of J.N. Meenan. An association called the Clinical Association of St Vincent's Hospital Dublin was established. The objects of the association were to promote and provide:

(*a*) Facilities for meetings and scientific discussion.

(*b*) The advancement and co-ordination of different departments, services and teaching.

(*c*) A medical and scientific reference library.

(*d*) Publication of medical and scientific papers.

Any member of the senior and junior staff of the hospital was eligible for membership of the association and meetings were held during the university term, on the third Tuesday of the month at 8.30 p.m., and special clinical meetings were held apart from the ordinary meetings. The new clinical association was formally launched at a dinner in J.N. Meenan's house in the spring of 1940. The association was destined to play an important and successful role in the life of the hospital. Basically it provided the forum at which all members of the staff could voice their opinions and bring their problems and difficulties to the attention of their colleagues. As the years went by the association became less and less clinical, but during the planning and building of the new hospital at Elm Park it played a vital role. It was at meetings of the association that plans for the new hospital were discussed by all members of the staff. Among its other successful duties was that of organising the annual dinner for the members of the medical staff.

CHAPTER 14

THE COMMUNITY

A t the annual dinner of the Clinical Association attended by members of the medical staff, the important toast of the evening is the 'Irish Sisters of Charity'. Thus those doctors who work in the hospital pay tribute to the congregation of sisters who founded and administer St Vincent's. Medical staff come and go, major advances are made in medical science, the social and political structures change, but the thread which links the small early-Victorian hospital to the large modern teaching hospital is the sisters who give their lives' work freely to the hospital and to its ideals.

The relationship between the medical staff and the community has always been good. The annals of the hospital reveal no serious dispute between nuns and doctors beyond the odd minor difference of opinion and the occasional small storm in a teacup. This is probably due to the fact that both groups basically share a common ideal which is the care and healing of the sick. Illustrating the care with which the community has respected the independence of the hospital staff, it is interesting to note that the sisters were forbidden to enter the Medical Boardroom.

When recounting the labours of the community in the hospital one vital point must be emphasised. In this antibiotic era it is easy to forget that working in a general hospital a century ago was a difficult and indeed dangerous vocation. Infectious diseases, and particularly tuberculosis, were rife in all hospitals of the period. The annals of St Vincent's are full of accounts of the deaths of young nuns who obviously contracted serious diseases during the course of their duties. A young sister, Sister Phillippa Morris, daughter of a Lord Chief Justice of Ireland, died in 1889, a short time after she began nursing in a ward. In 1901 Sister Elizabeth Reidy, ward sister for ten years, and Sister Mercedes Esch died within a few weeks of each other—and there were many others.

In describing the work of the sisters over the years the historian must be aware that the labours of many members of the community who gave great service to the hospital must go unrecorded. Even the hospital's historians will admit that the records of the hospital are somewhat impersonal. By virtue of their office the names of Reverend Mothers and ward sisters are well known. Two names are especially remembered with gratitude from the early days of the hospital: they are Sister Lucy Clifford and Sister Otteran Kier.

Sister Clifford was the daughter of the Hon. Thomas Clifford and Henrietta Philippina, Baroness de Lutzow. Sister Clifford's dowry bought no. 57 St Stephen's Green for the hospital. Although she did not spend a long period working in St Vincent's, as mistress of novices she had a great influence on the development of the congregation. She died in 1860.

Sister Otteran Kier came from Waterford and entered the congregation late in life. Soon after her profession she was appointed to the hospital. She was a ward sister for many years. She organised regular grants and subscriptions from guilds and confraternities, entitling them to send in patients from their organisations. She had many friends from all walks of life ranging from painters, coopers and the police to the Earl of Carlisle the Lord Lieutenant who visited her ward frequently. On Sundays and weekday evenings former patients and their families would visit her to report on their progress since leaving hospital. She died in 1873.

Many of the sisters laboured in the background, working in vital departments without which no hospital can function. They did not seek recognition for their work, but their monument is found in the fruits of their labour. Sister Asicus Doyle who died in 1943 worked for fifty years in the kitchens. Sister Salome Murphy who continued to work in the kitchens for many years although she had rheumatoid arthritis died in 1937. Sister Alexis who died in 1955 also worked in the kitchen. Sister Dismas Moore in charge of the private nursing homes died in 1942. Sister Pelagia Finnegan laboured in no. 58.

Sister Benedict Joseph Constable Maxwell—Mrs Maxwell—was a member of the Herries family, an old pre-Reformation English Catholic family who could trace their lineage back to the Norman conquest. She was the aunt of a Duchess of Norfolk, wife of the Premier Duke of England. She celebrated her Golden Jubilee in 1921, the first St Vincent's nun to do so. She spent the greater part of her life as a sacristan and died in 1930 aged eighty-six. On one occasion she told her rather startled sisters in the community that her nephew had been appointed Governor in one of his Britannic Majesty's dominions overseas. She rather hoped that a 'decent pension' would go with the job.

Sister Monica Joseph Bourke who died in 1953 was also sacristan for many years. Sister Teresa Augustine, ward sister and infirmarian, died in 1949. Sister Magdalen Alphonsus Bowater—Mrs Bowater—spent many years in charge of the Leeson Street private nursing homes. She died in 1936. Sister Alcantara Coleman—Mrs Coleman—worked in many parts of the hospital; she also spent many years in the X-ray department in the nursing home, but is chiefly remembered for her labours in the out-patients' department. This was in the old out-patients' before the new department was built. There was much poverty amongst the patients attending the out-patients' and she spared no effort to help the poor and the sick. She was permanently lame.

Sister Loyola Donovan—Mrs Donovan—died in 1955. She was well known to many generations of young nurses in whose welfare she took a great interest. She had been ward sister in St Laurence's until she became completely crippled from rheumatoid arthritis and confined to a wheel-chair. She was wheeled by porters Barney and Christy into the chapel for Mass and then to the splint room where she worked. Sister Loyola was one of the last sisters to whom the title Mrs was given. Sister Jerome Gordon died in 1968. She had spent twenty years in St Patrick's ward, but she also organised the sales of work and Violet Day collections for the hospital. She had spent many years also working in the hospital's out-patients' department.

Sister Fidelis Butler had been Ministress of the hospital for many years and during the temporary absence of Mrs Carew she was Reverend Mother at one stage. She died in 1960. Sister Mary Basil O'Donnell was also Ministress for a considerable period, as well as Sister Lorcan McDonagh. Sister Josepha Shortall was also in charge of the out-patients' for a significant period of time.[1]

It is clear from the history of the hospital in the nineteenth century that the Reverend Mothers who succeeded Mrs Aikenhead were worthy successors. They had constant problems to attend to as they guided the destiny of a young hospital in troubled Victorian Ireland. They had no easy task. The Reverend Mother was the supreme power in the hospital and all decisions were made by her. Mrs McCarthy, Mrs Margison, Mrs Seagrave and Mrs Cullen were able and formidable administrators.

Mrs Cullen (Mother Canisius Cullen) inherited the talents of her uncle Cardinal Cullen, Archbishop of Dublin, who was considered by many to be the leading Churchman in Ireland during the nineteenth century. Margaret Cullen was born in Liverpool in 1839 and was educated by the Society of the Sacred Heart first at Glasnevin and subsequently at Mount Anville. It was her uncle Cardinal Cullen who suggested to her that she should join the Sisters of Charity. She became Rectress of the hospital in 1882. She was Reverend Mother during a vital period in the development of the hospital and she guided it successfully into a new century. During her period of office provision was made for a new surgical ward in the hospital. The private nursing homes in Lower Leeson Street were founded and the nursing school was established. A new system of sanitation was introduced into the hospital which required the closing of the institution for many months.

She was a strict disciplinarian but very tactful and many a student had reason to remember gratefully her skill and diplomacy in settling difficulties . . . she was admired, almost venerated by her community but as cold as marble even to the suggestion of a compliment. She seldom praised anyone, but yet there was never any doubt about her approbation or displeasure. She was tender with the weak, and well knew how to cheer the despondent. To a Sister who, from long meditation on her grievances, real or imaginary, had made herself, and possibly others, miserable, she remarked, at the conclusion of a lengthy jeremiad on the part of the Sister: Did you ever hear what the dying terrier said to the pup? 'In all life's adversities, keep your tail up.'[2]

She was appointed Mother General in 1905 and died in 1911.

It was fortunate for St Vincent's that the next century provided leaders of a similar calibre. It is fair to say that for most of the first half of the twentieth century the hospital was dominated by one personality, Mother Bernard Carew—Mrs Carew. She had several periods of office as Reverend Mother, but whether in or out of office she influenced the affairs of St Vincent's Hospital and guided it safely through many crises. She was Reverend Mother from 1905 to 1918. This was in the period before religious superiors were confined to a period of office of six years. She was Reverend Mother again in 1924. She had to travel abroad in the course of her duties but was Rectress during the Centenary Year 1934, when she was also involved in the purchasing of Elm Park estate for the new hospital. She was Mother General of the congregation from 1935 to 1953 and died in 1954. Everybody was rather in awe of Mrs Carew, but she was fiercely loyal to all who worked in the hospital and always ready to help them in their difficulties. She had a commanding presence and a formidable manner. Many stories are told about her.

She was supposed to be deaf in one ear and she possessed a large ear trumpet which could be wielded from either ear. It was a matter of constant debate amongst the officials of the Department of Local Government and Public Health as to which was the deaf ear. It was customary for newly-appointed consultants to the hospital to present themselves to Mrs Carew when she was Mother General and living in Mount St Anne's, Milltown. She did not approve of young consultants having cars; therefore it was a prudent young consultant who left his car concealed in Milltown Road and walked up the drive to the convent.

Mother Theckla Maunsell who was Reverend Mother for two terms during the 1920s and the 1930s did not mince her words. The story is told that a distinguished senior member of the surgical staff rang the hospital a number of times one evening and could not get a reply. Exasperated, he sent a telegram to Mother Theckla requesting her to remove 'the corpse' from the telephone office. The next morning he was summoned to an unamused Reverend Mother. He was told that if he did not like the arrangements in the hospital he could leave, or to use the usual euphemism, 'could better himself in another hospital'. He was also informed that surgeons were ten a penny, but good night telephonists were very difficult to get.

Mother Theckla's second term of office expired in 1941 and she was succeeded by Mother Joseph Ignatius Austin. Her term of office was interrupted by illness and she was temporarily replaced by Mother Baptist Magan. She returned to duty after a year's absence. She died rather suddenly in office in September 1948. Of a rather austere personality she was a very able and conscientious administrator. Even the most minor matters received her full attention. Mother Baptist resumed duty as Reverend Mother in November 1948. Of a retiring and shy disposition, she had a very human approach to patients and staff. She made many significant improvements to the amenities in the hospital, especially providing the community with more suitable accommodation. She was succeeded by Mother Canisius O'Keeffe in 1954.

Mother Canisius had worked in the wards for many years and also as Ministress. Thus she was experienced in all the affairs of the hospital. St Vincent's made many important advances during her period of office. The building of a new block consisting of lecture theatre, casualty, cardiology and metabolism departments in Leeson Lane was initiated. The school of nursing, which had been located in cramped quarters, was re-established in 94 Lower Leeson Street. The Pembroke Nursing Home in Upper Pembroke Street—which had been vacant—was purchased for the hospital. Nurses' uniforms were modernised and brought more into keeping with modern hospital fashion. In the 1950s Mother Canisius also revived the annual prize-giving ceremony at which a member of the staff read a paper on some contemporary medical problem and nurses and medical students received their prizes and awards. In the evening, the annual dinner of the hospital was held in a Dublin hotel to which friends of the hospital were invited. The ceremony had been discontinued for many years. Also during her period of office delicate negotiations took place with the authorities of University College Dublin concerning the relationship between the hospital and the university.[3]

In 1960 Mother Paula Gleeson became Reverend Mother. She was to be the last Reverend Mother of St Vincent's on the Green and she had a particularly difficult term of office. The hopes and ambitions of all those who worked in the Green were now focused on Elm Park. It was her difficult task to keep the flag of the old hospital flying until the very last moment before the move and in this she succeeded admirably.

A roll call of the sisters working in the wards in 1957 would include:

Sister Francis Mary Lawn, St Brigid's;
Sister Agnes Ursula Byrne, St Patrick's;
Sister Padua Hannon, St Laurence's;
Sister Marie John Sexton, St Charles's;
Sister M. Ignatius Killeen, St Raphael's and St Vincent's;

Sister Vincent de Paul O'Donovan, St Anne's;
Sister Margaret Cecilia Curley, 60;
Sister Francis Borgia Berney, St Joseph's;
Sister Catherina O'Brien, 96.
Sister Stephanie Murphy was away studying home nursing;
Sister Rosaleen Foley was working in the Pembroke Nursing Home.

Other well-known ward sisters of the period were Sister Fidelma McDonnell who was ward sister in St Raphael's for many years; Sister Dolores McGucken in St Laurence's; Sister Pascal Guerin in St Laurence's; and Sister Claude de la Columbiere Meehan in St Vincent's.[4]

They all had their individual methods and characteristics. Medical students, house officers, student nurses and above all patients fell under their expert and at times autocratic direction. Student nurses and doctors received a training from which they benefited for the rest of their lives. Patients were given unremitting care and attention in their illness and assistance and advice in their family affairs. If recovery was not to be they were prepared to meet the inevitable with courage and devotion. In the early days the ward sister was nurse, social worker, family advisor and religious counsellor all in one. In more recent years Sister Carmel Mary Flannery undertook the organisation and running of a medico-social department to deal with the various social and economic problems of patients.

It is perhaps inappropriate to single out one sister, but mention must be made of Sister Francis Borgia Berney—'the Borge'. She justified the rather hackneyed description of being a legend in her own lifetime. She had a rather forbidding manner and had the disconcerting habit of calling patients by the number on the bed rather than by their names. She was superficially severe to her student nurses and doctors and even the most senior consultants were known to defer to her. Behind a rather forbidding exterior was a kind heart and total commitment to the welfare of her patients. All over the globe there are Vincent's-trained nurses and doctors who still recount with pride their sojourn with 'the Borge'.

Another legend in the hospital is Sister Ibar Redmond. To many generations she is imperishably associated with the out-patients' department and admissions. Small, even tiny, she would look at one sideways with large dark all-seeing eyes. Her voice was soft but every word she spoke was full of sympathy and common sense. Like Mrs Coleman and the other sisters in the out-patients' before her she helped in many unobtrusive ways the patients who thronged the dispensary. She thought not only of their physical welfare but also of their social and spiritual needs. As an admission sister who controlled the acceptance of patients into the hospital she had an almost impossible task. In a relatively small hospital, the pressure on beds was enormous. Many were the Homeric encounters she had with irate consultants who felt that their patients should receive priority in admission to a ward. The small frame showed no lack of fire and she gave as good as

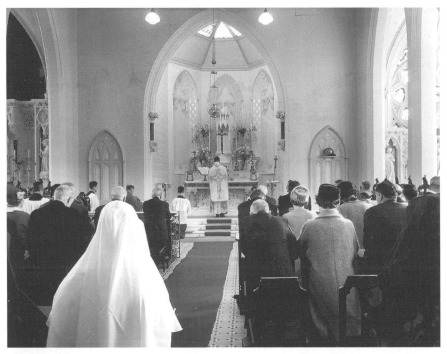

Hospital chapel, St Stephen's Green

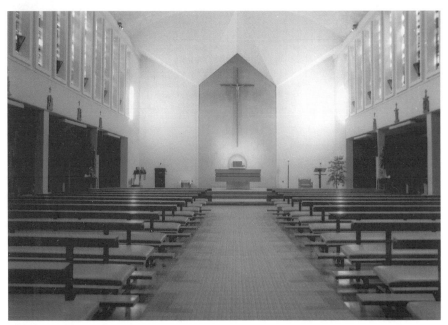

Hospital chapel, Elm Park

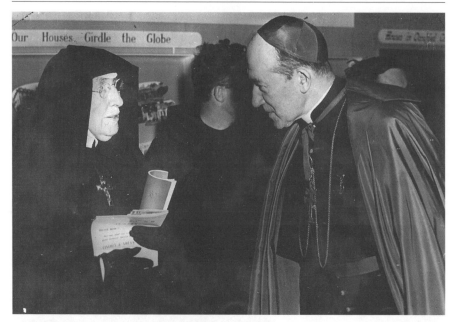

Mother Bernard Carew with Archbishop McQuaid

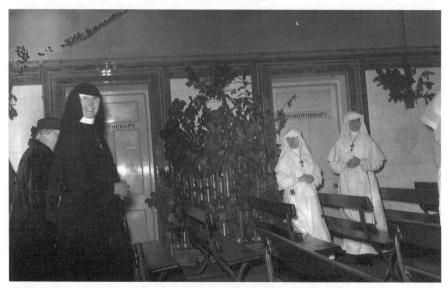

Christmas party, out-patients' department with (left to right) Mother Teresa Anthony, Sr M. Ibar, Sr M. Padua

she got from even the most formidable adversary. On hearing of her death one doctor was heard to remark that he was sure Sister Ibar was in heaven but he rather hoped she was not in charge of admissions. Sister Ibar celebrated her Golden Jubilee in 1964 and died in 1969. It has been reported that many people have seen Sister Ibar since her death wandering around the gardens at the back of 96–99 Lower Leeson Street. If so it means that the area is still in good care.[5]

Christmas is a special occasion in all hospitals and St Vincent's was no exception. Members of the staff and their families were invited to assist at Midnight Mass on Christmas Eve. This was in the days before there was general permission for Midnight Mass in all churches and it was a special privilege to be invited to St Vincent's. It was the highlight of the year when the community and staff worshipped together. The main altar of the chapel with its marble reredos and canopy was shining in the candlelight and garlanded with flowers. Visitors were ushered into seats at the sides of the altar and back of the chapel. The size of the chapel did not change from year to year but there was a constant increase in staff numbers. Nevertheless, there was always room for every visitor. In the choir the sisters knelt motionless in their prie-dieus, their long black cloaks trailing on the chapel floor. In contrast, the veils and aprons of the nurses' choir were shining white as they sang the *Adeste Fideles*. The peace of Christmas descended on the congregation. As the clock chimed the passing of the hours the chaplain celebrated the three Masses and distributed Holy Communion. The visitors then quietly withdrew.

On Christmas morning it was customary for members of the staff and their families to visit the hospital. They were received in the parlour by Mother Rectress and Christmas greetings were exchanged. The families then visited the wards of the hospital to greet the ward sister and her nurses and to admire the decoration in the wards, to which much thought and care had been given. Sister would be especially interested in the progress of the doctors' children. The older ones would be quizzed about their progress in examinations; the younger ones would be told, to their slight embarrassment, how much they had grown during the last year. It was altogether a happy family occasion. Patients who had to spend Christmas in hospital enjoyed the visit as well. They realised that their doctors were not demi-gods from some other world, but parents like themselves in most cases, with many of the same problems and difficulties.

For the last few years in the Green, while the attendance at Midnight Mass continued, the visit on Christmas morning was discontinued. Instead the visit took place on a Sunday afternoon before Christmas. This fitted in more conveniently with the domestic pattern of modern living. A few weeks after Christmas the staff and their families assisted at Quarant' Ore. Also many children of members of staff made their First Holy Communion in the hospital chapel.

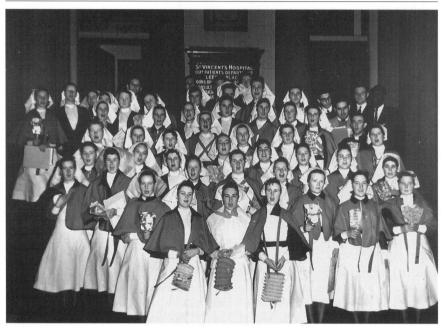

Christmas carols

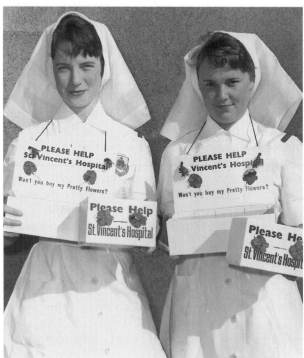

Violet Day

How does one sum up the relationship between the staff and the community? Perhaps it was best done by P.T. O'Farrell in *A Century of Service*:

> As a Vincent's man, he will never forget the Irish Sisters of Charity, who taught him the nobler side of his profession, by their example of undaunted courage, self-sacrificing devotion to the poor, and true compassion for those afflicted with the ills and misfortunes of mankind.

More than fifty years later this tribute is as valid as it was when it was written.[6]

CHAPTER 15

THE NURSING SCHOOL

There were many dramatic changes during the course of the nineteenth century, but none more dramatic than the changes which occurred in nursing. During the first half of the nineteenth century the profession of nursing did not exist. There was no system of training suitable young women who wished to become nurses. Many of the women, particularly in England, who looked after patients in lay hospitals came from the lower strata of society. They wore no uniform, had no training and were subject to little discipline. They were frequently disorderly. The nurse of the period is immortalised as Mrs Gamp in the pages of *Martin Chuzzlewit* by Charles Dickens.

Some modern historians are of the opinion that the picture of Mrs Gamp as a typical nurse of the period is exaggerated and there is no doubt that some of the mid-Victorian women who took up nursing came from respectable backgrounds. However, in general the standard of nursing during the first half of the century was deplorably low. The Governors of the lay hospitals were aware of the problems and undertook the Herculean task of improving the standards in their hospitals. In their struggle many of them were to take the example of St Vincent's Hospital as their ideal. Agnes E. Pavey in *The Growth of Nursing* states that the Irish Sisters of Charity had always been known 'for the beautifully finished technique of their nursing duties, for the order and completeness of their ward equipment and for attention to detail'.[1]

The nursing in St Vincent's was highly organised. The sisters looked upon nursing not only as a profession and that a necessary profession, but also considered the care of the sick and the destitute to be a vocation. There was great emphasis on training, as can be seen from the appointment of Mother Camillus Sallinave to take charge of nursing from the very first years of the hospital's existence. Mother Camillus was a born organiser, with a natural taste for nursing. Having mastered the system of the great French Hôpital de la Pitié she lost no time in putting it into operation, and with her genius for detail she soon established a very efficient system in St Vincent's.

Mrs Aikenhead's instructions to her sisters were full of common sense. 'Patients are to be received with kindness and courtesy'; the sick poor were 'to be served with respect, cordiality and compassion'; they were 'to be made happy'; they were 'to have comforts'. 'There is no charity without respect'; they were not to be fatigued with too many devotions; regulations were not to be too rigidly enforced when reason suggested, or consideration permitted, some relaxation. She expected the highest attainable efficiency, with intelligence and charity in its application.[2]

The fame of St Vincent's spread and nursing reformers like Florence Nightingale visited the hospital to see if they could gain knowledge from the experience of the sisters. In general, hospitals run by nuns had limited need for lay nurses. The nursing positions were adequately filled by members of the community. However, a small number of reliable nurse attendants were needed to work in the wards and look after the patients at night. The nurse attendants were trained and supervised by the ward sisters. In later years Sister Alcantara Coleman was particularly interested in their training. Many of them reached a very high standard. This can be judged from the fact that it was the quick thinking of a night nurse which saved the hospital from the effects of a disastrous fire in 1854.

The last of the old nurse attendants, Josephine Fortune, only died in 1935. She had been night portress for many years, when there was no longer a need for nurse attendants. She was known to at least three generations of sisters, doctors and nurses. She was eulogised in *A Century of Service*, by John Mowbray, a former student of the hospital.[3] It was said that she was as memorable a feature of the hospital as the granite pillars of the portico. She looked after the wards at night and had the task of waking the sisters to come to the bedside of any patient who was dying.

The lay hospitals had a more urgent need for training nursing personnel and in the latter half of the nineteenth century they took the initiative in opening schools.

The prototype of the nursing school in England was the Nightingale school of nursing opened under the inspiration of Florence Nightingale in St Thomas's Hospital, London in 1860; this school was for the training of matrons and senior nursing personnel. A school for training nurses had previously been opened in King's College Hospital, London. In Ireland the Adelaide Hospital nursing school for the training of young Protestant nurses preceded the Nightingale school by two years. It opened in 1858 under the direction of a Miss Bramwell, although it did not become functional for about another two years.[4] Dr Steevens' Hospital nursing school opened in 1866; as pointed out by KirkPatrick, in his history of the hospital, this school ran into religious difficulties. 'Any such institution was likely to be looked upon as suspect by a Roman Catholic community while it would have too much flavour of a Roman Catholic religious order to be acceptable to some Protestants.'[5]

Thomas Laffan, in *The Medical Profession in the Three Kingdoms in 1879*, gives an interesting picture of hospital nursing at that period:

> The nursing arrangements have material relation to the state of our hospitals. Despite the labours of a host of philanthropical persons during the last few years, the nursing arrangements of most of our hospitals are still most imperfect. In some of the London ones and some of our Dublin ones the nearest approach to perfection seems to have been attained. In those London ones referred to, the nursing is done under a combined arrangement of lady superintendent and women nurses.
>
> We can conceive no nursing that could equal the tender care of the intelligent wife or mother, but the nearest approach to this will, we think, be found in the above system. The nursing carried out under the personal direction and exertions of the Sisters of Charity and of kindred orders is, at least, not inferior to that to which we have above referred. Personal experience induces us to look with something like horror on the work done by nurses of the common sort. They are as a rule so neglectful; and in some instances so dishonest that there is no safety in entrusting life to their care. Nothing that we can conceive can bear a more important relation to clinical studies and clinical results than proper nursing.[6]

In the beginning of the 1890s the Catholic Archbishop of Dublin, Dr William J. Walsh, requested the Catholic hospitals in Dublin to organise schools for the training of young girls in the nursing profession. There were several reasons for this request. The rapid advances in medicine necessitated more facilities for treatment. Up to this time well-off people who could afford to pay for their medical attention were treated at home. To cater for this class private nursing homes attached to the hospitals were being opened. All these developments required more nurses, because even in this period there were not enough trained nurses to provide full nursing services in the hospitals and nursing homes. In addition during the previous thirty to forty years there had been a considerable increase in schools established for the education of young women. Now there was a large number of girls highly educated and anxious to use their talents in a suitable and beneficial fashion and to play a significant role in the community. On 7 July 1891 there was a meeting of the Medical Board of St Vincent's. Present were Mr McArdle, Dr Cox, Mr Tobin and Dr McHugh.

The meeting was called in obedience to a request of Mrs Cullen, Mother Rectress, that the Board should consider the desirability of the establishment by her of an institution for training nurses in connection with the hospital. The Board having considered the matter was of the opinion that the establishment of such an institution was a highly desirable step and in connection with it, and if possible in the same building, one or two wards for the reception of private patients should be opened. These views were then conveyed verbally to Mrs Cullen who subsequently attended the meeting and was informed verbally of the views held by the Board as expressed above.[7]

St Vincent's in common with the other hospitals acceded to the Archbishop's request and a training school was opened on a small scale in May 1892. Pavey commented, 'Although many of the older religious sisters viewed the development with some dismay the standard of the nursing school has continued to be in complete harmony with the traditions of the hospital.'[8] No. 65 St Stephen's Green, the corner house at the junction of Stephen's Green West and Earlsfort Terrace, was purchased for sleeping accommodation. The first lay superintendent appointed was a Miss Robinson who had done her training in the Adelaide Hospital. She filled the post for a period of approximately six months and then retired to join the religious of the Society of the Sacred Heart at Roehampton.

A Miss Campbell who had trained in the Edinburgh Royal Infirmary was then appointed superintendent and another lady, Miss Mason, who had trained at Sir Patrick Dun's Hospital, filled the post of night superintendent. Six trainee nurses, or probationers as they were called at the time, started the course. In the following year twenty-four probationers were admitted to the school. The annals of the period state that 'these young ladies were a great help to the sisters in their attendance on the sick poor and added considerably to the comfort of these poor afflicted creatures, in helping the doctors to carry out their work as to compete with any other institution of its kind in Dublin'.

Lectures in medicine and surgery were given by the medical staff to the probationer nurses and they were instructed in ward practice, care and management of patients by the sisters. At the end of each year each trainee sat a house examination. Those who were successful would be deemed to be proficient in the art of nursing and were awarded a hospital badge and certificate. In 1904 it was recorded that:

> The working of the training school for nurses during the last five years shows a gradual improvement, the outcome of many lessons learned in the school of experience. However on the whole the results have been satisfactory and the assistance of nurses in the wards has become a necessity for the efficient working of the hospital. In order to give the certificate required for the government appointments, it has been arranged that they shall spend the two years in training before being sent out to nurse for the benefit of the hospital. On the expiration of the four years of training the greater numbers have got good appointments on the nursing staffs in England. Three fill the posts of lady superintendents, six are well married, four have entered religious orders, two succeeded in joining the army medical service and others are doing good work as Jubilee nurses in country districts.[9]

In the early days there had been opposition to the concept of a nursing school, but this seemed to vanish as the nursing school proved its value. Miss Campbell retired in 1906 and was succeeded by a Miss Sutton. William Doolin remembers her as 'a daughter of the gods, divinely tall'. Miss Sutton might have been a daughter of the gods, but apparently she had a slightly sharp tongue. She told Doolin, 'Young man, when you die you will be found talking in your coffin.' Doolin described the nurses of this period as wearing absurd mob caps, with long strings tied in huge bow knots under the chin.

In 1909 sisters from many orders were admitted to the nursing school. Queries were raised by the local government board as to the qualifications of the nuns appointed to teach the probationers. It was decided that the ward sisters who were not certified should go up for examination. They had to attend lectures and study with the ward nurses. In May 1910 eight sisters presented themselves for oral and written examinations with the different grades of nurses. They passed successfully and received certificates which secured many long-desired advantages for them. At this time it was also decided that sisters coming to take up ward work in the future should receive training and obtain their certificates before taking charge of a ward.

With the marked increase in the number of probationers studying in the training school fresh accommodation had to be provided for them as a matter of urgency. In 1910 a new home was built at the back of the hospital, on Leeson Lane—a large redbrick four-storey building. On the first floor were the library, refectory, store-rooms, kitchens; on the second the matron's apartment, infirmary and linen-room. There were separate sitting-rooms provided for staff nurses and probationers and a large recreation room. The probationers' cubicles were on the third floor and the staff nurses had separate rooms on the fourth. The nurses' home was connected with the hospital by means of a bridge which crossed Leeson Lane, and with the private nursing homes on Lower Leeson Street by a metal stairs and bridge which was the gift of Dr Michael Cox. The building was completed in April 1913. The building cost in the neighbourhood of £17,000 and there was no money left to provide a lift. The fifth storey was added to the nurses' home in 1924.[10]

In those times the probationers received no material reward, but their parents paid a considerable fee for the privilege of their training. Miss Angela Halbert was matron from 1918 to 1946. Although small in stature she was a formidable lady. She was a strict disciplinarian but essentially fair-minded and was respected by her nurses. She stamped her personality indelibly on the nursing school. Geraldine McSweeney has written a comprehensive account of the day-to-day work of the nursing school.[11]

> In 1919 the Parliament of Westminster introduced legislation to standardise nurse training and the Nurses Registration (Ireland) Act became law. A General Nursing Council ensued and approved a three year training course with State examination, success in which was essential for registration in the 'General Register'. Participating

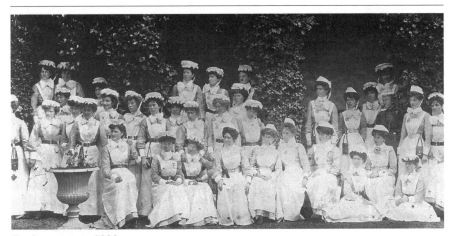

Student nurses, 1906

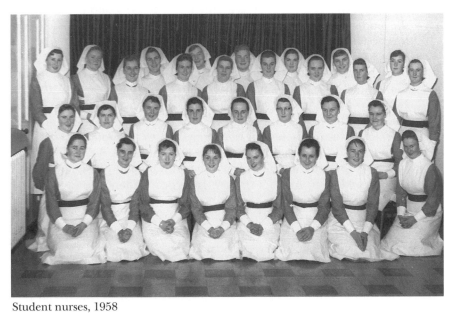

Student nurses, 1958

hospitals were inspected and approved as training schools. In Ireland, only the voluntary hospitals took their place in the scheme. St Vincent's was approved as a training school. This meant that probationers had to be educated according to the guidelines set out in the syllabus and at the end of three years training sit a State examination. Although the nurses became registered after three years, their training lasted four years, gaining experience as registered nurses for the last year.

Typical duties of the nurse at that time included dusting, scrubbing, long brushing of walls and ceilings, cupping, leeching and poulticing in addition to the obvious general care of the patient, e.g. bed-making, bathing, feeding etc. The hours worked were long and the off duty meagre. The day began with Mass at 6.30 a.m. and following breakfast the nurse was on duty in the ward from 7.30 a.m. to 8.00 p.m. with a two hour break in addition to allotted meal times. A half day off, commencing at 3.30 p.m., was granted once a week, and provided that the student did not obtain any black marks for lack of punctuality she was permitted one day off per month. The students went on night duty for a period of three months every so often. Night rounds with the night matron were carried out in candlelight—the student carrying the lighted candle—this practice continued until the early 1950s. The students worked from 8.00 p.m. to 7.30 a.m. with no nights off. At the end of the three months she got 2–3 days off if the staff situation was satisfactory, if not these days were added on to her holidays . . . There were open fires in each ward for heating purposes. These fires were also used to boil water and to toast bread. Often, on a Sunday a ward sister would sit in front of the fire and cook rashers and sausages for the patients' tea . . .

In 1950, the first steps were taken to dissolve the General Nursing Council (1919) and the Midwives Board (1918) and to set up our own statutory body for Ireland. The Nurses' Act of 1950 established An Bord Altranais to make provision for the registration, certification and training of nurses, including postgraduate training. New syllabi were issued and new conditions of training were laid down. The 1940s brought the introduction of a course of basic lectures in nursing at the beginning of a student's training. All other lectures were still attended during the student's time off. This system of formal education continued until 1956.

In 1993 on night duty the student nurse has seven nights on and seven nights off. On day duty there are two shifts of eight hours and the student nurse has two days off per week. It was during the 1930s that the students first received monetary remuneration—£2.00 per month. This increased gradually over the decades and in 1994 the salary of a first year student nurse is £4,959 per annum, a second year nurse £7,593 per annum and a third year nurse £10,746 per annum.

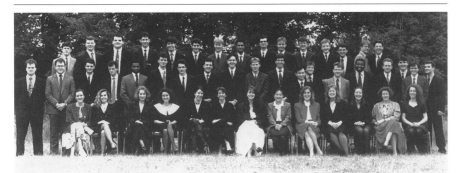

Resident medical staff, 1992

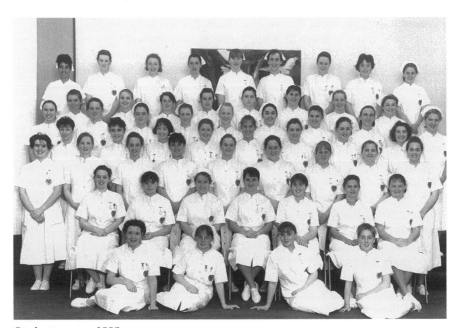

Student nurses, 1992

Annie Kelly succeeded as matron in 1946. She had been out-patients' and theatre sister. A Northerner, she performed her duties with typical common sense and directness. She was succeeded in 1968 by Emma McDonnell who had been assistant matron. She had a tall imposing dignified presence. She surmounted successfully the difficulties which arose during the change from the Green to Elm Park.

During the 1950s the education of student nurses became more comprehensive, and extra room was required for the development of the nursing school. Mother Canisius O'Keeffe established the Mary Aikenhead school of nursing in 94 Lower Leeson Street. 66 St Stephen's Green was decorated as a new residence for the nurses and for a short period a house was also rented at Lower Hatch Street, where nurses on night duty could sleep quietly, away from the noise of the hospital during the day.

In 1959 a new nurse's uniform more in keeping with modern medicine was introduced into the hospital. The uniform was all white, a coat frock with the congregational badge in blue, white shoes and the usual white veil. Seniority was indicated by a coloured stripe worn on the shoulder: blue for first year, yellow for second year and red for third year.

Miss Roseanne Cunningham was appointed nurse tutor in 1952, a position she held until 1955 when she became education officer of An Bord Altranais. Sister Frances Rose O'Flynn, having completed the nurse tutor course, was appointed principal tutor and remained in this position until 1969, directing nurse education with the assistance of Miss Bridin Tierney and Miss Marjorie Deegan. In 1964, the first clinical teacher, Mrs Rena Burke (*née* Murphy), was appointed. Her role was to teach the students practical nursing in the school and in the clinical area. Miss Brigid Barlow who returned to this country from Australia was night superintendent for many years before her retirement.

In other fields of nursing activity, Vincent's graduates were to be found in great numbers. Many of them served in the armed services at home and abroad. Several of them reached the highest position in their speciality. Annie Kelly was appointed matron of St Laurence's Hospital in 1968. She was succeeded as matron of St Laurence's and subsequently Beaumont Hospital by another graduate nurse of the school, Josephine Bartley. Ann O'Neill was appointed matron of Dr Steevens' Hospital and Kate Sheeran was appointed matron to Castlebar Hospital. Finola Harrington became matron in Teach Ultan. Bridin Tierney was appointed research officer of An Bord Altranais and Eilish Fulham became Superintendent, Public Health Nurses, Co. Kildare. Many Vincent's nurses also found fame outside nursing. Jenny Dowdall was a member of Seanad Éireann and was also the first woman Lord Mayor of Cork. Eileen Kennedy became a solicitor and subsequently a District Justice. Moira Lysaght became very well known for her historical writings and broadcast talks on many aspects of Irish literature and culture.

Although the conditions for student nurses improved over the years,

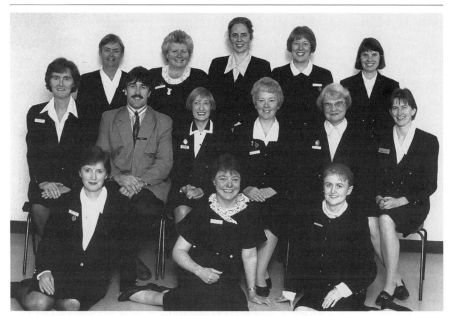

The Nursing School, 1994. (Back row, left to right) Mrs A. Malone, Miss M. Killeen, Miss H. Kevelighan, Miss L. Browne, Ms L. Crawley; (middle row, left to right) Miss M. Maume, Mr T. Kearns, Miss G. McSweeney, Sr A. Curry (principal tutor), Miss H. Marchant, Miss C. O'Reilly; (front row, left to right) Miss S. Byrne, Mrs M. Nicell, Mrs J. Burke

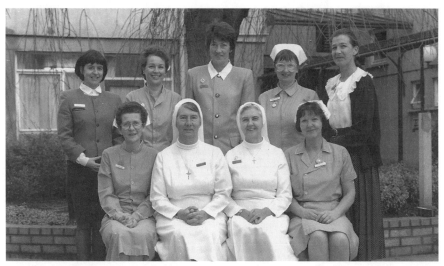

Department of Nursing Staff, 1994. (Back row, left to right) Ms Fiona Tyndall, Ms Margaret Murphy, Ms Pauline Doyle, Ms Valerie Feehan, Ms Stephanie MacDarby; (front row, left to right) Ms Petronilla Martin, Sr Philomena Farrell, Sr Agnes Reynolds, Ms Mary Murphy

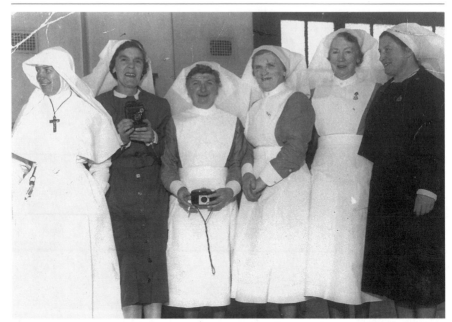

(Left to right) Sr Carmel Teresa, Emma McDonnell, Irene Hayes, Lil Fleming, May Maguire, Annie Kelly, at 96 St Stephen's Green

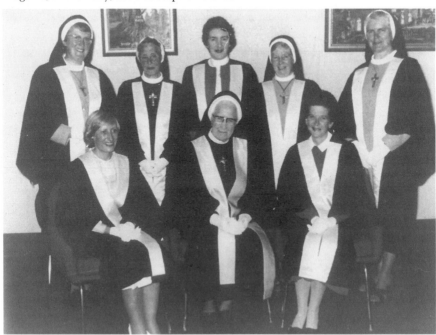

Fellowship in Nursing RCSI, 1984. (Back row, left to right) Sr Pauline Campbell, Sr Marie John Sexton, Miss Josephine Bartley, Sr Joseph Cyril Fortune, Sr Margaret Vincent Dockery; (front row, left to right) Miss G. McSweeney, Sr Canisius O'Keeffe, Miss Petronilla Martin

nursing remained a demanding vocation. Discipline was strict and had to be strict. Adherence to regulations, some of which might appear to be antediluvian, was essential. Crises involving danger to patients' lives could arise at any moment and had to be dealt with by the well-trained nurse. On a less dramatic note, student nurses had to learn practical nursing skills which were becoming more complicated all the time.

They had to show a sympathetic and helpful interest in all the patients' troubles. In *A Century of Service* one former nurse mentions how difficult it was for her to come on duty and listen to patients' sorrows and worries when she herself was recovering from a devastating family tragedy.[12] All these problems faced the nurses of the period and in changed circumstances could basically still arise for the modern nurse. Not alone had the student nurse to be always sympathetic and kind to her patients, but she also had to maintain a well-groomed appearance in the wards and in out-patients'. One could always single out a Vincent's-trained nurse by her deportment in uniform.

Rules regarding relationships between the student nurse and other members of the hospital staff were strict. Under threat of extreme penalty she was not allowed to talk to a house officer or student in the hospital except in the line of professional business. There are stories told of student nurses being sent home for transgressing this rule. No figures are officially available, but one has a feeling that such stories may have been somewhat exaggerated. There is certainly no doubt that many romances which were to last for a lifetime began in St Vincent's Hospital. Nothing gave the members of the community more pleasure than to see one of their nurses marrying one of the medical graduates of the hospital and over the years this was a frequent occurrence.

Several graduates of the Mary Aikenhead school continued their vocation by becoming members of the congregation of the Irish Sisters of Charity or other religious orders. Many of them have spent their whole life in the service of the hospital.

No. 58 was ruled with a silken rod by Fifi Kiely. In the theatre of 96 there was Miss Wallace, tall, grey and strict, succeeded by Pearl Phelan (Sister Joseph Ignatius). The ground floor and first floor of 96 were the territory of the two Lils. Lil Fleming held kindly but firm sway over the ground floor and its elegant appendage 'Bella Vista'. She was proud of the high standards of her hospital and indeed there are many successful consultants who learned more medicine from Lil Fleming than they ever did from a medical text book. An equally famous Lil, Lil Tuohy, governed the first floor. Behind a rather shy and austere manner she had a rich and warm personality. There must be many patients who owe a deep debt of gratitude to Lil Tuohy for her support in times of illness and crisis.

Presiding over the second floor one would meet Nancy McDermott (Mrs David Coyle). On the third floor were Tessie Deegan, Aggie Dunne and Molly Rouse with her imperturbable manner, beaming and radiating confidence. On the top floor, Frances Osborne (Sister Teresa of Avila), Maura Smart, Irene Hayes, and the soft Kerry accent of Rosie Clarke mingling with the clipped Northern accent of May Maguire. Away in Pembroke Street May Walshe was looking after the affairs of the Pembroke Nursing Home, Jenny Powell was working in the lab, Kitty McBride and Beatrice Byrne were organising the nurses' home, Carmel McCarthy was the sister in the orthopaedic department and Blanche Connolly and Hester Gleeson were in charge of the central sterilising unit.

Members of the community associated with the running of 96 were Sister Canisius O'Keeffe, Sister Paula Gleeson, Sister Catherina O'Brien, Sister Frances Mary Lawn and Sister Padua Hannon.

One ex-patient of the home, Mrs Pansy Cannon, broke into verse praising the virtues of the staff of 96 in a poem entitled: '96—From the One Who Got Away!'[13]

If ever you're ill in Dublin town and need to be cared and nursed,
Get yourself into 96 and then you're over the worst.
Sister Cath'rina is the one to see—She'll ferret you out a bed,
And you tell your doctor firmly, you're going nowhere instead.
Now we'll start down low where the rooms are large,
The prices are high and Lil Fleming's in charge.
She'll take you in hand, and females or males,
In no time at all you'll be back on the rails.
Go up the stairs and Lil Tuohy you'll meet,
Now the likes of her it is hard to beat.
Take her advice and do what you're told,
And after a week you'll feel new and not old.
Now climb two flights and you're up on the third,
Aggie Dunne is in charge and you're 'out of this world',
She'll spoil you and care you, and make you her pet,
And you'll get the attention you never had yet.
Now up to the top and here is Miss Smart,
Who'll take you at once to her dear kindly heart.
But what of the doctors they term it you're 'under'?
Well for me it's Harold Quinlan who's stolen the thunder,
Gussie Mehigan's my surgeon, he's really a dear,
I was just crossing the Jordan when he hauled me back here,
But I know he'll admit that without Dr Griffin,
I'd be playin' a wee harp instead of her spiffin'.
Then, too, Jack Molony who ignores all my groans,
And makes me do handstands for arthritic bones.
Down in the kitchen, Sister Dominique holds sway,
I'd like 'Baked Alaska' each day on my tray.
Miss Byrne and Miss Casson bring menus to choose,

They're always so nice you just couldn't refuse.
Elsie's my girl with her well laden trays,
The standard of food would really amaze.
Mrs Heylen's the Sec.—she brings round the accounts,
And smiles at you sweetly as you face the amounts.
Miss Tyrrell's the physio who comes every day,
To flatten my tummy—God keep it that way!
The X-ray is gas! 'Breathe in, and breathe out',
Do they really and truly know what it's about?
Thanks Dr Cantwell and also Miss Snee,
For all the indignities you've done to me!
In the hall there's Cecilia and Christy's there too,
To them and all others my praises are due.
Now I've left someone out—on purpose 'twas done,
Could I ask Mother Rectress to join in the fun?
Yes, friends, I believe I could, and I do,
Because she'd enjoy it, and so it's her due.
And what of the chaplains? The Prods and R.C.
Blessings on both—they were so good to me.

Moira Lysaght has left an entertaining and an informative account of her years spent as a probationer nurse in St Vincent's during the late twenties and early thirties. She ran into some choppy weather from the beginning. First she had to solve the intricacies of dressing in the nurse's uniform. Subsequently, due to a misunderstanding with a patient in one of the wards, she was hauled up for interview by Miss Halbert, the matron, and then for a further interview with the Reverend Mother Mrs Carew. After a short sojourn in St Joseph's ward she was transferred to St Patrick's. St Patrick's was under the care of Sister Jerome, whom she described as a woman of strong character and the dread of the indolent and the inefficient. Sister Jerome told Miss Halbert that Moira Lysaght was the best probationer she had had for a long time. From St Patrick's she went to St Laurence's where she had a very happy relationship with Sister Ibar.

At this period the parents of probationer nurses had to pay an entrance fee of £60. Nurses' allowances were nothing in the first year, £10 in the second year, £12 in the third year and £15 in the fourth and final year. The period of training was four years; the State Registration was at the end of the third year.

Time off was two hours on two mornings each week plus one long evening from the end of the three o'clock dinner (if one were lucky) or at the end of the four o'clock one; otherwise one had to go to matron's office for permission and if a button was missing from one's sleeve one was greeted with 'No time off nurse, go and spend the time sewing on your buttons.' Once a month there was a whole day off with theatre leave which meant that you could stay out until 11 p.m. and on Sunday one had a half day. Night duty lasted for two consecutive months with two whole days off at its termination. Discipline was very strict, time off being refused for the slightest transgression. Moira Lysaght emphasises that Miss Halbert was not a type of ogre. As time went on one detected a sense of humour that lay beneath that stern exterior and one came to respect her absolute absence of favouritism.

During the nurses' qualified year they went on special duty cases in the private nursing homes in Leeson Street. The hours of duty were '4 to 4', which meant you went on from 4 p.m. to 4 a.m. or vice versa when the other special took over.

The relationship between the nurses and doctors including the senior staff men was very cordial.

The uniform in Moira Lysaght's day in St Vincent's consisted of a drill material, greyish-blue in colour, a long-sleeved dress with tight bodice and voluminous skirt. Over this was worn a starched white apron with wide straps over the shoulders, white linen pull-on sleeves extending above the elbow— with advanced training these gave place to starched white cuffs. A wide red webbing belt encircled the waist of the probationer until she became a registered nurse, when it was replaced by a stiff linen counterpart. Surmounting all from the very start was a white starched fly-away veil. In the fourth year, already qualified but not yet entitled to the hospital certificate, one was posted to the nursing home or onto 'the Mat' which meant going out on private cases. For the latter the uniform was a grey gaberdine belted coat and an unattractive brimmed hat of grey felt. A silver St Vincent's Hospital badge was pinned on the coat. It was received (through purchase) after one had qualified.

In December 1924 there was a red letter day—the first nurses' dance in the history of St Vincent's Hospital. This came about because there was a lot of food left over after an entertainment the previous evening in the out-patients' department. Mother Rectress, Mrs Carew, agreed to dispense her charity at home instead of abroad in the disposal of the food surplus. It is said that in the petitioning of Mother Rectress a younger staff man was turned down, and it was either Dr Dargan or Dr Meenan who performed the miracle.

At one stage Moira Lysaght was charge nurse of the out-patients' department which meant the overseeing of all the clinics, medical, surgical, gynaecological, dental and eyes combined with personal executive duty in the ear nose and throat department, the domain of P.J. Keogh and Albert Fagan. She was then appointed theatre sister. There was only one general hospital theatre at that period, with a small one off it for minor surgical treatments and anaesthetics. Her predecessor had been Mary Gleeson (Sister Mary Paula). At the end of her year of theatre duty she went again on 'the Mat', going on special cases in the nursing home or to patients in their own homes.

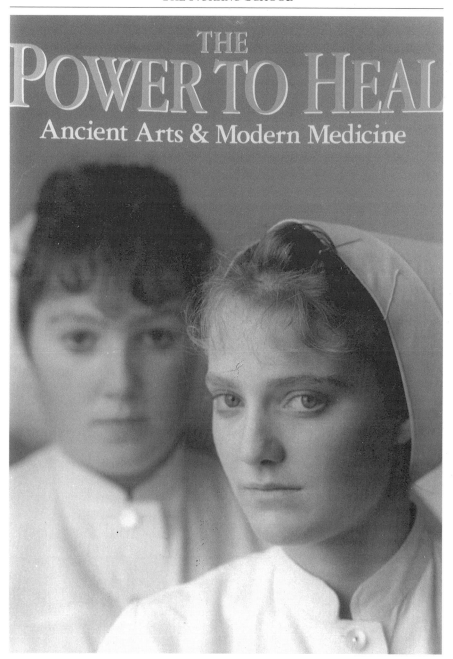

The Power to Heal

Moira Lysaght bid farewell to St Vincent's Hospital in February 1931, having qualified as a State Registered Nurse in September 1928. She summed up her recollections of her four years in St Vincent's Hospital thus:

> The principal point that floats down the years is not so much about standing and heroic feats performed in the medical and surgical field as the cheerful, kindly co-operative atmosphere that existed throughout the hospital from the staff men down to the stretcher bearers but especially between the nurses and their charges. For the well-being of the patient give me a kindly nurse who has a sense of humour rather than her opposite number with all the rigid discipline and efficiency at her fingertips.[14]

Nancy McDermott (Mrs David Coyle) also has fond memories of her time as a probationer and subsequently as a staff nurse in the nursing homes. Time off was short, it was a long day, 7 a.m. to 8 p.m. unless time off was due. It was hard but it was the same for every probationer. She makes the point that in her time there was no pre-nursing school. So it was straight into the wards and very disconcerting to find many pairs of eyes observing you:

> Miss Halbert was a wonderful person, a great teacher, very keen in her judgements at all times and always determined that her nurses would be at the top of the proficiency scale. She was a very difficult act to follow. She took the students for classes and was prone to pop a question on a day dreamer, e.g. 'What membrane separates the outer from the inner ear, nurse?', calling her name. 'The Titanic.' Miss Halbert, 'Oh dear dear, that ship went down years ago.'

Elm Park was bought during her time in training. That dream is now a reality, but for Nancy and her contemporaries their hearts will always be in the old building; and the dreams of being back on duty in St Patrick's, St Laurence's or St Joseph's persist though fifty years have passed.

In 1990 the well-known publishing firm of Prentice Hall Press published a large beautifully-illustrated book, *The Power to Heal*, which dealt with the diversity of health, healing and medicine around the world. For the illustration on the dust cover the publisher had chosen two student nurses from St Vincent's Hospital, Siobhan Magner and Carol Burke, who had trained 1988–91. This illustrates beyond anything that words can say the reputation of the Mary Aikenhead school of nursing around the world.

CHAPTER 16

THE WINDS OF CHANGE

No hospital is an island and an institution like St Vincent's with its healing and teaching functions could not operate in isolation. It was profoundly influenced by the social and political changes unleashed by another war to end wars. As R.J. Rowlette has stated, 'Any hospital system if it is to keep pace with the changing needs of the country it serves, must be in a constant state of development. It must be a live organism and in common with other living things it must adjust itself continuously to its environment.'[1] The old social order damaged by the First World War was destroyed by the second conflict. The system which had operated in the voluntary hospitals since their foundation was no longer adequate; people were demanding medical services as a right rather than as a charitable gift.

The Beveridge Report published in 1942 in the United Kingdom, with its emphasis on social and medical insurance from the cradle to the grave, was a political catalyst. Soldiers returning from the wars were determined not to go back to the old pre-war days of social injustice, and elected a Labour government. The 1948 National Health Service Act provided for a comprehensive health service for the entire population.

A small neighbour like Ireland could not escape the effects of these changes. Many Irish people had worked in the factories in England, and on returning to Ireland demanded the same standard of social services. The fact that compared with England, Ireland was a relatively poor and undeveloped country was not taken into consideration. Irish politicians learned from their English colleagues that there were votes in health. The scene was set for confrontation between the government of the day and the medical profession and the voluntary hospitals. Over the next forty years conflict periodically erupted, as more and more of the population were given free medical services, whether the facilities were available or not. The increased costs meant that the voluntary hospitals had to be subsidised by the State to provide the services. This resulted inevitably in the erosion of the hospitals' independence—a process that is still continuing.

The establishment of the Irish Hospitals Sweepstakes fund was of enormous assistance to the voluntary hospitals, but their financial problems were by no means solved. As detailed in chapter 11 payment of funds from the Sweepstakes was tightly controlled by the Hospitals Commission. Originally it had been planned that the fund would be used to pay for capital development of the hospitals, but over the years more and more of the money available went to pay running costs.

The deficit in the voluntary hospitals increased significantly in the next decade. This was due to several factors. There was an increase in the demand for hospital services. The rapid developments in medicine and medical technology required more expensive equipment and personnel. The numbers of medical staff and ancillary services rose sharply in St Vincent's and in other hospitals during the 1930s and 1940s. Funds from charitable sources fell off considerably, as the general public thought that the hospitals had adequate funds and did not need any further charitable contributions. The Second World War halted the flow of Sweepstakes funds. The Sweepstakes were confined to Ireland and no funds came in from abroad. They were resumed after the war, but as the years went on and hospital deficits spiralled, the Hospitals Sweepstakes funds were insufficient to pay the debts. By the end of the 1960s the State paid for most of the voluntary hospitals' annual deficit of £5,000,000. According to Barrington the Sweepstakes fund had become little more than an accounting mechanism.[2]

Meanwhile, the rapid increase in the cost of hospital care was creating grave problems. In 1942 hospital treatment benefit was extended to a small group of suitably-insured persons. It was obvious that the old system was breaking down. Although there was no lack of charity in the voluntary hospitals, financial considerations were becoming paramount. After the war the stage was set for confrontation between the State and workers in the health service.

In 1947, the Minister for Health Dr James Ryan (a former Vincent's student) published his proposals. Persons with incomes up to £500 or rateable valuation up to £50 were eligible for hospital services with some token payment. The Fianna Fáil government fell before the proposal could be implemented.[3] In 1948, Dr Noël Browne became Minister for Health in the first coalition government. The medical profession admired his efforts to eradicate tuberculosis. However, the introduction of the famous Mother and Child scheme caused a rapid deterioration in the relationship between the Minister and the profession.

Dr Browne also pursued what Barrington has described as 'a massive hospital building programme'. The plan included the building of sanatoria and new hospitals for St Vincent's and St Laurence's in Dublin. The hospitals would be paid for by Sweepstakes funds. Dr Browne also stated that 'the amount of Sweepstakes funds which would be paid towards the deficits of the voluntary hospitals in 1950, 1951 and 1952 would be no more than was paid in 1948'. 'The Dublin consultants establishment were incensed by what they considered an act of piracy by the Minister.'[4]

Many members of the staff of St Vincent's were members of the Irish Medical Association and took an active part in the negotiations between Dr Browne and the association. The ensuing struggle was a major cause of the downfall of the coalition government and the return to power of a Fianna Fáil government with Dr Ryan again as Minister for Health. By the exercise of much diplomatic skill Dr Ryan produced the Health Act of 1953. By the terms of this Act persons with incomes up to £600 per annum and rateable valuation up to £50 were eligible for hospital and specialist services. History repeated itself and a new coalition government had arrived before the Act came into force—and some provisions of the Act were postponed until March 1956.[5]

The extension of the hospital services to the majority of the population at nominal or no charge, with local authorities paying the voluntary hospitals and the consultants for their treatment, meant that the hospitals would be even more dependent on public funding. In accordance with the terms of this Act, members of the staff of the voluntary hospitals were now paid for their work in the general wards and also for conducting out-patient specialist clinics. Many senior members returned to the out-patients' department and conducted clinics in their own speciality. The consultant was now paid a fixed amount for an out-patients' session of usually three hours duration.

The method of paying the consultant for treating patients in the wards was rather more complex. The senior members of the staff would naturally have more beds than their junior colleagues and thus would treat more patients. A system was devised by which the monies paid by the local authorities for in-patient care was put in a pool and was divided up amongst the consultants according to the amount of beds that they had. In most hospitals the system works surprisingly amicably. The system which had characterised the voluntary hospital ethos for over two hundred years was now at an end. No longer did the consultants treat the patients in the wards and the out-patients without charge and make their livelihood from the 'rich sick'. Society had become too egalitarian for such a system to continue. However, it must be admitted that over the years the voluntary hospital system had served the country well.

In January 1955 negotiations began with the new Minister for Health, Mr T.F. O'Higgins, with the object of introducing a Voluntary Health Insurance scheme, 'which would enable citizens to insure themselves and their dependents voluntarily against the cost of hospital specialists, maternity, dental services and medical appliances'.[6] Prominent in these negotiations were Oliver FitzGerald, T.C.J. O'Connell and P.N. Meenan of St Vincent's. The negotiations were successful. Legislation to set up the Voluntary Health Insurance Board was introduced by Mr O'Higgins and subsequently supported by his successor Mr Sean McEntee.

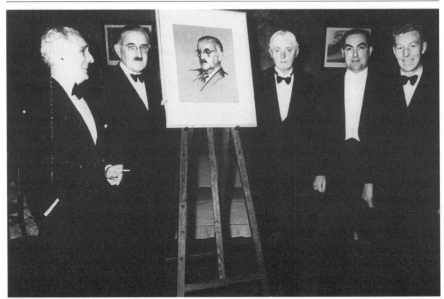

Annual Dinner of the Clinical Association, 1948. (Left to right) William Doolin, Harry Meade, J.N. Meenan, T.C.J. O'Connell, James Maher

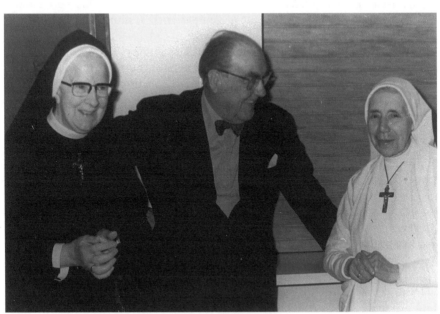

(Left to right) Mother Canisius, T.C.J. O'Connell, Sr Borgia

In 1967, another member of the staff of the hospital, Patrick FitzGerald, was to play an important role in the development of health services. The then Minister for Health, Mr Sean Flanagan, appointed a 'Consultative Council on the General Health Services', and appointed FitzGerald as chairman. The FitzGerald Report recommended the development of two regional hospitals, one based at St Vincent's on the southside and the other at the Mater on the northside of Dublin. Two general hospitals were to be established at St Kevin's and at Blanchardstown. All the other Dublin hospitals were to be re-grouped around these hospitals.[7] In many ways these recommendations in the FitzGerald Report were not too different from those of Mapother a hundred years previously!

The Health Act of 1970 further weakened the control of the owners over their own hospitals. The Act established Comhairle na nOspidéal,[8] a body to advise on the number and type of consultant appointments in all voluntary and Health Board hospitals. An applicant for a position had to have a senior degree and to have pursued specialist studies for many years. From now on a hospital had to obtain approval from the Comhairle before it appointed any specialist to its staff.

In the fifties there had been another threat to the independence of St Vincent's and other teaching hospitals. This threat came from abroad. At the beginning of the decade, the American Medical Association had found it necessary to impose restrictions on foreign-trained doctors who wished to practise in the United States. This obviously had serious implications for Irish-trained medical graduates. In September 1953, representatives from the authorities in the United States who controlled medical education were invited to visit the medical schools in the Republic and their associated teaching hospitals. The object of the visiting committee was to secure information for the licensing bodies in the United States as regards comparability of programmes of the medical schools in other countries with those of the United States of America.[9]

Historically medical schools in Ireland evolved in a different way from the medical schools in the United States. The voluntary teaching hospitals, while associated closely with the relevant authorities who examined and conferred degrees, were basically quite independent and made their own appointments to the staff. St Vincent's was a teaching hospital closely associated with the medical school of University College Dublin. The UCD medical school had no control over the appointments of the medical staff in the hospital who taught their students. Appointments to the medical staff at the hospital were made by the Mother General, on the advice of the Reverend Mother and senior members of the staff. While no system is perfect, this method of appointment to the staff had worked well for the hospital over the years. It has been recorded that in the 1880s when the young Michael Cox was appointed to the staff of the hospital against considerable opposition on the grounds that he was too young and inexperienced, the appointment turned out to be an excellent one. Another example of some of the good points of the system was that in the 1940s several bright young graduates were offered places on the hospital staff before they went abroad for postgraduate work; this was done to make sure that they would come back to their hospital and not be lost to the hospital and to the country. Professorial and other appointments to the medical faculty at University College Dublin followed a rather byzantine system. The medical faculty, academic council, governing body of the college voted in turn for candidates but the final choice lay with the senate of the National University.

The visiting medical committee from the US issued a diplomatic report on the state of the Irish medical schools. However, while paying the routine obeisances to the great days of Irish medicine, the committee made its meaning quite clear. Its findings were well summarised by Murphy. The committee considered that the medical schools in the country were inadequately staffed; they found that clinical teaching methods differed from those in the American schools. The pathology departments of teaching hospitals had not sufficient access to post-mortem material, were not integrated into teaching programmes of the medical school and, more importantly, the medical schools had no control over appointments in the teaching hospitals. The American visitors were not prepared to make a final decision on the Irish medical schools until new and improved methods and administrative procedures, some of which were then under consideration, had been put into operation. They advised that at this stage the medical schools in the Republic should not be recognised in their international list.[10]

Over the next few years there were changes in the relationship between the UCD medical school and its teaching hospitals which helped to resolve the problem. A representative of the medical faculty of UCD sat on the hospital selection committee which appointed members to the staff of the hospital. The UCD representative had the function of ensuring that the new member of the staff would be suitable to teach students in his or her particular speciality. The first occasion that a representative of the UCD medical faculty sat on a selection committee in the hospital was for the appointment of Fergus Donovan as a surgeon in 1953.

Following an agreement between University College Dublin and St Vincent's in 1957, university departments of medicine and surgery were established in the hospital. These departments were headed by professors appointed by the college, assisted by lecturers and tutors. They controlled the administration of teaching in the hospital. Similar arrangements were made with the other teaching hospitals affiliated to the UCD medical school. These arrangements worked satisfactorily, but of course they diluted the power of the hospital authorities to appoint their own medical staff. The relationship between the hospital and UCD has always been harmonious —although it might be suggested that the college authorities have been rather niggardly in granting some form of academic recognition to many of the hospital staff who teach UCD students.

In January 1956 D.K. O'Donovan spoke on the duties and responsibilities of a general hospital in modern society, at the annual prize-giving ceremony of the hospital.

> One of the most desirable accomplishments of a general hospital is to gain the complete confidence of the population served by it. This may nowadays seem too evident to emphasise. But more than a century ago when this hospital was founded, the admission of a patient was very often the last resort to the alternative of death, and indeed it was often an expression of the patient's desire to receive spiritual succour. We still emphasise that the spiritual aspect of an illness must receive prior attention, but it is a comforting thought that admission to hospital is now more a matter of fact, less frightening and a less irrevocable step in the life of the patient.[11]

He emphasised that it was the duty of the hospital to alleviate the natural fear that patients would feel on entering hospital and to gain their confidence. Patients should be educated in the natural course of their disease. 'We must guard against going to the other extreme of converting patients into self-centred neurotics. Nevertheless, it is true to say that too often in Irish hospitals patients are admitted and discharged without having received any reasoned account of their condition.'

He stressed that clinical research in the hospitals must be governed by the strictest ethics. He noted that physicians were now running their own out-patients' departments, a revival of an old discarded system. He emphasised that the role of almoners, health visitors and social workers should be closely integrated with the work of the hospital. 'We are still searching for such an ideal; let us hope it will be accomplished without further delay.'

He pointed out the problems arising from the increasing number of specialities. He said that there was a real danger that the individual patient might feel lost if he was passed around between too many specialists. He mentioned the possibility of patients being admitted overnight for treatment of their condition and then going out to work during the day. 'The idea of treatment and rest overnight in hospital to enable one to do a day's work will grow, as the organisation of daily life becomes more complicated and enforced absence from work becomes more disrupting for one's colleagues.' These words of O'Donovan anticipated the concept of short stay wards which are an integral part of a hospital's function today. He quoted the Oslerian definition of teaching hospitals: 'To care for the sick, teach medicine and nursing and add to the general sum of knowledge.'

O'Donovan foresaw the hospital of the future as a 'combination of the lay hospital of today, the happy convalescent home, a school for technical instruction of patients and the home of retreat for spiritual help'. At the meeting where O'Donovan expressed his vision of the future the then Minister for Health Mr T.F. O'Higgins said:

> It is, of course, of primary importance that the standard of care and treatment available in the hospital should be of a high level and in this connection I think it can be justly claimed for the populations they serve. The record of St Vincent's Hospital is one of which it can be justly proud and I am confident that the Sisters of Charity and the medical staff of the hospital will continue to play a vital part in the medical life of this city.

In 1958, centenary celebrations in honour of Mother Mary Aikenhead were brought to a fitting conclusion by High Mass in University Church St Stephen's Green. The Mass was presided over by Most Reverend Dr Norton, Bishop of Bathurst, and attended by An Taoiseach Mr de Valera and Mr J.A. Costello. In his sermon Fr Patrick Fitzsimons former chaplain to the hospital said, 'You have received a great heritage, a great tradition, a work rooted and founded in charity, the driving force being the love of God. You must add still further jewels to the already glittering crown. I know you are proud of your great traditions, I know you will hand them on to your successors more gilded than ever.'

CHAPTER 17

WOMEN DOCTORS

A meeting of the Medical Board was held in St Vincent's on 19 October 1885: present Dr Cox, Dr Quinlan, Dr Mapother and Dr McArdle. The question of receiving lady students was introduced by Dr Mapother who proposed the following resolution which was passed unanimously:

> That looking to the circumstances that female medical students are now admitted to the Diplomas of the Royal University and of the College of Physicians and Surgeons and that several such female students are now in actual attendance in the Medical School of the Royal College of Surgeons St Stephen's Green, that they be permitted to attend here under proper restriction during the present winter session.

The secretary was directed to communicate this resolution to the Mother Rectress and in doing so to point out 'the great field for female medical practitioners now existing in British India and the great want of proper facilities here for their hospital education'.

A further meeting of the Medical Board took place on 13 April 1886: Dr Quinlan in the chair; present Dr Cox, Dr McArdle; Dr Mapother absent in England. Dr Cox presented the application of a female student, Miss Mary Josephine Hannan, Riverstown, Killucan, Co. Westmeath, recommended to him by the Very Rev. William Delany, LL.D., S.J., President of the Catholic University College Stephen's Green and member of the senate of the Royal University. 'Fr Delany especially recommends this case to the Medical Board of St Vincent's Hospital. The lady is a recent convert, and of the best social position being a niece of Lady Wolseley's, twenty-seven years of age and is a medical student of the Royal University of Ireland.' Dr Cox was directed to write to Fr Delany informing him that under the circumstances this female student would be permitted to attend, and that suitable and special arrangements would be made for her attendance and instruction. It would have been a brave Medical Board that would have refused Fr Delany, who was one of the most prominent educationalists in the country.

The Medical Board met on 5 October 1886. Present: Mr Tobin in the chair, Dr Cox and Dr McArdle. A letter from the Superioress dated 5 October 1886 on the subject first of lady pupils, second on the management of the dispensary, was read. As regards lady pupils it was decided to advise the Superioress to the following effect: 'that the Board considers it inadvisable that lady pupils should go round with the general class but that if such pupils presented themselves in sufficient numbers to form a class, the Board would be prepared to make special other arrangements for their instruction'.

A meeting of the Medical Board was held on 25 November 1886, all present, Mr Tobin in the chair. A letter from the Superioress was read as follows: 'I beg to inform you that having submitted the resolution at the Medical Board dated 5 October 1886 anent lady pupils, to His Grace the Archbishop, His Grace is of the opinion that it is inexpedient for the present at least that classes for lady pupils should be opened in St Vincent's Hospital.' Signed M. Cullen, Superioress. Proposed by Mr McArdle and carried, Dr Quinlan dissenting, that 'we accept Mrs Cullen's views as regards lady pupils in its entirety'.

The Medical Board met on 16 December 1886, Dr Quinlan in the chair, to consider a further application from Miss Hannan for re-adoption as pupil to the hospital. 'The secretary was directed to inform her that the Board must adhere to its previous decision.' Signed Michael F. Cox.[1]

The case history of Miss Hannan is typical of the opposition which aspiring lady doctors experienced in their quest for medical degrees during the last part of the nineteenth century. Miss Hannan subsequently qualified in the Royal College of Surgeons in 1890. She worked for a time in India at the Dufferin Hospital, Ulwar State, Rajputana. She returned to Europe but finally settled in the Transvaal at Pretoria where she lived for many years.[2]

Antagonism to women doctors was widespread in the medical profession. Possibly not all members of the medical profession were as hostile to women doctors as Sir William Jenner, physician to Queen Victoria. He is reported to have raised his hands to heaven and testified that he had but one dear daughter and he would rather follow her bier to the grave than allow her to go through such a course of study as medicine. [3] Dr Walter Rivington in *The Medical Profession* (1879) seemed to advise cautious opposition to medical women:

> Without professing ourselves to be at all enthusiastic in favour of a medical career for women, we think that by frame, temperament and mental condition, woman is not adapted for medicine, far less for surgical practice. We think that it is not for the members of our calling to do more than exercise a private influence against the destination of

young women to the medical profession . . . It is not however the office of our profession to lead the van of any public crusade against the admission of women within the ranks . . . There was nothing and could be nothing very dreadful in opening the stores of medical knowledge to women . . . To move heaven and earth metaphorically speaking to endeavour to exclude a few ladies from the medical profession never seemed either a wise or a dignified procedure. We say a few because we feel convinced that the movement must always be of a limited character; women's disabilities are too many to allow more than a few to adopt the medical profession as a livelihood.[4]

The view of Dr Rivington who was surgeon to the London hospital must have met with general approval in Ireland because he received the first Carmichael Prize of £200 awarded by the Royal College of Surgeons in Ireland for his essay.

Thomas Laffan, lecturer in anatomy in Cecilia Street, in his account of the medical profession in 1879 stated grudgingly that the admission of women into the profession had been accomplished. But he added that, 'Women doctors will never constitute a numerous class so there need not be much fear of their ever doing much material mischief to their male rivals. The cost of their education will always be sufficiently high to make it more profitable to invest in matrimony . . . We hope the day is far distant when any hospital or school will be guilty of the impropriety of allowing mixed classes within its walls.'[5]

Opinion amongst the staff of St Vincent's Hospital appears to have been mixed. Mapother must have been a late convert to the women doctors' cause, because he wrote in 1868, 'If a supply of men to undertake the duties of pharmaciens cannot be had because they ambition medical practice, let the art of the apothecaries be handed over to females, who while they are by nature unfitted for medical or surgical practice are in every way suited for the manipulative art of dispensing.'[6]

Dr Quinlan was more in their favour. It will be noticed that he dissented from the decision of the Medical Board to exclude Miss Hannan from clinics in the hospital. It is also to be noted that subsequently, when women students were admitted to Cecilia Street, he offered to surrender his pharmacy laboratory and specimen room so that they could be fitted up as a waiting room and dissecting room for the use of the lady students.

Over the next twenty to thirty years women gradually infiltrated the male-dominated medical profession. St Vincent's had its quota of medical pioneers. An important event in the history of the hospital occurred in 1899 when Miss H.A. Hall, who subsequently practised in Manchester, won the junior prize. She was the first woman to win any of the prizes in the hospital. A typical example of the new women graduates who were coming onto the university scene was Blanche J.C. Griffin who took an active part in student politics in Cecilia Street in her student days. Also known as Bawn, she was medical editor of *St Stephen's*, the journal of the Catholic University medical school. She qualified M.B. in 1910 and was house surgeon in 1911. Hospital records refer to many women students and house officers in the hospital during the 1920s and the 1930s. These included the following: Marcella B.M. Kelly (1918) (Mrs Swan), Weston House, Sligo, became assistant medical officer, Mental Hospital, Powick, Worcester; Annie Scully (1921), St Patrick's Road, Drumcondra, won the Bellingham Medal in 1920; Annie Brereton (1923) (Mrs Keelan) won the Junior Prize in 1921 and the McArdle Prize (ex-aequo) in 1923, and she also qualified B. Mus.; Maggie Josephine McColgan (1924), Culduff, Donegal, won the Junior Prize in 1922, and was assistant medical officer, Donegal; Ita Brady (1923) was Co. MOH, Dublin and school medical officer; Ann Sullivan (1923), Streete, Co. Westmeath; Jessie N. Cooke (1923), Hunslet Road, Leeds; Catherine Mary Barry-McKenna (1924), 367 Hackney Road, London; Catherine Portley (1924), Janesboro, Limerick; Maeve Halligan (1924), Glasnevin; Kathleen Magdalen Lynch (1924) (Mrs Brindley); Josephine McGovern (1925), Liverpool; Kathleen Kennedy (1925) won the Junior Prize in 1923 and the McArdle Prize in 1925—she was daughter of Denis Kennedy, surgeon to the hospital; Mary Farrington (1925) was pathologist to the Children's Hospital Temple Street; Alice Mary Lemass (1925), Dublin, sister of Taoiseach Sean Lemass; Catherine Purcell (1927), Naas, Co. Kildare; Catherine Cunningham (1928), Carrick, Co. Donegal; Eileen Kennedy (1933) won the Junior Prize in 1931 and subsequently became ophthalmic surgeon in Co. Clare—she was daughter of Denis Kennedy; Tess O'Donnell (1936), Carndonagh, Co. Donegal, mother of President Mary Robinson; Mary Winifred Meagher (1934), Ferbane, Co. Offaly, sister of Dr Declan Meagher.

The increase in the number of women graduates in the first half of the twentieth century can be gauged from the figures in the President's Reports on the medical school of University College Dublin, where the greater part of the Vincent's students studied.[7]

During the early 1920s, due to the increase of women students in the hospital, half of no. 60 St Stephen's Green was taken over as a women's residence. This arrangement only lasted for a couple of years, as no. 60 was used subsequently as a semi-private nursing home. By 1940 women students had asserted their ability beyond any doubt. In the final medical examination of summer 1940 there were three first class honours, two of them gained by women students of the hospital—Philomena Guinan, later ophthalmologist to the hospital, and Nuala Sheehan (Mrs O'Conor Donelan), later consultant paediatrician to the Children's Hospital in Temple Street. By 1940 women in the hospital had achieved equal academic status and prestige. However, the subsequent increase in the number of women consultants in St Vincent's has been hardly spectacular. In 1993 there were eighty-two consultants on the staff of the hospital of whom nine were women.

Year	Male Medical Students	Female Medical Students
1915–16	284	51
1916–17	386	67
1917–18	414	81
1918–19	421	97
1919–20	517	101
1920–21	487	109
1921–22	375	84
1922–23	375	90
1923–24	324	64
1924–25	251	35
1925–26	196	33
1926–27	189	27
1927–28	173	28
1928–29	187	20
1929–30	215	22
1930–31	260	33
1939–40	655	144
1940–41	679	186
1944–45	731	208
1948–49	611	185
1949–50	593	168
1959–60	402	192

CHAPTER 18

LAST YEARS ON THE GREEN

It would have been understandable if the last two decades of hospital life on the Green had been a period of conservation and marking time. What was the point of expanding in the old hospital when in a few years it would all be located in the pastures of Elm Park? It just didn't happen that way. The period 1950–70 was as active and expansive as any period before or since in the history of the hospital. Amongst the staff the old order was changing rapidly. The senior members of the staff who had guided the hospital through tempestuous years were now retiring. They had steered St Vincent's safely through a period of unparalleled strife. They had to cope with the effects of two World Wars, the Anglo-Irish conflict when warfare literally came to the doorstep of the hospital, perhaps worst of all a bitter civil war, and finally the birth pangs of a new State.

James N. Meenan died in 1950 and Harry Meade died in 1952. Doolin died in 1962. P.T. O'Farrell and J.F. Cunningham retired from practice in 1960. Molly Gunn, senior radiographer in the department of radiology for many years, died in 1960. Gerry, who gave many years to the hospital as porter, died in 1962. A new generation of consultants had to deal with the changes which came with the second half of the century. These changes were probably not as traumatic as those of the first half but they were just as challenging and potentially dangerous to the welfare of the hospital.

D.K. O'Donovan was appointed Professor of Medicine St Vincent's Hospital in 1952 and Senior Professor of Medicine UCD in 1958.[1] Over the next twenty years many honours came his way including Honorary Fellowship of the Royal College of Physicians of London, chairman of the Medical Research Council and chairman of the Academy of Medicine and dean of the faculty of medicine in UCD. He had the onerous task of keeping the medical curriculum for students up-to-date. Despite the many demands on his services he also ran a first class endocrine service in the hospital.

In 1954 Patrick FitzGerald was appointed Professor of Surgery (St Vincent's). After a close contest with his friend and colleague T.C.J.

164

O'Connell, FitzGerald won by one vote in the senate of the National University. In spite of the close race there was no bitterness between the two candidates and they remained firm friends. It was possibly a little embarrassing for the hospital to have such a galaxy of talent on its staff. FitzGerald was subsequently appointed senior Professor of Surgery in UCD in 1958. He was a specialist and a pioneer in vascular surgery in which he achieved a worldwide reputation. Like his predecessor in the chair of Surgery he was appointed President of the Association of Surgeons of Great Britain and Ireland in 1966–67. During his professorship he established an experimental surgery department at Woodview, University College Dublin in 1962. The twelfth annual meeting of the International College of Angiology was held in Spain in October 1978, a few months after his death. One of the four days of the meeting was dedicated to his memory.

O'Connell was a man of many and diverse talents. He had a special interest in cardiac and abdominal surgery. He played a key role in Irish medical politics and he played a major part in the organisation of the Voluntary Health Insurance Board together with his colleagues O. FitzGerald and P.N. Meenan. He also took a deep interest in sport, particularly rugby football. He was an accomplished raconteur. His after dinner speeches were received with as much relish as the choicest food and wines. He made surgical history by being the first surgeon to perform a mitral valvotomy in the Coombe Hospital upon a woman who was in labour and suffering from heart failure. Raymond Davys gave the anaesthetic. She survived and had several more babies. D.K. O'Donovan has also called attention to the many other contributions which O'Connell has made to gastric and thyroid surgery and sports injuries. His pioneer work in the establishment of a Blood Transfusion Service has been noted. According to O'Donovan, O'Connell summarised his view by quoting Hippocrates, 'What you should put first in all the practice of your art is how to make the patient well: and if he can be made well in many ways one should choose the least troublesome.'[2]

After the retirement of T.T. O'Farrell, J. (Jock) McGrath was appointed Professor of Pathology in UCD and was also dean of the faculty of medicine. He had been Professor of Medical Jurisprudence and State Pathologist. Unfortunately he died in 1957 at the height of his career. He was a man of many talents and his early death was a major loss to Irish medicine.

In 1958 P.N. Meenan became Professor of Microbiology as applied to medicine. He was a pioneer in the study of virus diseases in this country and set up a virus reference laboratory in University College Dublin. He was subsequently dean of the faculty of medicine in UCD for a period of ten years. Oliver FitzGerald was appointed Professor of Therapeutics in 1958. His clinical sphere of interest was in gastroenterology. He was appointed chairman of the National Drugs Advisory Board, set up by the government to evaluate the efficiency and safety of new drugs before they were made available to the public on prescription. He read widely and had a vast knowledge of medical literature. He demanded perfection in everything he did and was a living example of the old adage that if you want to get something done ask a busy man.

In 1957 the university departments of medicine and surgery were formally established in the hospital. The departments consisted of professor, lecturer and tutor and a definite allocation of beds and laboratory space. Frank Lavery, who was Professor of Ophthalmology in UCD, was appointed to the hospital in 1953. Liam O'Connell was appointed whole-time haematologist in 1954. Frank Duff, who specialised in urological surgery from 1957, achieved international recognition for his work. He was a pioneer in many aspects of urological surgery. He was President of the Royal College of Surgeons in Ireland from 1972 to 1974. He was always most courteous and helpful in his relationship with his colleagues and was held in high esteem by everybody who worked in the hospital.

At the other end of the spectrum there was no shortage of able young men and women coming on the staff. New appointments to the hospital had to be made with the realisation that the hospital would be moving out shortly to Elm Park, with more facilities for the development of the various specialities. Francis P. Muldowney was appointed physician in 1960. He was to become an international authority on metabolic diseases.

On the surgical side there were many important appointments. J.A. (Gussie) Mehigan after a first class undergraduate career became assistant surgeon. Another young surgical graduate, Joseph P. McMullin, was surgeon to St John's and Elizabeth's Hospital in London. He was invited back to the hospital by Patrick FitzGerald in 1955 to assist him in organising the surgical department. McMullin accepted the invitation and played a key role in the future development of the hospital. Fergus Donovan took up appointment as the first neurosurgeon to the hospital in 1958 and Joseph Gallagher became the first whole-time orthopaedic surgeon in 1959. Dan Kelly became assistant urological surgeon in 1966 and Seamus O'Riain was appointed plastic surgeon in 1969.

Dermot Cantwell joined the expanding X-ray department in 1959. Robert P. Towers, whose speciality was histology, became assistant pathologist to the hospital in 1955. He subsequently became editor of the *Irish Journal of Medical Science.* John Harman was appointed to the staff in 1958 and became Professor of Pathology in UCD in the same year. He died in 1982.

On the medical side, Risteard Mulcahy was appointed assistant physician in 1950 and subsequently cardiologist. He was to gain national and international recognition for his work in the field of preventive cardiology. In 1960 Jack Molony was appointed physician in physical and rehabilitation medicine. James Fennelly was appointed physician with a special interest in oncology in 1968.

Thus, at the beginning of the 1960s Vincent's had a large and talented staff. The physicians were Quinlan, O'Donovan, O. FitzGerald, E.L. Murphy and the assistant physicians were P. Brennan, R. Mulcahy and F.P.

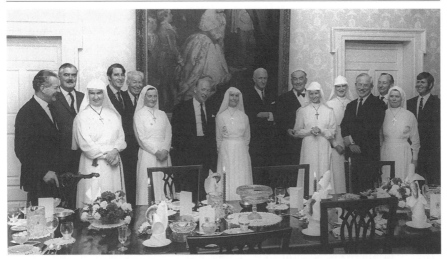

Centenary Dinner Medical Board, 1969. (Left to right) P. Brennan, P.N. Meenan, Sr Stephanie, F.A. Duff, J. Maher, Sr Catherina, P. FitzGerald, Mother Paula, H. Quinlan, T.C.J. O'Connell, Sr Marie Therese, Sr Carmel Mary, O. FitzGerald, D.K. O'Donovan, Sr Joseph Ignatius, J. Harman

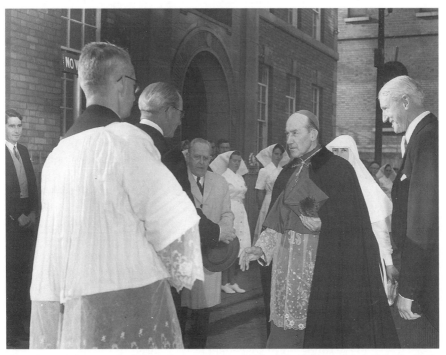

Opening of the new building, Leeson Lane, 1961 with (left to right) F.A. Duff, Fr Mulvey, J. Cunningham, Sean McEntee, Minister for Health, Archbishop McQuaid, Harold Quinlan

Muldowney. The surgeons were F.J. Morrin, T.C.J. O'Connell, P. FitzGerald, F. Duff and the assistant surgeons were J.G. Maher, J.A. Mehigan and J.P. McMullin. The neurosurgeon was F. Donovan. J.K. Feeney was senior gynaecologist and C. Coyle was his colleague in the department. The radiologists were Denis O'Farrell and S.J. Boland and the assistant radiologist was D. Cantwell. The ophthalmologists were P. Guinan and F. Lavery. The dermatologist was F.O.C. Meenan. The consultant paediatric cardiologist was A. McDonald. The pathologists were P.N. Meenan, R.P. Towers and L. O'Connell. The anaesthetists were O.J. Murphy, G.R. Davys, M. Nash and D. O'Leary. The psychiatrist was F. McLaughlin and the orthopaedic surgeon was J. Gallagher. The dentist was N. Martin and the otorhinolaryngologists were A. Fagan, B. O'Brien and O. McCullen.

In 1961 many specialised clinics were conducted in the hospital: cardiology R. Mulcahy, chest diseases H. Quinlan, gastroenterology O. FitzGerald, neurology/psychiatry F. McLaughlin and E.L. Murphy, rheumatology D.K. O'Donovan, diabetes D.K. O'Donovan, orthopaedics J. Gallagher. There were at this stage 243 nurses in the hospital and the total number of beds including private beds was 304. There were fifteen pre-registration interns, one university medical tutor, one medical registrar, one anaesthetist and one blood and electrolyte registrar. The number of intern patients treated in 1960 was 3,368.

During the early 1960s the hospital had to bear the loss of two members of staff at the height of their powers. E.L. Murphy died prematurely in 1962; and in 1963 his colleagues in the hospital were also shocked by the sudden death of Charles Coyle. He had been Master of the National Maternity Hospital as well as gynaecologist to St Vincent's. He was a loyal and wise colleague to his many friends both in and out of the hospital. Brennan was appointed to the Medical Board after the death of E.L. Murphy. He continued to be a valuable consultant in all branches of medicine.

In 1964 Declan Meagher was appointed consultant gynaecologist to the hospital. Kevin Feeney was appointed Associate Professor of Obstetrics and Gynaecology in UCD in 1962. Apart from his skill in his professional work, Feeney was remarkable for his loyalty to his hospitals and to his colleagues. He was devoted to the interests of the two hospitals to which he was appointed, St Vincent's and the Coombe Hospital. He also wrote widely on the history of the two hospitals and compiled a very comprehensive history of the Coombe Hospital. Amongst his accomplishments, Feeney was a successful writer of detective novels. However, nobody solved the mystery of his *nom de plume.*

With the enormous increase in staff and specialities more space had to be provided and this was difficult in the cramped quarters of the hospital on the Green. Every single bit of space had to be utilised to the maximum. This was achieved with great ingenuity and skill. The developments in the Mary Aikenhead school of nursing have been recorded in chapter 15. In 1957–58 the ground floor of the old residency of no. 55 St Stephen's Green was turned into a ward for neurosurgery. Twenty beds were established in the ward, under the supervision of nurse Carmel O'Donoghue.

Because of the new rule of the Medical Registration Council that newly-qualified doctors had to intern in hospital for at least a year before being put on the medical register, and the fact that the students had to spend more time in the hospital, there was an urgent need for a new residence. In 1958 a new residence was built behind the hospital, at the top of Leeson Lane, at the back of 60 St Stephen's Green. The cost of the new residence was £12,209. New equipment and space had to be found for the physiotherapy department, and an electromyographic department had to be organised in the out-patients' department at a cost of £229.

The conversion of 94 Lower Leeson Street into a nursing school resulted in an immediate shortage of beds for private patients. It must always be emphasised that the income from the treatment of private patients went to subsidise the work of the main hospital and its public patients. It was at this time that the Pembroke Nursing Home in Upper Pembroke Street came up for sale; it was purchased by the hospital and converted into a private nursing home for St Vincent's. This was a convenient arrangement, because it took only five minutes to walk up Quinn's Lane from the back of the hospital, through the archway, and into Pembroke Street.

Undoubtedly the major event of the 1960s was the opening of the new unit St Peter and Paul's, consisting of a large and very handsome lecture theatre, a new casualty department, a cardiac unit, consisting of twenty-two beds, and a metabolic unit, consisting of thirteen beds and laboratories. It was opened in October 1961. This unit was built at the back of the hospital, in Leeson Lane facing the out-patients' department. A library was also incorporated in the building. The metabolic unit was under the directorship of Frank Muldowney and the cardiac unit was under the directorship of Risteard Mulcahy. The new unit cost approximately £80,000 to build. In his speech at the opening ceremony Mr McEntee, Minister for Health, emphasised that no funds from the Hospitals Sweeps had been given for the construction of the unit, but all the monies had been provided by the Irish Sisters of Charity from their own resources. Mr McEntee said that he would hope to allocate some financial assistance to run the laboratories.[3] He added that in the case of the Elm Park venture planning had now reached the stage when it would be possible to invite tenders for the superstructure within a matter of months.

At the end of the decade three members of the staff who had contributed much to the welfare of the hospital died. They were F.J. (Pops) Morrin, S.J. (Vesty) Boland and O.J. (Ossy) Murphy. In 1957 the St Vincent's Hospital Pools was launched to run a weekly football pool in aid of the hospital. Mr David Coughlan was first chairman of the company. The pools brought in a considerable amount of money for several years.

During the nineteenth century the main treatment of the hospital patient was carried out by the doctors and the nurses with the help of an auxiliary staff. Operations were relatively uncomplicated and medical treatment simple. Up to comparatively recent times the number of staff involved in the running of the hospital was small. The science of medicine and surgery was in its infancy. Patients were admitted for treatment at the request of a patron of the hospital or because of necessity. The details of the patient's stay in hospital were recorded in a large ledger under the appropriate headings of name, address, disease and outcome. Examining these records a century and a half later, one conjures up a vision of a young nun sitting at her desk inscribing laboriously in copperplate handwriting with her quill pen by candlelight the details of the short life and death of a young man or woman—or more happily, writing the word 'cured' in the final column. Patients were admitted to the out-patients' department or dispensary purely because of their needs. There was no guiding rule except necessity.

This situation changed with the advances in medicine and science and with different social circumstances. The hospital patient was now subjected to an ever-increasing battery of complicated tests and treatment. No part of the human body was inviolate from investigation and the surgeon's knife. The patient was being exposed to a continuous flood of new and powerful drugs; many of these drugs also had a potential for serious side effects and the patient had to be carefully monitored. All these procedures had to be accurately catalogued in the patient's chart for present and future treatment.

Attending the out-patients' department or on admission to hospital patients were questioned about their private life and their financial and social situation. With increasing involvement of the State in hospital affairs, the eligibility or entitlement of patients to hospital treatment had to be established. They had to conform to the many rules laid down by the Department of Health. Again, as the State took over the payment of many of the expenses of the voluntary hospitals, patients who were attending hospital felt that it was their taxes which were supporting the hospital and naturally expected more service from the staff of the hospital. The advances in medicine and science, the running of a hospital, keeping up-to-date with the provision of modern equipment and ever-increasing staff numbers resulted in an enormous increase in the amount of money that had to be given as subsistence to the hospitals. Hospitals were under constant pressure to keep their costs down to a minimum. For these reasons administration assumed a vitally important role in the modern hospital.

In 1968–69 there were approximately sixty-four people on the administration staff in St Vincent's. They included accountants and assistant accountants, secretaries in the accounts department, salary officials, medical records officers in the medical records department and filing clerks. The various departments like pathology, radiology, pharmacy had their own offices and administrators. There was a purchasing officer to buy food; the schools of radiography and nursing had their own officials, as also the out-patients' and the private homes. The telephonist department, one of the most vital departments in any hospital, had to be suitably staffed. Answering the telephone in the hospital or in out-patients' or in the casualty department demanded careful interpretation and it was a most responsible job—mistakes in a department like this could so easily lead to a tragedy.

In St Vincent's in the 1960s the backroom girls and boys were playing an essential and ever-expanding part in the running of the hospital. The administrators may feel a little bit aggrieved at times that their work in the hospital is not appreciated as much as it should be. In the Annual for 1968–69, it is noted that, 'You will never see a bust or statue erected to a hospital administrator, we are only the backroom boys.' There is a certain amount of truth in this, but possibly it is a sign that the affairs were so efficiently administered in the hospital and the departments functioned so smoothly, the efficiency of the administrators was not adequately recognised. It is only when things start going wrong that one realises the enormous role that administrators play in the work of the hospital. Perhaps the best tribute to the contribution of the hospital administrator is that there is now a course in hospital administration leading to a diploma for those who have completed it successfully. Hospital administration has come a long way from the single nun laboriously writing details of patients into a large ledger to the all-embracing computer technology of today, but the object remains the same—it is all for the care and treatment of sick people.

The ladies' committee was particularly active in the 1950s and 1960s. The first secretary was Mrs Mairead Meenan who was succeeded by Eileen Monahan. The committee helped to produce funds for many projects in the hospital and this work continued after the move to Elm Park. In 1969 the secretary of the Clinical Association, Dan Kelly, requested Dr Livina Meenan, the then president of the ladies' committee, to sponsor the equipping of the new library in Elm Park. A sizeable sum of money was collected by the committee for this purpose. Mention must be made of the exhibitions of prize-winning dolls organised in aid of the hospital by Bernadette Maher, sister of James, Nora and T.J. Maher. Exhibitions of the dolls were held in Vincent's on the Green and subsequently in the assembly hall in Elm Park. They attracted widespread interest.

The annual general meeting of the Irish Medical Association was held in St Vincent's from 28 June to 2 July 1965. This was the first time in the history of the association that such a meeting was held in a Dublin hospital. St Vincent's was chosen because of the excellent lecture theatre and other facilities which were available. To mark the opening of the meeting Mass was celebrated in the hospital chapel by the chaplain Fr Mulvey and was attended by delegates of the Irish Medical Association and members of the hospital staff; it was also attended by the Minister for Health, Donagh O'Malley.

The AGM was held in the new lecture theatre and a reception was held subsequently in the out-patients' department for the attending delegates and their guests. During the following day the lecture theatre was occupied with the presentation of scientific communications or with specially-organised symposia. Two of the largest surgical wards were vacated to house a scientific and medical exhibition, organised by Philip Brennan. The meeting was a great success and appreciation was expressed by the Irish Medical Association for the full co-operation and splendid hospitality dispensed by the authorities of St Vincent's, Mother Rectress and community, and the nursing and medical staff. The clinical milieu, the continuing routine activities of a busy hospital and the presence of an active medical and nursing staff on the scene were undoubtedly factors which attracted colleagues from other hospitals in other parts of Ireland to the meeting.[4]

In retrospect it can be seen that this was the last salute of the old hospital on the Green to Irish medicine, a cause to which it had contributed so much over so many generations.

CHAPTER 19

MEMORIES

Before the final move to Elm Park many former medical students of the hospital must have paid a sentimental journey to the Alma Mater on the Green. As they wandered through lofty wards with elegant ceilings or strolled down the main artery of the hospital, the long corridor, many memories of their salad days must have flooded through their minds. Around every corner they would recall those who had worked with them, friends and colleagues now scattered all over the world, the medical staff who imparted their knowledge of medicine and surgery to the students, and all those in the background who organised the workings of the hospital. Some of them would still be there but many would have gone to their reward.

Let us accompany one of them as he climbs slowly up the steps through the main portico and into the main hall. There he comes under the careful scrutiny of Mrs Aikenhead and Archbishop Murray, vigilant as always. He is greeted by Michael Hanly, hall porter, tall and slim as befits an ex-army man, immaculate in his green uniform. Perhaps at this stage he might recall Gerry who took over the door in the evening times, always clad in a dark suit with a white shirt and black tie. Gerry knew all who worked in the hospital and was jealous for its reputation, but sometimes, possibly if he was a little tired of answering those who were always asking for the way out, his answer would be short, 'Follow the breeze, mam.' He might remember Josephine— Josephine, last of the assistant nurses, who took over as night portress. When she opened the door at night she would hide behind it so that she could say truthfully the next morning that she could not see what condition Dr X or Mr Y were in when they returned.

Our visitor then proceeds in from the hall and straight in front of him he sees the holy of holies, the Medical Boardroom, formerly the office of Mary Aikenhead. Even now he would still be afraid to peep in. He turns sharply to the left and into the students' waiting room. Unchanged since his day, the passage of time is marked only by the increase in the number of medal winners whose names are displayed on the boards around the room. There

173

is still the pervading smell of cigarette ash and as usual no fire in the grate. Here he had waited for the clinician to emerge from the Boardroom to lead him and his colleagues up to the wards for a clinic—and then the supreme ordeal as he waited to be taken to the ward for his final medical or surgical clinical examination.

From the students' room he passes into no. 55 St Stephen's Green, the old residency, the former home of house surgeons and students during their internship. The old residency is a shadow of its former self. The ground floor is now the Mary Aikenhead ward for neurosurgery, the first floor is part of St Benedict's ward and the third floor part of the convent.[1] In the garden at the back of the residence in his time there was a home for porters and a piggery abutting on Leeson Lane. Now the new more elegant residency is to be found in Leeson Lane where it joins Lower Leeson Street behind no. 60 St Stephen's Green.

But the old residency has a history and a mythology of its own. It was widely believed that many a promising medical career was wrecked by a night of too much celebration in the residency. The flash points would be the night the final results came out or the memorable occasions when Vincent's won the Hospitals' Rugby Cup. Then a night of festivity might end sadly before the disciplinary committee of the Medical Board. On one occasion the *casus belli* was the winning of the inter-hospital relay race by the St Vincent's team. During the celebrations damage was done to the furniture and fittings and there was an amount of noise which caused considerable annoyance to patients and staff. The Board called the resident medical officers before them to give some explanation of the incident. The officers contended that the proceedings were conducted with decorum until the residency was invaded by a rowdy mob, mainly students, over whom they failed to obtain control until a late hour. One wonders whether the resident medical officers had missed their vocation and should have been barristers. The Board reprimanded them severely for not exercising their authority and for not having taken sufficiently drastic steps to have the intruders removed.[2]

It is well established in the folklore of the hospital that on one occasion a young doctor drove a flock of sheep up the main corridor. This procedure did not apparently damage his future career as he went on to become a distinguished surgeon on the staff of the hospital. There is only one point of dispute concerning the episode: that it was pigs and not sheep that were driven up the corridor—this is a reasonable opinion to hold as the raw material for driving pigs was readily accessible in Leeson Lane. Bob O'Connell also recounted another porcine story:

> In 1927 I came to St Vincent's Hospital as a medical student. I had just passed my Third Medical and was encouraged to go there by Professor John Cunningham whom I had met in 1925. At that time there were few formalities about entrance. One applied and one got in. There

Francis J. Morrin, surgeon
1924–68

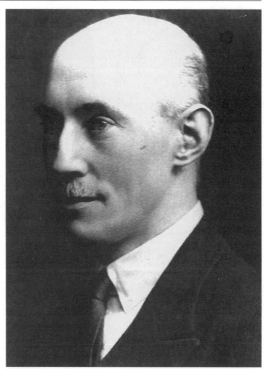

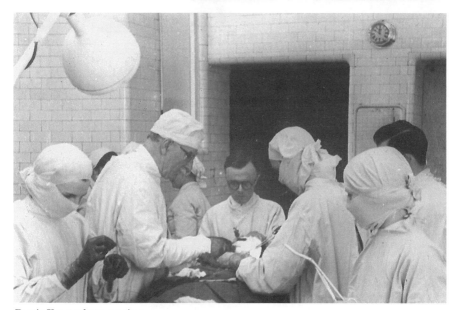

Denis Kennedy operating

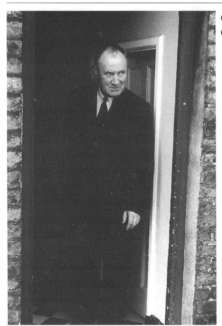

Gerry, porter at St Vincent's, St Stephen's
Green

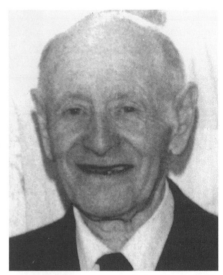

John FitzGerald,
laboratory porter,
Pathology Department

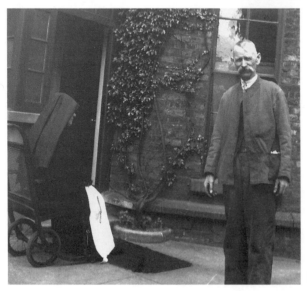

Barney and Mrs Donovan

were six house surgeons and about twelve students in residence. The Residency was unique. It was an old Georgian house beside the hospital and had changed very little from the time it had been built. We slept in dormitory-like rooms—six or seven in each room. One was lucky if companions came in quietly and early at night. It was the tradition to have Residency parties and a lot depended on the personnel. We were lucky in the late twenties as we had a rather quiet crowd. Some extraordinary parties went on until the very early hours in the morning and invariably brought down the wrath of the Board upon all our heads. My home was in Dublin and I sometimes took the opportunity of going there when things looked a little bit dangerous. At that time pigs were kept in the mews behind the hospital. It is unnecessary to say that this fact constituted a supreme temptation to the 'gentlemen' who occasionally introduced the pigs to the delights of the Residency. After one such episode there was serious trouble. One of the pigs escaped in the morning time, unfortunately broke his leg, and had to be despatched by the local butcher. The Rev Mother at the time was Mrs Carew. She took a poor view and imposed a stiff financial settlement upon the Residency. As I was at home on that particular night, and considered blameless by my companions, I was sent by them to plead with Mrs Carew, who had charged seven pounds for the pig. They said that as they did not get the pig—which they could have eaten—they thought that it was unjust that they still had to pay the seven pounds. I well remember the formidable interview which I had in the office. Mrs Carew took a large wooden hearing aid out of her bib and held it out to me. I felt like a hypnotised rabbit as I stared into this affair and stumbled a few words about the 'Gentlemen' in the Residency. 'The what', she said, as I hastily corrected this description to 'the boys'. She looked steadily at me for a moment or two and then asked 'What is all this about?' When I told her she announced that she would not take a penny less than Five Pounds for the pig and 'that was all about that'.[3]

St Vincent's took a great interest in the Hospitals' Rugby Cup competition which is one of the oldest competitions in rugby. St Vincent's Hospital football club was founded in 1885. The object of the club was to play the game according to the rules of Rugby Union. The colours of the club were black, green and red. The club consisted of students (present and past) whose names were on the books of the hospital and of the staff of the hospital as *ex-officio* members. A senior member of the staff was president and other members vice-presidents. Management of the club was left in the hands of a committee consisting of a captain and six members. The annual subscription was two shillings and six pence. The committee was authorised to award caps for good play at the end of the season. The committee also had the power, subject to the approval of a general meeting, to expel any member who might in any way make himself objectionable.

For the season 1888–89 Dr Quinlan was president and Messrs. McArdle, Gaffney, Robin, Drs Cox, McHugh, Byrne and Redmond vice-presidents. Dr F.B. Nowlan was captain and the committee was P. McGann, B. Byrne, G. Hickey, J.J. Jerrard, W. Keane and D. Ryan. Hon. secretary was B. Byrne, hon. treasurer W. Keane. The captain and secretary of the second team was T.C. Cummins. Twenty-two fixtures were listed for the season 1888–89 including matches against Bective Rangers, Trinity, Santry School, Rangers, Claremont, Clontarf, Monkstown, the Adelaide and Meath Hospitals, University College St Stephen's Green and University College Blackrock.

It was recorded that Denis Kennedy in his student days was a formidable figure in forward rushes; in the first year that Vincent's featured in the Hospitals' Cup Final, Robinson, an Irish international playing for the opposite team, broke away and was vigorously tackled by Reggie White. Robinson scrambled over the line for a try but his 'togs' remained in White's hands. T.J. Crean's achievements have been described elsewhere. J.N. Meenan was picked for the team in 1903–04. In a trial match he tackled so forcibly that he broke his collar-bone and had to cry off. Vincent's won the cup for the first time in 1912–13 under the captaincy of J.B. Minch, an Irish international. The victory was suitably celebrated with a dinner in the Gresham Hotel, Mr Tobin in the chair. A former captain of the club, Paget Butler, was to die in the First World War. The cup was won again in 1928. Two members of the team, Sean Lavan and Theo Phelan, represented Ireland in the Olympic Games. The first St Vincent's Rugby Club dance was held in the same year and became a distinct social success.[4]

By 1993 St Vincent's Hospital had won the Dublin Hospitals' Cup twenty times—the biggest number of victories for any of the hospitals. The competition is one of the oldest rugby competitions in the world and has been run since 1882. The Dublin Hospitals' Cup trophy is without doubt the oldest sporting trophy in these islands and the most valuable. The solid Hunting Trophy dates back to 1812 and was made in England by the silversmith Paul Storr. The trophy was purchased by the Dublin Hospitals' Football Union in 1881 from Waterhouse of Dame Street at an expense of £50. The Dublin silversmith who recently restored the trophy commented that it was the finest sporting trophy in the country and estimated its value at over £50,000.[5]

Our visitor makes his way back through the students' room to the main hospital. On the left is the ornate staircase, leading up to what was now St Joseph's ward. On his right is the main front parlour. If he looks inside the parlour he will find little change. The large picture of Miss Jane Bellew being received into the congregation by Dr Murray, with Mrs Aikenhead by her side, still dominates the room. Coming out of the parlour he turns left down the main corridor, thinking of the times he had to dash down it to catch up with the tail of the clinic before it disappeared into one of the wards at the end of the corridor. Hanly is striking the big gong, summoning

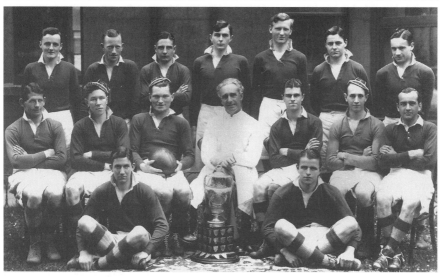

St Vincent's Hospital, St Stephen's Green RFC, winners of the Hospitals' Cup, 1936. (Back row, left to right) D. O'Brien, D.J. Curran M.B., H.A. Doyle, G. Hickey, P.J. Morrissey, R.A. Sheehan, B.L. McCormack M.B.; (middle row, left to right) G.B. Macaulay, J.G. Maher M.B., B. Cullen (captain), W. Doolin F.R.C.S. (president), J.F. Houlihan, A.P. Barry M.B., J.P. O'Riordan; (front row, left to right) V.F. Sherry, J.J. Moloney

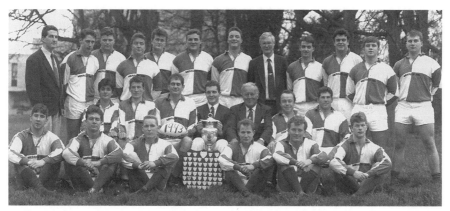

St Vincent's Hospital, Elm Park RFC, winners of the Hospitals Cup, 1993. (Back row, left to right) Conor O'Leary, Brian Burns, Turlough O'Donnell, Barry Browne, Dr Brian Maher, Robert Hannon (hon. sec.), John Quinlan, Dr M. Crowe (DHFC Committee), Dr Mark Lucey, Dr David Brophy, Ross Morgan, Brian O'Brien; (middle row, left to right) Ronan Kilbride (PRO), Feargal McCourt, Michael Molloy (playing captain), Dr John Carey (captain), Mr D. Kelly (president), Rory O'Donoghue (treasurer), Paul O'Brien; (front row, left to right) Brian McManus, Ian Norton, Oran Rigby, Emmet Andrews, Niall Hughes, Michael O'Brien

a member of the community. One stroke for Mother Rectress, two for Sister Ministeress and in ascending number of strokes down to the most junior member of the community. If he has to summon junior members of the community very often, it is no wonder that Hanly is slim.

Halfway down on the left hand side he sees the casualty department, the old 'dog house' and beside it the steps up to St Brigid's ward. He recalls the days and nights when as an intern on duty he would be called to the 'dog house' to solve some acute medical or surgical problem. He would hope that the problem would not be too serious, that he would be able to cope with it himself and not have to ring up one of the consultants and take him from his fireside to the hospital. On the other side of the corridor is the X-ray department on the site of the old theatre and students' gallery.

Near the end of the corridor he could turn left into the main hospital theatre. In the old days at the bottom of the corridor one could take the left turn up to St Patrick's or the right turn up to St Laurence's, or one could go down the stairs to St Charles's or St Teresa's, that old historic area of the hospital which years before had been the site of the out-patients' department. He re-traces his footsteps up the long corridor to the front of the building.

At the top of the corridor he slowly climbs the winding granite staircase (built originally between nos. 56 and 57 St Stephen's Green), up to the front floor of the hospital. At the bottom of the stairs, the large circular clock still records the passage of time. Halfway up he might recall the hospital chaplains who served him and the hospital so faithfully over the years. It could not have been easy for a young priest to deal with the many problems that confronted him in his daily routine: Mass to be celebrated, the sick and dying to be strengthened and comforted, possibly pastoral help with the problems of many employed in the hospital, and also a fatherly eye to be kept on the young students and doctors in the hospital to see that they did not do anything silly which might endanger their careers. Depending on his time in the hospital he might recall Fr Robinson, Fr Kenny, Fr O'Donoghue, Fr Fitzsimons, Fr Brady, Fr Mulvey, Fr Deering, Fr Dooley, Fr Farnan and Fr Staunton S.M.

On the first floor he finds St Joseph's and St Benedict's with their exquisite plasterwork. On moving along the corridor parallel to the front of the house he reaches St Elizabeth's, St Agnes's and St Vincent's wards. On the next floor he visits St Anne's front and back with its gynaecological theatre and St Camillus's and St Gabriel's, and then at the Earlsfort Terrace end on the second floor—another feat of architectural ingenuity—St Michael's and above St Raphael's.

Coming down the stairs again at the top of the long corridor he turns sharply left, passing on his right the other parlour and Mother Rectress's office. On his left is the entrance to the community recreation area and dining-room. Now he enters no. 58 and experiences the hushed calm of a private nursing home, the narrow stairs thickly carpeted. He might look into the 58 theatre to see if there are any operations going on. Then up the staircase he literally passes through the wall into no. 60, the corner house. No. 60 St Stephen's Green has had a chequered career. For many years it was the home of Mr Tobin, then for a short period in the early 1920s it was a residence for women medical students. Now, it had been a semi-private nursing home for many years.

If he is not too exhausted at this stage, our visitor descends the stairs of no. 60 to the ground floor, crosses the garden at the back of the hospital and goes through the passageway down to Leeson Lane. There he finds the new residence, the mortuary and at the bottom of Leeson Lane, facing up Quinn's Lane, the new block. He goes across the lane to St Mary's nurses' home and 96 X-ray. The two bridges across the lane are still intact and busy with the clatter of people constantly coming and going. He would probably be glad to see that Mr Fitzpatrick the shoemaker is still going strong; he had looked after the feet of many generations of Vincentians. He might drop in for a chat and for reminiscences of the old days in Vincent's.

He should pay a visit to the out-patients' department. Entering the main hall of the building he would see the patients sitting outside the various clinics. He could listen to the chat as they waited to see their doctors. Their conversation might give a more accurate account of the state of Irish medicine than any medical journal. The visitor could recall his own days in the OPD, helping the assistant physicians and surgeons to deal with an unending stream of patients.

He might possibly recall the number of 'chronics' with whom he dealt. Many patients attended over the years and after an unspecified incubation period passed into the peculiar state of morbidity known as the 'chronic'. The chronics would perform a function rather like that of a Greek chorus. Sitting outside the consulting room door they would comment on the doings and fortunes of nuns, nurses and doctors. The chronic was always a respected person in a clinic. It was a considerable therapeutic triumph to hear a chronic say that he or she had not been worse since their last visit. Of course no chronics worth their salt would ever admit for one moment that they were better. Alas, as our visitor was aware, due to the advances of modern medicine the chronic was fast becoming a rarity. This was a pity, for the chronic was a source of education to the young consultant and a source of chastisement to his senior.

At the back of the out-patients' he knocks at the door and enters the pharmacy, the domain of the pharmacist Dr John Shiel. If he is lucky he may get a sample of one of the most famous products of the pharmacy. It is a mixture known as 'pink pearl' and it lived up to its name for it was a pearl of great pharmacological value and a sure protection against all the ailments which affect the human body.

Leaving the out-patients' our visitor turns around the corner and strolls up Quinn's Lane, running parallel to Lower Leeson Street, in the direction of Upper Pembroke Street. He would not forget to break his journey at the pathology department at the back of the out-patients'. He climbs up the narrow steps, goes through the main laboratory to the small laboratory at the back and pays his respects to John. John FitzGerald was porter in the laboratory for many years and showed generations of students how to do that important chemical test which was a necessary part of any doctor's skills. John also had other interests. He was what in modern parlance is known as a 'film buff'. In the 1940s when the cinema was at the height of its popularity John would go to the pictures regularly. Afterwards he would meticulously write down his impression of the film, its plot, its stars. John expected the highest standards, and not even the brightest star of the screen was immune from his criticism. If one was planning to go to see a particular film it was a wise move to obtain John's opinion first. He was probably as good as or better than any high-powered film critic of the time.

A stroll up the lane through the archway and across Lower Pembroke Street and he is at the Pembroke Nursing Home, now run by St Vincent's. A quick look into the operating theatre on the first floor might find an operation in progress. A climb up the stairs to the top reveals a tall Georgian house not quite as grand, but basically of the same design as 96. On the way back he might encounter Ned Dunne. Ned had been keeping the chimneys of the hospital and surrounding areas free of soot for many years. Dressed appropriately in black, wearing a pillbox type of hat with a flap at the back slightly reminiscent of the French Foreign Legion, he carried lightly the brooms which were his symbols of office. Ned had a fine figure and a kindly face. It was well known that Ned used to give out bread to the poor in the OPD.

Re-entering the main hospital one wonders as our visitor walks slowly up the corridor, out the main door and down the steps, whether he would remember many of those working in the background to run the hospital where he was trained. Some he might have met, some had long gone but their work remained. Did he remember Barney Burke the boiler man, with the droopy moustache? Barney's main job was wheeling Mrs Donovan around. When he died his remains were carried out through the front of the hospital—a rare privilege.[6]

There was 'ould' Dick O'Neill, ex-British army, wardsman in the male wards; he had the disconcerting habit of asking new patients where they came from. While talking to them he would be engaged in cutting his plug tobacco into slices with a knife. He would then point the knife at the nervous patient and say, 'I will do you tomorrow morning at ten o'clock.' No doubt 'ould' Dick reassured the patient he was only joking. Bob O'Connell remembers him putting his two arms under a huge woman lying on the stretcher and lifting her up to place her on the table. 'Come to me me darlin' girl—you are the full of me arms of Irish love.'[7]

Then there was Pat O'Reilly, a Longford man, and George Wallace of 96,

Nan Moore outside the X-ray
department

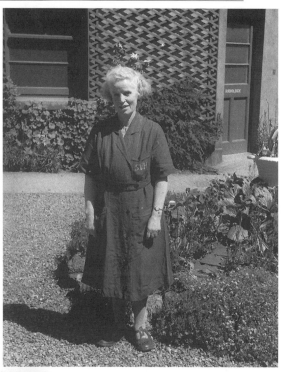

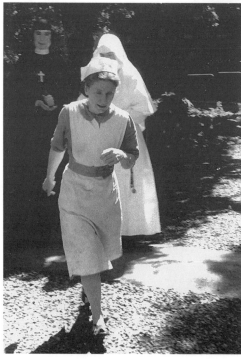

Maisie Kenny outside the nurses'
home

Alice Graham from the laundry, Bert Palmer electrician and plumber, the resident carpenter Tom Murphy, and Billy Parkinson who was in charge of the piggery. Kitty McSharry was cook in St Mary's and Maisie Kenny was on the domestic staff there. Jack Jones was the painter and Annie and Bridie Reynolds were on the staff of no. 58. Who could possibly forget Nan Moore, Connie Ryan, Edith, Julie, Christy Bannon, Christy Kenna and Jenny and the linen-room staff? He may have a special thought for Mary King, night telephonist for thirty years.

Our intrepid visitor must be rather weary after his odyssey as he steps on to the pavement in Stephen's Green. He might feel a little thirsty and he may remember that his teachers emphasised to him the importance of treating dehydration energetically. A visit to Doc Hartigan's around the corner may be prudent. There he might sit in the Doc's consulting room sipping a beverage laced with appropriate electrolytes. In the advancing twilight he might see faint pictures of old friends and colleagues now practising their art throughout the world, and recall dreams of hope and promise frozen in time when he and the world were young.

CHAPTER 20

THE ROAD TO ELM PARK

In terms of physical distance the road from St Stephen's Green to Elm Park is only a few miles. In terms of the establishment of a completely new hospital the road was long, arduous and winding; it was marked by many rough passages, innumerable culs de sacs and economic and political potholes. On the road there were many milestones marking success, sometimes disappointment, but always hope. Over the years many members of the staff were involved in the building of the new hospital. They gave generously of their precious time without any material reward. They sat for long hours on numerous committees. They endured frequent disappointment and frustration. It is sad that many of them did not live to see the fruits of their labour and enter the promised land. The story of the building of Elm Park is a rather complex and tortuous one. It was characterised by long periods when nothing was happening interspersed with periods of intense activity.

In July 1934 fifty acres of land at Elm Park were purchased by the Irish Sisters of Charity as a site for their proposed new hospital. Following the purchase a sub-committee of the Medical Board was set up to survey the situation with the hospital architect Mr Ralph Byrne.[1] The committee consisted of: Mother Rectress and members of the community; Medical Board members, D. Kennedy, J.B. Magennis and T.T. O'Farrell; medical staff members, R. White, J.B. McArevey and P.J. Keogh. An office was set up in the hospital known as the Elm Park office with a senior nurse, Miss Teresa Austin, to collect and correlate information about the hospital building and design. A sections committee of the medical staff was set up to discuss the various needs for each section: a. medical, b. surgical, c. pathological, d. gynaecological, e. laryngological, f. dental, g. ophthalmological, h. radiological (therapeutic and diagnostic), i. nurses' committee. In the interim the lands purchased were leased to the re-established Elm Park Golf Club which had its club-house in Nutley House, formerly the residence of Mr Francis Ellis.

Due to the Second World War and its aftermath there were no developments from 1939–47.

In 1947 a new building committee was established consisting of Mother Rectress and members of the community; chairman F. Morrin; members H. Meade, J. Cunningham, T.T. O'Farrell, D.K. O'Donovan, O. FitzGerald, P. FitzGerald; solicitor, Arthur Cox; and hon. secretary, T.D. O'Farrell. This committee recommended to the Mother General that Professor J.V. Downes and Mr F.B. Meehan be appointed architects. Many meetings between representatives of this committee and the Department of Health took place.

It was decided to visit the recently-finished Bergspital in Berne, Switzerland. The chairman and Denis O'Farrell inspected the building with the hospital architects, and many of its modern features were incorporated in the Elm Park design.

After a meeting with the Department of Health in November 1948, it became clear that the Department was not willing to provide teaching facilities, stating this was a matter for the university and the Department of Education. However, a change of policy produced a compromise and minimal teaching facilities were sanctioned. Following this the hospital authorities were informed that £1,000,000 would be granted to build and equip a 550 bed hospital. This was considered insufficient by the architects and medical staff. After further prolonged discussion £1,350,000 was granted to equip and build a 450 bed hospital.

During the period 1948–55 many meetings were held between the building committee and representatives of the Department of Health. At this time the latest hospital to have been built in these islands was the Westminster Hospital which was built ten years previously; so the committee had little to guide it. The basic principle of having linked buildings with a central service corridor on two levels to connect these various blocks had been adopted during this period, as based on the best advice then available —and this has indeed stood the test of time.[2]

In 1956 a tender was signed between the Irish Sisters of Charity and Messrs. Wall Brothers for the initial site development work including all piling and foundation beams, main sewerage and drainage, water mains and road foundation. On 20 January 1956 the first sod was turned in Elm Park by Fr Fitzsimons, chaplain to the hospital, in the presence of Mother General, Mother Rectress and members of the community.[3] The first tender was completed and all work ceased in 1958.

The building committee was re-formed in 1958 under the chairmanship of J. Cunningham, with J. McMullin as secretary. During the next three years this committee held monthly meetings at which the recommendations of various working parties and sub-committees were considered.[4] In his capacity as secretary, McMullin tried to keep liaison going between the sub-committees, the main committees and the architects by sitting in on all their deliberations. These working parties went over the existing plans, room by room, floor by floor, altering, improving and re-organising each section of

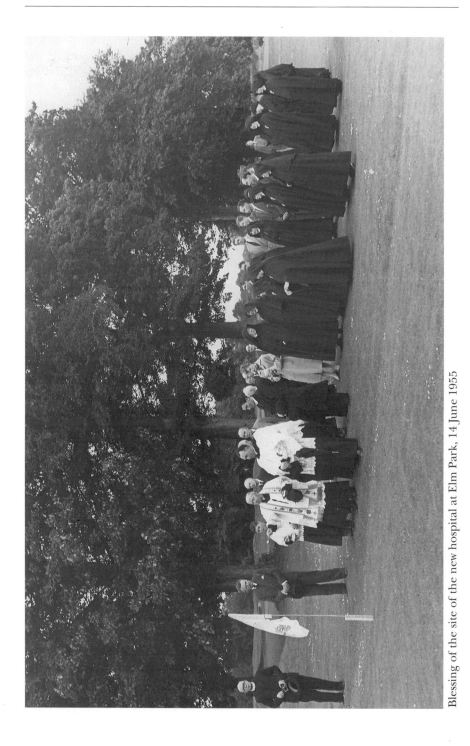

Blessing of the site of the new hospital at Elm Park, 14 June 1955

the building in turn. During this period the casualty (accident and emergency) department was re-planned. The original plan for the area had also included a very large pharmacy, which seemed to be necessary at the time.

Space was found for the electro encephalogram department and a physiotherapy building was added to the existing plan. There was no out-patients' department in the plan as it was thought that the hospital would continue to use the out-patients' department in Stephen's Green. This was shown to be impracticable and a new out-patients' department was added to the existing plan. The entire theatre floor was altered to provide for changed ideas of what constitutes the ideal theatre suite. Intensive care units, the metabolic unit, the pulmonary laboratory, the surgical laboratory and a centrally-sited sterile supply area were all incorporated in the existing framework of the hospital. This required a good deal of give and take from all sections, the loss of a ward here and a staff room there and so on.

In July 1960 a deputation met the Minister for Health, Mr McEntee, in the Custom House. Among those present at this meeting were the Mother General, Mother Canisius, J. Cunningham, J.V. Downes, F.B. Meehan, B. O'Brien, J. McMullin, Arthur Cox; Mr Murray, Mr White, Mr Hargadon and others from the Department of Health.[5] At the meeting the Minister stated that he was in a position to offer St Vincent's Hospital £1,500,000 towards the building of the new hospital. He pointed out that there were many other applications for grants from the Hospitals Sweeps funds, particularly from the provinces, and he also pointed out that the revenue from the Sweeps was not guaranteed. He agreed that hospital building costs had risen and the present rate was about £1,000 per bed. There would have to be some reduction therefore in the size of the hospital and economies would have to be effected. The final decision was that the hospital was to go ahead with the greatest speed, produce a plan and submit it to the Department on the basis of £1,500,000 for a 250 bed hospital.

In 1964 Messrs John Sisk were appointed general contractors and work on the superstructure of all the main buildings was re-started. All structural work on these buildings was completed by December 1965. It became obvious that it would be very difficult if not impossible to reduce the size of the hospital from 450 beds to 250 on the existing foundations. The Department of Health finally gave sanction for the completion of the full 450 bed hospital in its original form.

In 1966 the building committee was re-named. From now on it was known as the co-ordinating committee. Its main job was that of acting as a watch dog on the sub-committees which were at this stage beginning to order equipment.[6] It also had the task of working out the logistics of the eventual move from Stephen's Green to Elm Park.

Commissioning of the new hospital began in 1968.

Commissioning is described as the process of bringing the complex of buildings into use. In simple terms it covers all the activities essential for that purpose. It includes not only the obvious task of taking over completed buildings and associated engineering plant and services, but the detailed preparation within a master plan of the schedules for equipping and staffing the new hospital. It also involves a major effort for the researching and preparation of the general administrative policies under which the new hospital will operate and the essential detailed working procedures in every section and department, which will govern its day to day functioning.[7]

Commissioning of the new hospital raised serious financial problems in January 1968. These problems were solved by the generosity of Sir John Galvin who became very interested in the hospital and its problems. He offered to be responsible for the commissioning of the new St Vincent's and for the transfer out of the old hospital to the new one.[8]

Sir John Galvin was born in Tasmania. He served with the British army during the Second World War and after a dramatic escape from Singapore came to London to the Foreign Office. After the war, he returned to the Far East where he worked with General MacArthur as advisor on the economic reconstruction of Japan, and with Chiang Kai-shek on the national military war council of China. After an active business career, spent chiefly in controlling engineering, building and mining works in Malaysia, India and China (where his kinsman Bishop John Galvin began the missionary activities of the Columban Fathers), Sir John came back to Ireland to complete the education of his family, which now includes a graduate of the Dublin College of the National University of Ireland. He had of course visited Ireland since boyhood.

The responsibility for organising the commissioning was entrusted to Mr James N. McHugh, a civil engineer who had been associated with Sir John and his business affairs in the East.[9] In January a commissioning executive group was set up to provide a central unit where all matters relating to commissioning could be studied. The tasks fell under the following headings, (a) building services, (b) plant and equipment, (c) staffing, (d) procedures and methods, (e) other items.

The first meeting of the commissioning committee was held in the building on 25 January 1968.[10] Present were Rev. Mother General; Mother M. Aquin Jordan First Assistant Bursar General; Mother Paula Mother Rectress St Vincent's Hospital; Mother Canisius; Sister Agnes Carmel; Professor P.N. Meenan hon. secretary Medical Board; Mr McHugh; Mr O'Malley of Downes, Meehan and Robinson, architects; Mr McCambridge, building site supervisor; Mr W.R. Plunkett; Mrs R. Verner, secretary. Mr Gerard Smith, hospital secretary, subsequently joined the commissioning committee. It was decided to utilise the services of a group of hospital consultants of international repute to advise and comment on a number of matters related to the detailed planning of the commissioning of the hospital.

From July Messrs. Llewelyn-Davies, Weeks, Forestier-Walker & Bor were appointed to advise on a wide variety of problems.[11]

The most urgent need at this stage was the building of the nurses' home and the schools of nursing and radiography.[12] The original plan of the nurses' home consisted of two linked tower blocks, both of them twelve storeys high. The final plan consisted of one tower block. Permission was granted by the Department of Health, the first sod was dug and work began on the nurses' home and the schools of nursing and radiography.

In September 1968 Mother Canisius O'Keeffe was appointed first Rectress of the hospital.[13] On 7 October three Sisters of Charity arrived: Sister Francis Jude Cullinan, Sister M. Cephas MacDonald, Sister Teresa Paul Cullen. They made history by being the first Sisters of Charity to sleep in the new hospital. On 8 October Mother Canisius, Sister Otteran Harrington, Sister M. Bernard, Sister Anthony Mary O'Neill and Sister Joseph Miriam took up residence. The first batch of nurses, thirty in all, also took up residence in the medical hostel in October.

On 11 October 1968 the new community took formal possession of St Vincent's Hospital. Until such time as the convent was ready the sisters lived temporarily in the medical hostel (subsequently the residency). At the end of October the sisters took over the convent's sleeping quarters and the refectory was transferred to the convent parlour. Midnight Mass was celebrated at Christmas in the convent refectory. It did not pass without incident. Apparently the night watchman had locked the big entrance gate on his way out, forgetting that a Jesuit priest was due to celebrate Midnight Mass. When the priest arrived to find the gates locked there was no way of communicating with the oratory as the phone lines had not yet been laid down, but being a resourceful chaplain he climbed the gates of the hospital, and fortunately landed safely on the other side.

In January 1969 three quarters of the department of pathology moved out to the new hospital. They were the first medical personnel to work in the new hospital. Sir John Galvin was anxious that a section of the grounds should be laid out for the private use of the community and he offered to pay the cost. Plans were drawn up by a well-known landscape architect, Mr Victor Van Boven. Work at the back of the convent began in January 1969 and was completed by the end of August of the same year. A number of trees were made available from Sir John Galvin's garden, some of them fifteen to twenty years old. All the trees recovered after transplantation with the exception of an old almond tree which died off.

In February 1969 thirteen working parties comprising the various departments of the hospital were set up to advise on the staffing and equipping of the new departments. The last floor of the nurses' home was completed in July 1969 and the topping out ceremony took place. Over the months groups of nurses continued to arrive from the old hospital. Until

Sir John Galvin

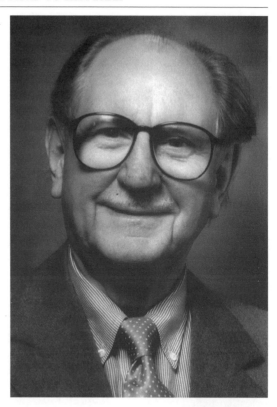

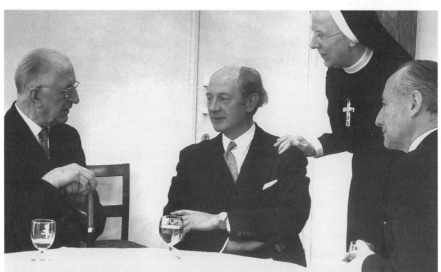

(Left to right) President de Valera, An Taoiseach Jack Lynch, Mother Canisius, D.K. O'Donovan at the opening of the new hospital

the nurses' home was ready for occupation temporary arrangements were made to house them on the fourth floor of the hospital as well as in the medical hostel.

The chapel and convent were solemnly blessed in August 1969 by the Archbishop, Most Rev. John Charles McQuaid.[14] Amongst those present who received the Archbishop were Mr Michael Devlin, K.S.G. K.M., who presented the community with a cheque for £30,000 to cover the cost of the chapel building. Mr Devlin's connection with the hospital had begun three years previously. Coming from Mass one Sunday in Killiney Parish Church he was talking to Dr Boland, senior radiologist to the hospital; he remarked on the high steel scaffolding erected in the Elm Park grounds and asked what was the building. He was told it was the new St Vincent's Hospital and he responded that he would like to make a donation to it. He was subsequently introduced to Mother General and gave his generous contribution to the construction of the chapel. The chapel itself was placed under the protection of St Michael. The sculpture of St Michael the Archangel which was mounted on the chapel gable wall was also the gift of Mr Devlin, the artist being Mr Richard Enda King. To commemorate the occasion, a gold communion plate engraved on one side with the Archbishop's crest and the other side with the crest of the Sisters of Charity was presented to His Grace by the architects. The tabernacle in the chapel is of burnished bronze and incribed within on a gold bar are the following words: 'This tabernacle was donated in loving memory of Mrs Bridget Cox and of her devoted husband Arthur Cox who was subsequently ordained priest and died in Zambia aged seventy-four years.' Arthur Cox was the son of the Right Honourable Dr Michael Cox, physician to the hospital for many years. He was one of the most distinguished solicitors in the country and was for many years legal advisor to the Sisters of Charity. After his wife's death he was ordained to the priesthood and went to work on the missions in Zambia. He died in Zambia from injuries received in a car crash.

In October 1969 Mr L. Trotter who was a member of the staff of Messrs. Llewelyn-Davies and Associates was appointed administrator to the hospital. Mr Trotter under the direction of Mr McHugh was responsible for commissioning the new hospital.

The first patients from St Vincent's Hospital St Stephen's Green to be admitted to St Vincent's Hospital Elm Park arrived on 23 January 1970. This was a significant date as it was on 23 January 1834 that the Irish Sisters of Charity took over the Earl of Meath's house on the Green. The ward chosen for admission was St Anne's ward, under the care of Sr Agnes Ursula Byrne. Twelve patients were admitted, all of whom were transferred from various wards in the old hospital. There were six male and six female patients; all were medical patients as the operating theatres were still unfinished. Patients were received by Mother General, Mother Canisius, Mother Paula, P.N. Meenan, chairman of the Medical Board, J.A. Mehigan, secretary of the

Medical Board, and the secretary of the building committee, J. McMullin.[15] There was considerable public interest in the move and television cameras were active photographing the event, even though a strike had commenced on that very day in Telefís Éireann. The first patient to enter the hospital was Connie Ryan, a member of the staff of the old hospital for over forty-two years. In the evening Archbishop McQuaid arrived and toured the wards and departments of the hospitals and visited the patients.

The hospital kitchen and cafeteria were opened in February 1970. In March 1970 a second ward opened—St Charles's ward.[16] A management course was organised by Mr Trotter, administrator. There were sixteen participants and the course continued for three days. Fr Thomas Fox C.S.S.P. was appointed chaplain in May 1970. St Rita's Staff Hostel opened on 10 June 1970 to provide temporary accommodation for seventeen nurses. The top floor was used for the nurses and the bottom floors by the supervisors and girls. The first anaesthetic in the hospital was given by Dr Denis O'Leary in the treatment room of St Charles's ward on 7 July 1970. Central Stores opened in September.

The first two patients for surgery were admitted on 21 October 1970 and first operations were carried out on 23 October by J. McMullin; R. Davys was the anaesthetist. Sister Joseph Ignatius Phelan was appointed superintendent of the theatre and she and Sister Marie Therese Claire and Sister Columbiere were also part of the theatre team as the equipping of the whole suite of the eleven theatres and their auxiliary rooms proceeded.

The pharmacy department opened on 26 October 1970 under the direction of Mrs Fitzpatrick and two assistants, Mrs FitzGerald and Mrs Lambe.

CHAPTER 21

THE MOVE TO ELM PARK

I t would appear that according to the best newspaper tradition the London *Daily Mirror* had its eye on St Vincent's Hospital in Dublin. The following note appeared in its edition of Monday 2 November. 'On Sunday 1 November 1970 St Vincent's Hospital performed its trickiest operation for more than a century . . . moving lock, stock and scalpel.' These few words summed up admirably the final days of St Vincent's Hospital St Stephen's Green and its removal a few miles away to become St Vincent's Hospital Elm Park. 'It was the last act in an operation unique in the history of Irish medicine.'

When the news came that the final move to Elm Park would take place in the summer of 1970 it was received in the hospital with mild interest and much cynicism: we had heard this one before. There had been so many false dawns in the history of the coming into operation of Elm Park. However, during the early months of the summer of 1970 when more and more departments began to move out to Elm Park it was recognised that this was the real thing. Kevin Connolly has described the reaction of the junior staff of the hospital during those hectic summer months:[1]

> J.A. Mehigan newly appointed secretary of the Medical Board was in charge of the patients' move and he had as his helpers two members of the junior hospital staff, Dr John Bugler (John the Park) and Dr John O'Sullivan (John the Green). The two Johns insisted that provided everything was planned in advance the move itself would be a non-event. Everything certainly was planned minutely, down to the last detail. Mehigan had gone over to Addenbrook's Hospital in Cambridge which had recently moved from one site to another. There he studied the way in which the authorities in Cambridge had managed their particular operation and gained much valuable knowledge from their experience. The commissioning executive group under the directorship of McHugh had set up a sub-committee to look after the patients intake fully six months before the move and

Trotter and Mehigan drew up a plan based on the experiences elsewhere.

The patients' transfer committee under the chairmanship of Mehigan began to meet regularly in both hospitals and the numbers and variety attending each meeting grew and grew as more facets were pulled in. There was also another committee under the chairmanship of Dermot Cantwell the radiologist, dealing with the move out of the departments. Cantwell began to arrange to transfer all equipment not needed at the Green. Bulletins and memorandums began to fly between various departments.

A notice telling us how many days to D day appeared at the front hall in the Green as well as at Elm Park. The Department of Health and other organisations involved in the move and admissions were informed about our plans and D day rapidly approached. Sunday was chosen because there would be less traffic problems and no non-acute cases were admitted for three weeks before D day. Ten days before the move most urgent cases were admitted to other hospitals, thus on the day of the move itself there were only seventy-three patients to be transferred.

A rehearsal was carried out on the Sunday before the final move.

On Saturday 31 October the hospital of St Vincent's on the Green was closed to all patients and the casualty department on Leeson Lane closed its doors at midnight. As in all the best traditions Sunday 1 November 1970 dawned bright and clear. There were quite a number of onlookers waiting on the Green to see the drama unfold. The press were there in strength, there were TV cameras on the roofs and reporters from the various papers all over the place. As press officer, F.O.C. Meenan had the unenviable task of seeing that the TV cameras and the reporters did not intrude too much on the safety, comfort and privacy of the patients. Radio Éireann was also present in the Green in the early morning and later in Elm Park when Joe Linnane talked to Mother Paula and other members of the staff about their feelings at the time of the move.

The transfer was reported by the *Irish Independent* on 2 November 1970:

> A fleet of twelve Order of Malta ambulances took part in the first event of its kind in Irish medical history yesterday when seventy-three critically ill patients were transferred three miles to the new St Vincent's Hospital Elm Park Dublin from the 136-year-old hospital in St Stephen's Green. The entire transfer took nearly four hours but was carried out with military precision thanks to detailed advanced planning. The plans were originally begun months ago under the direction of J.A. Mehigan, honorary secretary of the Hospital Board.
>
> Nurses and staff doctors travelled in the ambulances with some of

the patients when this was considered necessary. In one case a senior consultant staff member accompanied a patient who was suffering from respiratory failure. The ambulances were fully equipped to deal with any emergency that might occur in the three mile trip across town. A Garda motorcycle escort accompanied each ambulance on the trip and Gardaí along the route diverted traffic and manned traffic lights. Merrion parishioners were asked not to park their cars along the route while at Mass. 'There were absolutely no hitches during the transfer but we were ready to deal with them if they occurred,' Mr Mehigan said yesterday.

Each patient wore a coloured tag, and a similar tag bearing his name, ward and condition was attached to his belongings. The colour of the tag decided what door the patient would enter at Elm Park, what lift would be used, what ward would be allocated and what bed would be ready for the patient. Many of the patients were post-operative cases and a special cardiac ambulance was used to transfer heart patients. Some ambulances were brought from Belfast, Limerick and other areas.

As the last patient left the St Stephen's Green Hospital, the doors were ceremoniously closed in the presence of Mother Teresa Anthony, Mother General of the Irish Sisters of Charity. The Mother Rectress, Sister Paula and other nuns will continue to live there and to take care of the patients in the private nursing homes in nearby Leeson Street.

Most of the cases moved yesterday were either stretcher or wheelchair cases and many needed special equipment necessary for their treatment with them at all times. The casualty and emergency unit at the St Stephen's Green hospital which closed at midnight on Saturday will re-open at 9.30 a.m. today in Elm Park.

Mother Canisius, Mother Rectress of Elm Park and Dr John Bugler supervised the intake of patients at the new £5 million hospital. 'All the patients arrived perfectly well and perfectly comfortable,' Mr Mehigan said yesterday afternoon, relaxing after the task was over. The Elm Park hospital complex is the first voluntary general teaching hospital to be commissioned in Britain or Ireland since the Second World War. The £5 million was provided from Irish Hospitals Trust funds and from voluntary contributions. The new hospital provides 454 beds and will employ 1,100, including a nursing staff of 435. Elm Park will be officially opened by the Archbishop of Dublin Most Rev. Dr McQuaid on 27 November.

Amongst those who made the great trek from St Stephen's Green to Elm Park were two bowls of goldfish.

On arrival the patients were greeted by Mother Canisius O'Keeffe, Rectress of Elm Park, and her community, doctors, nurses, administrators, including Mr McHugh, chairman of the commissioning group who were the

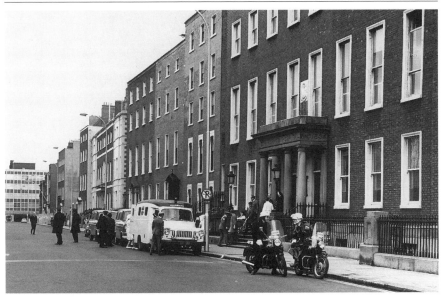

Leaving St Stephen's Green

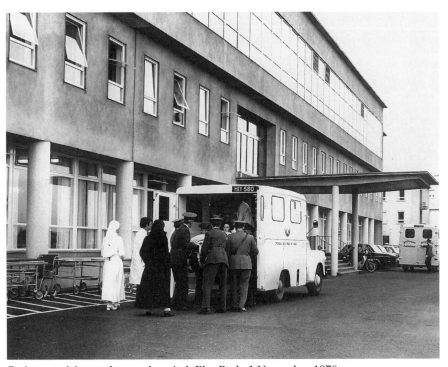

Patients arriving at the new hospital, Elm Park, 1 November 1970

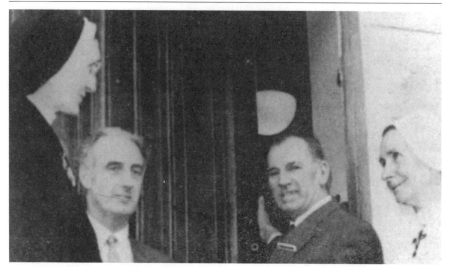

Last closing of the door of St Vincent's Hospital, St Stephen's Green, 1 November 1970, with (left to right) Mother Teresa Anthony, J.A. Mehigan, Michael Hanly, Mother Paula

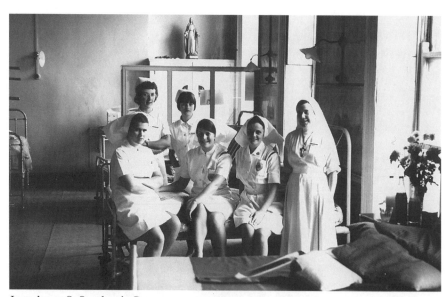

Last day at St Stephen's Green

first to commence work on the transfer in January 1968. Secretarial staff, innumerable journalists, television and cameramen, public relations men, porters and guards were present. Everything went extremely smoothly, without any hitch or discomfort to the patients. It was all completed in under three hours. Naturally in Elm Park there was a feeling of pleasure and gratification that the operation had gone so smoothly, without any problems or adverse effects to the patients, and that now after so many years St Vincent's Elm Park was a reality.

It is understandable that back at the Green the mood was rather subdued —one cannot forget over a hundred years of service in a few hours. There was an air of sadness as Mother Paula assisted Mother General to close the main door of the old hospital, marking the end of 136 years of service. Mother Paula and a small community were to stay on in the nursing home which was continuing to function. Now that the crowd had dispersed and the action was out in Elm Park, Sister Paula expressed her feelings as she toured the old hospital, now silent:

> The stillness that prevailed left us numb; the long corridor that only a short time previously was full of gay young nurses and doctors was silent except for the thud, thud, thud of the Securicor officer on his rounds; what a sad reflection on our society today, that it was deemed necessary to protect the hospital right away with Securicor. We immediately set to work and toured the entire hospital, locking doors here, windows there. We first visited the Chapel. How regal it looked that November morning, standing there in all its gothic glory. The sanctuary lamp seemed to burn particularly bright, and the Master we felt was very near, while Our Lady smiled on us from beneath her glittering halo. Memories came floating by—memories of all the sisters who once filled the priedieux now empty, and the altar rails where so many of our doctors made their First Communion.
>
> After a fervent 'thank you' to the Lord for allowing us to transfer our hospital with all its traditions intact, and with the spirit of Mary Aikenhead still so active after the passage of well over a century, we re-traced our steps—down the stairs we went past the famous circular clock to the Board Room, now the headquarters of Securicor. The room, once Mother Mary Aikenhead's office, could tell many a tale. It looked forlorn as its furniture and portraits had already gone to their new home in Elm Park. How many hospital problems were solved here by many great men. The students' room was still intact except, instead of a babble of voices, all was now hushed.
>
> The elegant parlours, scenes of so many functions, First Communion breakfasts, Christmas parties when Santa held court, looked as stately that day, with their antique furniture, Adam mantlepieces and beautiful flowers as surely they did when the Earl himself was master of the house.

On the grand stairs with its wonderful stuccoed ceiling, one could almost see the charming ladies in their crinolines and their dashing escorts in their powdered wigs, gliding up to St Joseph's ward, once upon a time the front drawing-room. How sad the ward looked now bereft of all its patients. This was the first ward Mother Mary Aikenhead opened with twelve beds. How very many patients must have gone through its doors, restored in body, renewed in soul, animated with courage to begin anew life's struggle. How many too during the same passage of time, to whom restoration to bodily health was denied, have been prepared to pass through the portals of death with soul prepared to meet their maker.

Everywhere we went, wards, theatres, X-ray rooms, told their own tale of dedication. Since its foundation, numbers and numbers of generous souls gave their thoughts, their devotedness, their skill to make St Vincent's the great hospital it is today. After weeks and weeks of hard work we finally said 'goodbye' to the old hospital and took up our abode in 94 Lower Leeson Street, the former school of nursing. From there we administer the private nursing homes and St Mary's nurses' home.

Faithful to its motto *Caritas Christi urget nos,* St Vincent's gave one hundred and thirty six unbroken years of service to the sick from all parts of Ireland. Let us hope that whatever may be the future of the new St Vincent's that in years to come, one will find its traditions intact. 'The old order changeth and giveth place to new', but the spirit is unchanging for it is rooted and founded in Charity. The staff could now enter their new hospital which took £5 million and the sweat and toil of generations of Vincent's staff and their friends and associates to build.[2]

On Thursday 26 November 1970 the *Irish Independent* described the new hospital:

The New St Vincent's Hospital has 455 beds with a high degree of advanced medical and surgical specialities. There is a fully equipped casualty department, an out-patient department, clinical laboratories, a lecture theatre and library. The clinical laboratories, metabolic/renal and radio isotope departments will ultimately occupy a new building being planned, together with the main lecture theatre and library.

The hospital has eleven operating theatres and extensive diagnostic facilities. Two of the operating theatres have overhead viewing domes for the use of students. An internal television circuit from the theatres is also proposed for teaching purposes.

More than three hundred students are being provided for, comprising some two hundred and ten medical students—seventy in each of three clinical years—as well as seventy pre-clinical students and twenty-five dental students who will attend for one special term.

The new hospital also accommodates the Mary Aikenhead school of nursing, the school of radiography and facilities for the practical training of dieticians and certain classes of para-medical workers. A staff training centre has been established for training hospital administrative, clerical and other staff with the co-operation of the College of Commerce Rathmines.

There is a nursing staff of 430 out of a total staff complement of about one thousand. The wards mainly comprise 6 bed units with some 3 bed and single rooms. There are 82 beds per floor divided into two nursing units each of 41 beds.

A central kitchen and a staff cafeteria service provides a peak service of 1,000 main lunchtime meals over a 24 hour period. There is also a snack bar for those not requiring the cafeteria main meal service. A staff coffee lounge and rest room are almost completed. The main supply services route is by means of a subway running beneath the main building. It is almost 400 yards in length and supplies are transported by electric vehicles. The subway is linked to the nurses' building and all service buildings.

The nurses' home accommodates 250 nursing staff while the staff hospital accommodates 70 people. The accounts, medical records and allied patient services are being designed for computer use. In the planning of computerisation the hospital administration are collaborating with the Medico-Social Research Board.

The operating theatre suite in the new hospital is the most up-to-date in these islands, reflecting the most advanced thinking in the field of surgery. Effective steps have been taken to eliminate the danger of infection—a major hazard in the operating theatre —through an elaborate system of sterile barriers. The operating theatre zone is fully sterile and no one may enter the area without first passing through a 'twilight zone' involving a complete change of clothing in the changing and shower rooms attached to each 'Link'. These 'links' give access to the theatres and are used, respectively, by surgeons and registrars, nurses and patients, and students. A red line across the threshold of each doorway leading into the sterile zone is an effective reminder that only those who have gone through the 'twilight zone' can enter.

The New St Vincent's Hospital Elm Park was officially opened on 27 November 1970. There could not be a greater contrast than between the opening of St Vincent's Hospital St Stephen's Green and the opening of St Vincent's Hospital Elm Park. On 23 January 1834 Mother Mary Aikenhead with her small band of nuns drove up in their carriage to the door of number 56 St Stephen's Green; they slipped quietly inside to start writing

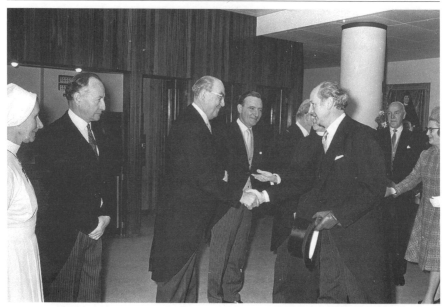

Arriving for the opening of the hospital, An Taoiseach Mr Lynch and Mrs Lynch, with (left to right) Mother Paula, D.K. O'Donovan, T.C.J. O'Connell, J. McMullin, J.N. McHugh

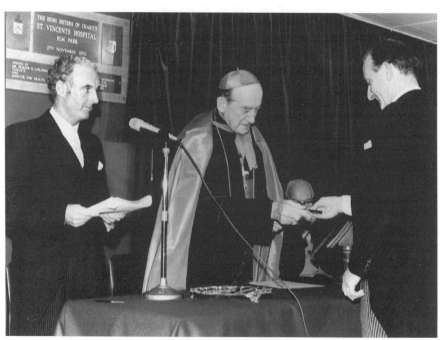

Archbishop McQuaid presenting a medal to J. McMullin, J.A. Mehigan (left)

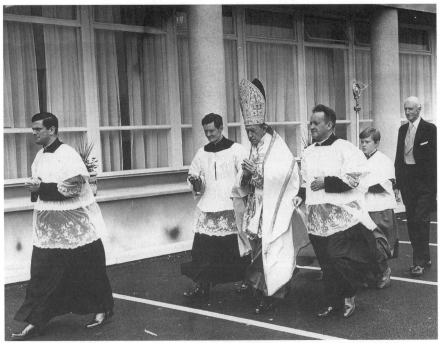

The hospital is blessed by Archbishop McQuaid, accompanied by H. Quinlan.

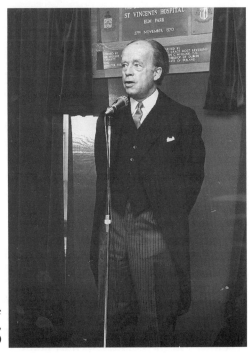

Minister for Health Erskine
Childers opening the new hospital,
27 November 1970

the first chapter in a proud history. On 27 November 1970 St Vincent's Hospital Elm Park was officially opened amid pomp and ceremony and in the presence of leaders of State and Church. The ceremony took place in the main hall or concourse, a side wall of the concourse having been removed to give additional accommodation. A dais and a special altar for the celebration of Mass had been erected in the concourse. The altar was prepared for Mass against the splendid backdrop of crimson velvet curtains which spanned the entire west wall of the concourse.

At 10.48 a.m. the Archbishop of Dublin the Most Rev. John Charles McQuaid arrived, to be followed by An Tánaiste Mr Erskine Childers, Minister for Health, and Mrs Childers, and the Taoiseach and Mrs Lynch. The distinguished guests were greeted in turn by Mother General, Mother Canisius and Mother Paula, Professor D.K. O'Donovan, Professor P.N. Meenan, Professor Oliver FitzGerald, Mr T.C.J. O'Connell, Mr J. McMullin, Mr J.N. McHugh and Mr L. Trotter, after which they joined the reception party to await the arrival of His Excellency, the President of Ireland, Mr de Valera, who was met by D.K. O'Donovan. The President entered the concourse at 11 a.m. precisely.

Mr McHugh, chairman of the commissioning executive group, started the proceedings by inviting the Tánaiste formally to open the new hospital. Mr Childers mounted the dais and drew aside a small curtain to reveal a wall plaque commemorating the opening of St Vincent's Hospital Elm Park. Trumpeters of the no. 1 Army Band sounded a fanfare and spotlights illuminated the plaque.

After robing, the Archbishop proceeded from the concourse to bless the hospital. He passed through St John's ward, the lecture theatre and tutorial rooms. He then went out to the front of the hospital, leaving by the west door and returning up the front steps and through the main entrance. Concluding prayers were said at the altar. The Archbishop then presided over Mass which was celebrated by the Right Rev. Monsignor Barrett, Parish Priest of Monkstown. The first lesson was read by Mr F.B. Meehan of Downes, Meehan and Robinson, the architects, and the second lesson by Mr J. Sisk, the building contractor.

After Mass the principal guests took their places on the dais for the speeches. The first address was given by the Archbishop who thanked all those who had contributed to the new hospital and to the day of celebration. He noted that 'Many regret the passing of the old St Vincent's at St Stephen's Green. Its warm and dignified façade must ever be in memory a contrast with the stern rectangles that house the new hospital. But the emanating spirit will be none other than that of the old St Vincent's.'

The Minister for Health paid tribute to the Irish Sisters of Charity and reminded the gathering that the sisters controlled over two thousand hospital beds in Dublin alone as well as providing a wide range of services elsewhere in the country such as home visiting, orphanages, homes for the

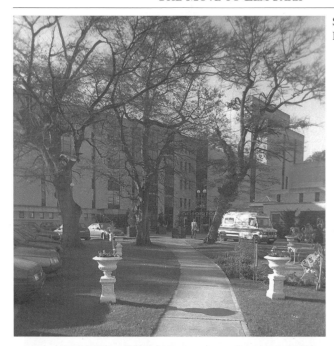

St Vincent's Private
Hospital

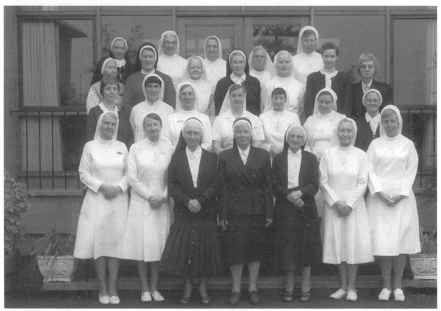

The community, St Vincent's Hospital, Elm Park, 1994. (Back row, left to right) Srs
Lorcan, Malachy, C. Rita, Josepha, Maureen; (third row, left to right) Srs Ursula,
Manus, Teresita, Marie de Montfort, Ignatius, Maureen, Dolores; (second row, left to
right) Srs A. Marie, Cecilia, Philomena, Margaret, M. Therese, Hilary, Ita; (front row,
left to right) Srs Agnes, T. Avila, F. Mary, J. Cyril, C. Colette, Rosario, Baptist

blind, homes for women and girls, youth clubs, meals for the poor and care of the mentally handicapped. Mr Childers drew attention to the large capital investment in building and equipment and to the fact that the cost of running hospitals was now by far the largest component in the nation's total health bill. He went on to urge that as the resources of the country were limited, the new hospital should be administered as economically as possible because if one sector of medical endeavour got more than its share, it would be at the expense of other sectors which would get less than they needed.

Mr McHugh referred to the history of the move from the old St Vincent's in St Stephen's Green and briefly outlined the development of the new hospital. He spoke of the gratitude owed to the Sisters of Charity for their generous contribution to the new hospital, and to those members of the staff of the hospital who had been involved in the many activities before and during construction. He paid tribute to all who had been involved in the new building.

P.N. Meenan, chairman of the Medical Board, went further back in history to describe the origin of the new hospital when the Elm Park site was purchased in 1934, the centenary year of St Vincent's. He drew attention to the close proximity of University College Dublin on its developing campus at Belfield and the potential for co-operation which this offered.

After the speeches the Archbishop presented commemorative medals to eight representative members of the hospital staff: Harold Quinlan, longest serving member of the medical staff; T.C.J. O'Connell, longest serving member of the surgical staff; J. McMullin, honorary secretary of the building committee and consultant surgeon; Ms Emma McDonnell, previous matron; John FitzGerald, pathology department and in the service of the hospital for nearly forty years; Ms Connie Ryan and Ms Maisie Kenny (each of whom had been in the service of the hospital for more than forty years). A similar commemorative medal was subsequently presented to every member of the staff.[3]

CHAPTER 22

BRIGHT MORNING

After the celebrations there was little delay in organising the hospital to work at full capacity. St Vincent's Hospital Elm Park might not have been the most elegant of edifices; nevertheless it was an impressive sight with its spread of buildings and lofty nurses' home occupying eleven acres overlooking Dublin Bay; situated between the main route from the city to the south-east and the main road from Dublin to the port of Dun Laoghaire; and also near the medical school of University College Dublin which was the largest medical school in the country. Moreover, situated as it was there was infinite room for expansion. An indication of its strategic situation can be gauged from the fact that a helicopter pad was constructed on the grounds in front of the hospital so that badly injured patients could be rushed to the hospital or to other hospitals in the vicinity; and the great of the land could come and go to all parts of the country.

There was a spirit of optimism and enthusiasm among the staff. The dreams of many generations had become reality. There would be no more working in the cramped surroundings of Georgian buildings, or the inadequate functioning of departments at the end of long corridors or in the next available corner. The world was now their oyster. They were the envy of their colleagues in other hospitals. Nevertheless, the enthusiasm was tempered with caution and a sense of reality.

All who worked in the hospital realised that because much had been given to them much was expected of them. They appreciated that they had been given £5 million of tax payers' money and it was their duty to use that money to the best interest of the people of the city and also of the country. They realised that they would have to render an account of their medical services. New difficulties and new challenges lay ahead which had to be confronted and solved. In fact these new challenges and problems lay just over the horizon. In the sixties and seventies the whole fabric of social and medical progress was in ferment.

There was an unending torrent of medical discoveries and new techniques coming from medical centres all over the world. The cost of these new techniques was escalating at a staggering rate. Even the wealthiest of nations were beginning to realise that they could not afford a comprehensive medical scheme for their citizens from the cradle to the grave. This was especially realised in a relatively small and poor country like Ireland. No hospital, however well-equipped, could provide a complete range of all medical specialities.

The old system, whereby one hospital would have an expensively-equipped department in one particular speciality and another hospital not so far away would have an equally well-equipped department in the same speciality had to change. It was the function of the newly-established Comhairle na nOspidéal to decide how the specialities would be divided between the various hospitals. In each major teaching hospital all the larger specialities would be represented; the more specialised ones had to be distributed among the hospitals according to needs of the populations. In other words the seventies and eighties were to be an era of choice.

The pattern of medicine itself was also changing. Diseases caused by infection, malnutrition and poor social standards had been largely wiped out. There was a sharp increase in the standard of living and there was over-indulgence in alcohol, nicotine and other drugs of addiction. Various forms of cancer were growing more common; carcinogenic factors were being increasingly pin-pointed. It was becoming apparent that the concept of preventive medicine must play a prominent part in the medicine of the future. Psychiatric problems, many of them due to the stresses of modern life, were on the rise. With an ageing population, disease of the elderly and care of the old and infirm were becoming more and more of a problem.

An increasingly literate and well-educated population was demanding the highest standard of medical services. As has been noted, politicians were rapidly becoming aware that there were votes in medicine with the result that any political party that tampered with the standard of medical services to the community did so at peril to its reputation in Dáil Éireann and the country. This possibly led to the problem that politicians at times promised in their election manifestos more medical services than there were facilities for in the country.

Hospitals run by religious orders were facing new problems. Due to the marked decline in the number of vocations to the religious life, religious orders found it difficult to staff their hospitals with members from their own communities and had to depend more and more on lay workers. Another difficulty was that a section of the community considered because the voluntary hospitals were now almost completely subsidised from government funds, the religious orders should not be allowed to impress their own particular ethos on the hospitals which they owned and managed. They may perhaps have forgotten that if it was not for the religious orders there would be much less education and fewer voluntary hospitals in the community.

One of the first challenges to be faced in the new hospital was the need to devise new methods of administration. Obviously the old system which had operated in the Green would not be capable of handling the administration of a large modern hospital. Chronologically the first step was the re-organisation of the Medical Board. The centenary of the first Medical Board occurred in October 1969. The original members of the Board were F. Quinlan, William O'Leary, E.P. Mapother and Robert Cryan. In 1969 the members of the Board were P.N. Meenan, secretary; D.K. O'Donovan, P. FitzGerald, O. FitzGerald, T.C.J. O'Connell, F. Duff, J. Maher, H. Quinlan and P. Brennan. Mother Canisius and Mother Paula took the opportunity of making more appointments to the Medical Board so that it could be more representative of the staff.[1]

The Board could not be entirely confined to the senior physicians and surgeons. The specialities which were playing an increasing role in the work of a modern hospital demanded adequate representation at Board level. The new members were R. Davys, K. Feeney, Sir John Galvin, F. Lavery, J.N. McHugh, J.P. McMullin, J. Mehigan, R. Mulcahy, F. Muldowney, B. O'Brien and T.D. O'Farrell. Three members representing the Clinical Association were appointed for a three year term. Mother Canisius and Mother Paula attended the meetings when they wished to do so.

The first meeting of the enlarged Medical Board in Elm Park was held on 3 March 1970. Sister Francis Joseph Lang was appointed secretary manager of the hospital and took up duty in Elm Park on 14 October 1970. Sister Francis Joseph was no stranger to the hospital. Her early years were spent as a nurse training in the hospital and later she became a ward sister. In 1957 she was commissioned to open the new Orthopaedic Hospital in Kilcreene, Co. Kilkenny and later the Arthur Davidson Hospital in Ndola, Zambia where she spent the years 1963–70.

In 1972 the congregation of the Irish Sisters of Charity established a Board of Management (the Board), to manage the affairs of the hospital on behalf of the congregation. The duties and functions of the Board are set out in the constitution.

The first chairman of the Board would be appointed by the Superior General of the congregation and hold office for a period of three years, a vice-chairman would be elected by the Board and would also hold office for a period of three years. Both chairman and vice-chairman, neither of whom would be a member of staff, would be eligible for re-election.

The Board would consist of no more than twenty and no fewer than eight members. The Reverend Mother Rectress of the hospital would be *ex-officio* member of the Board. From among the sisters of the congregation, two would be appointed to membership of the Board, one at least of whom would be engaged in active nursing. Three members of the consultant staff would be appointed to membership of the Board, two of whom would by election be nominated by the Medical Board, the third of whom would be nominated by the entire medical staff. One member of the governing body

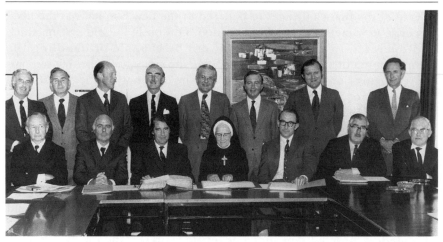

Medical Board, 1973. (Back row, left to right) J.A. Mehigan, J. Gallagher, F. Muldowney, R. Davys, P. Brennan, D. O'Leary, D.G. Kelly, D. Cantwell; (front row, left to right) D.K. O'Donovan, F.O.C. Meenan, F.A. Duff, Mother Canisius, R. Towers, P.N. Meenan, O. FitzGerald

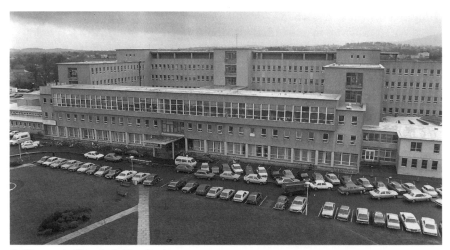

St Vincent's Hospital, Elm Park

of UCD selected by the Superior General of the congregation would be appointed. The members of the Board would hold office for three years.

The Board would appoint a full-time secretary manager when the need arose, responsible to the Board and whose conditions of employment, jurisdiction, obligations and remuneration would be determined by the Board. The Board would also have the power to appoint such other administrative officers to the staff as would from time to time be considered necessary for the effective administration of the hospital.

The constitution also provided for an executive council directly responsible to the Board which would consist of the secretary manager, the matron, a sister of the congregation and two members of the medical staff. The function of the executive council was to regulate and to keep under constant review the day-to-day administration of the hospital within the terms laid down by the Board and to deal with such other matters as may from time to time be deputed to it by the Board. Proposals or recommendations from any department or source in the hospital would be first submitted to the executive council, but the executive council would not have the power to veto any such proposal or recommendation from the Medical Board.

A new medical board was also established, responsible to the Board of Management through the executive council; appointments would be made to the medical board on the recommendation of the Reverend Mother Superior for the time being of the hospital. The membership of the medical board would not exceed thirty and would include the Professors of Medicine and Surgery, nor would there be more than one representative of each of the following departments within the hospital: anaesthetics, gynaecology, pathology, radiology, ophthalmology, otorhinolaryngology. Three representatives of the medical staff would be elected by the Clinical Association.

Members of the medical board would be appointed for three years and would be eligible for re-appointment. The chairman of the medical board would be appointed for three years and would be eligible for re-appointment for one further term of office. The medical board would appoint a secretary who would hold office for two years and be eligible for re-election for one further successive term of office, and would also appoint a registrar who would hold office for not more than three years and would be responsible for the finances of the medical board. The medical board would also establish its own executive council responsible to the medical board consisting of not more than nine of its members of whom the chairman and the secretary would be *ex-officio* members.

The medical board would make recommendations to the Board of Management on medical education, medical policy and development, medical staffing and appointments, interns, house officers, registrars, medical students and financial affairs of the medical staff. There would also be a sub-committee of the medical board to deal with matters relating to medical students and interns.

The first chairman of the Board of Management was the Hon. Mr Justice Brian Walsh, a distinguished judge of the Supreme Court. The first vice-chairman was Mr Denis Crowley, a prominent Dublin businessman.

Innumerable committees were set up to deal with the many aspects of the hospital's work. The consultant staff had to play their part as members of various committees. The medical board had to be represented on the executive council of the hospital, on the Board of Management and on the executive council of the medical board. Many of these committees met weekly. There were also committees to run the out-patients' department, records and the residency. The physicians and surgeons had their own sub-committees of the medical board. There was a committee also to deal with the running of the surgical theatres.

Particularly important was the committee of the medical board to supervise medical education in the hospital. Twice yearly the executive of the medical board met to appoint newly-qualified doctors as interns to the hospital, and also house officers and registrars. This was a difficult task as the number of well-qualified applicants was frequently greater than the number of posts available. It often involved long sessions—sometimes almost all night—the last few places being particularly difficult to fill. All the committee work had to be done in addition to the consultants' routine work in the hospital; it was onerous and time-consuming.

The duties of the chairman and secretary of the medical board were especially arduous. The chairman had to preside at all meetings of the medical board; he/she was *ex-officio* a member of all board sub-committees and represented the views of the medical staff at meetings of the Board of Management. The secretary of the medical board also had to attend the various meetings, keep the records and summon meetings. All officers of the medical board had to be concerned with the difficulties which arose in the daily life of the hospital. One former secretary of the board calculated that on an average morning it would take him about half an hour to get from one end of the main corridor of the hospital to the other, as he was constantly ambushed by his colleagues pouring out their woes to him.

The medical board received great assistance from the medical board secretariat. This was originally organised by Elizabeth Carroll and carried on by Gretta Moore, Mona Farrell and Eimear Couse. The members of the consultant staff shouldered administrative burdens willingly in the interest of the hospital and they were actively helped by their colleagues in the nursing school and administration.

From the 1980s all members of the consultant staff of the hospital were eligible for appointment to the medical board. Those who worked in the hospital were especially appreciative of the many distinguished lay men and women who in the midst of a busy professional or business life found time to sit on the Board of Management and give their expert advice on the many problems facing the hospital.

During this period a new post, indicative of the times, was created in the

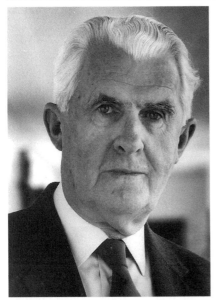

Mr Justice Brian Walsh, first chairman
of the Board of Management, 1973–89

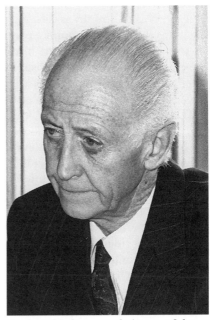

Prof. M. McCormac, chairman of the
Board of Management, 1989

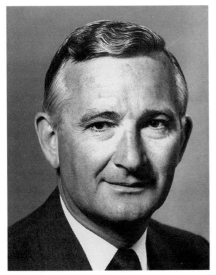

Prof. Noel Whelan, chairman
of the Board of Management,
1991

hospital. It had been quickly realised after the move that big hospitals like St Vincent's were big news. There was an almost insatiable desire among the general public for information on medical matters. News of some new treatment or some wonder drug would bring requests from the press for background material. Some distinguished person might be admitted to the hospital; the press would be on to the hospital in a matter of minutes to find out how the patient was progressing—and sometimes they would be on before the patient was actually admitted. If there was a strike involving essential services the hospital would be bombarded by the media with questions as to how it was carrying on.

It was decided to appoint a press officer and to direct all inquiries to him. It was his duty to acquaint himself with all that was happening in the hospital and to be ready to dispense accurate and up to date information to the media. The press officer realised that, within reason, the general public was entitled to the news of what was happening in one of its big hospitals, but at the same time one must guard against violating a person's confidentiality. F.O.C. Meenan was appointed the first press officer.

By the mid-seventies the number of people working in the hospital was close to eleven hundred, including fifty-four medical consultants and over eighty other medically-qualified personnel: almost five hundred nursing personnel and four hundred and fifty back-up staff, quite apart from the student population in the various teaching departments. The attendance at the out-patients' department increased yearly and in 1975, 51,226 patients attended. Accident and emergency attendances in 1975 numbered 40,206. The total number of admissions in 1975 was 11,985. The following list of specialist services provided in the hospital was like a roll call of modern medicine and an index of the facilities and services that a big modern hospital was required to provide for the population:

general medicine
general surgery
anaesthesia
cardiology
dental surgery
dermatology
endocrinology
gastroenterology
genito-urinary surgery
geriatric medicine
gynaecology
haematology
metabolism and nephrology
neurology and neurosurgery
nuclear medicine
oncology
ophthalmology

orthopaedics
otorhinolaryngology
plastic and facio-maxillary surgery
preventive medicine
psychiatry
respiratory medicine
rheumatology and physical medicine
thoracic surgery
vascular surgery

> In a hospital with students in the wards, the patients are more fully looked after, their diseases more fully studied, and fewer mistakes are made' (Osler). At St Vincent's Hospital, undergraduate teaching is carried out by the clinical staff, who are co-ordinated by the dean of medicine, the Professors of Surgery, Medicine, Experimental Medicine, Therapeutics and Psychiatry. These are assisted by the lecturers and tutors in medicine and surgery. Sixty medical students are accommodated in rotation during their six year training course. During any particular year, 200 students of all years are attending the hospital. Weekly seminars and conferences are held in medicine, surgery and the various specialities. Daily teaching rounds and tutorials are given to smaller numbers of students. Postgraduate teaching has been amplified in the past two or three years by the introduction of the national training scheme of the Royal College of Surgeons in Ireland and the Royal College of Physicians of Ireland in surgery, medicine, anaesthetics, gynaecology, ophthalmology and radiology and other specialities.
>
> There is no need for detailed comment on research. The medical literature down the years and the prominence of our medical staff at scientific meetings both in this country and abroad indicates the St Vincent's contribution. Suffice it to say that active clinical research is being carried on not only by the service medical staff but also by four full-time medical research workers at St Vincent's, in addition to the basic research being carried out in the adjacent departments of experimental medicine and surgery at Woodview, University College Dublin.

The establishment and expansion of so many specialised departments posed the question of how to staff them adequately with appropriately-trained young doctors. Fortunately there was no problem. As in the thirties and forties there was a constant stream of young men and women graduates returning to Ireland after intensive postgraduate studies in centres of excellence abroad, particularly in the UK and the United States. Fully trained, they were ready to bring the latest scientific expertise and knowledge to the service of their speciality. In fact there were so many suitable graduates for each post that it was difficult to make a choice between them. In addition to routine work, active clinical research studies were pursued in all departments.

The obvious catchment area of the hospital was the south city and south county, together with the counties of Wicklow and Wexford. This area provided a large number of patients for the hospital, but of course many others came from outside the Eastern Health Board area.

There were 125 medical beds in the hospital, staffed by D.K. O'Donovan, Oliver FitzGerald, Frank Muldowney, Philip Brennan, James Fennelly, Muiris X. FitzGerald, who was appointed to the staff in 1971, Marian Rice, appointed anaesthetist in the same year, and Andrew Heffernan, who was appointed in 1972. Because of the special interest of the individual physicians there were no general medical beds specifically classified as such, but each medical unit took in its own complement of general medical cases. Most acute and emergency medical cases admitted were therefore dealt with by the various physicians, while special problems were admitted electively under each specialist.

There were 100 general surgical beds staffed by Patrick FitzGerald, T.C.J. O'Connell, J.G. Maher, J.A. Mehigan, J.P. McMullin and T.V. Keaveny, who was appointed to the staff in 1971. In 1974, 2,957 general surgical operations were carried out.

The cardiology department was under the care of Risteard Mulcahy. Four hundred patients with acute coronary disease were treated in the hospital in 1974. Pioneer cardiology work in the fields of rehabilitation and cardiac disease prevention were carried out. Brian Maurer was appointed second cardiologist in 1974. He was a grandson of Denis Kennedy. He also had an appointment with the Federated Dublin Voluntary Hospitals. Close liaison between St Vincent's, the Federated group and the Mater Hospital enhances all aspects of diagnostic cardiology and cardiac surgery. At this period there were twenty beds in the cardiac department.

Dental surgery under Nicholas C. Martin had significantly increased its activity since the transfer of the hospital to Elm Park. This department worked closely with the plastic surgeons.

The dermatology unit under the direction of F.O.C Meenan had expanded considerably since the opening of Elm Park; there were ten beds available for dermatology patients. The out-patients' skin department has grown rapidly over the years and has been a very useful and valuable part of the services of the hospital. Special attention was given in the unit to the association of dermatology with systemic disease.

Professor D.K. O'Donovan had set up a pioneer endocrine unit in the Green in the 1940s. The unit transplanted very successfully to Elm Park and it continued to expand. The bed complement in the unit was twenty-eight, of which ten beds were seconded to Professor O'Donovan as Professor of Medicine. The prime interest of the unit was the study of thyroid disease, diabetes and para-thyroid disease and its related complications. Special emphasis was laid on the liaison between the endocrinological department, the speciality of genito-urinary surgery and the metabolic unit.

216

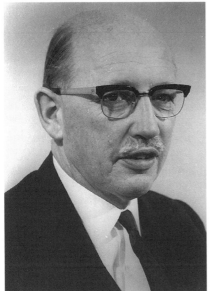

P. FitzGerald, surgeon 1940–78

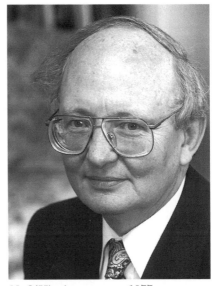

N. O'Higgins, surgeon 1977

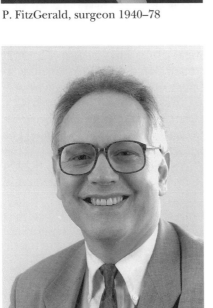

M. X. FitzGerald, physician 1971

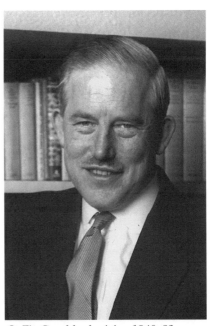

O. FitzGerald, physician 1940–83

Another very important and successful unit was that of gastroenterology which also had operated in the Green. The unit was directed by Professor Oliver FitzGerald who had a special interest in gastroenterology medicine. By 1976 over five thousand endoscopic examinations had been carried out in the theatre. The surgical aspect of the gastroenterological service was run principally by J.A. Mehigan and J.P. McMullin. There was also close liaison between the unit and the research department of experimental medicine of UCD at Woodview.

St Vincent's was one of the first hospitals on these islands to develop the speciality of genito-urinary surgery under the pioneer work of Frank Duff and subsequently Daniel G. Kelly. The unit had a special interest in and carried out much research in uro-dynamic work.

The gynaecological department was particularly active under the directorship of Professor J.K. Feeney. Brendan Murphy and A. Keane, who had associations with the major maternity hospitals, helped to provide a very active service catering for a wide spectrum of gynaecological problems.

There was also a modern and advanced department of metabolism under the direction of Professor Frank Muldowney—another of the departments which had its origins in the Green. The work in this department was of a highly specialised nature and was continuing to expand. Some of the services provided were unique and available only in St Vincent's. Professor Muldowney was in charge of the department of nephrology also. Through this department he worked in close contact with the Meath Hospital in relation to dialysis and other services of nephrology. The department also had close links with the Charitable Infirmary in Jervis Street.

The department of neurology was directed by E.A. Martin who came on the staff in 1971. Martin was also neurologist to the Adelaide Hospital. The two departments worked closely with each other, and also with the department of neurosurgery directed by Fergus Donovan. During 1974 there were 437 neurosurgical admissions, 784 out-patients were seen, and 153 brain operations were performed.

The oncology department under the direction of Dr James J. Fennelly was a unit of twenty beds with a busy out-patient service. The department worked in close association with St Anne's Hospital and St Luke's Hospital. The treatment of malignant disease and leukaemia by chemotherapy was rapidly expanding and promised great developments. A unique and essential facility was the establishment of an isolation unit where patients could be protected from infection when undergoing treatment. The establishment of four new units was indicative of the changes in the social and medical problems of the day.

The department of psychiatry under the direction of Noel Walsh was opened in March 1970. Walsh was appointed Professor of Clinical Psychiatry in UCD. The rapid expansion of this branch of medicine was necessary due to the great increase in psychiatric and psychological problems among the population. A new unit in the hospital to treat twenty-four in-patients and twenty out-patients was at this stage under construction.

An ageing population was posing its own problems and geriatric medicine was becoming an essential department in the spectrum of medical services. A whole-time geriatrician, Denis Keating, was appointed in January 1975. A special geriatric evaluation unit was constructed consisting of twenty-eight beds and facilities for twenty-five day-patients.

A scientific meeting to mark the opening of the psychiatric and geriatric units was held on 2 April 1976. Close on two hundred people including participants from Canada, England and Ireland attended the meeting. The importance of the development of these two units could be gauged from the fact that the opening address was given by Mr Brendan Corish T.D., then Minister for Health.

George Duffy was appointed director of the new department of nuclear medicine in 1970. The Department of Health recognised the need to expand nuclear diagnostic techniques and provided the department with sophisticated but necessary equipment. This department was the first diagnostic nuclear medicine unit in the country outside the cancer hospitals. At this stage the department of nuclear medicine was located on three floors of the hospital with space for growth and expansion urgently needed.

In 1975 there was another significant development in the hospital. The department of preventive medicine was established under Geoffrey Bourke and Noel Hickey. Noel Hickey was responsible for the day-to-day direction. An important role was assigned to this new department. Its function would be to co-ordinate the work of the different departments, to ensure the proper utilisation of limited resources, to commence a scheme of medical audit, to encourage development in preventive medicine and in the fields of continuing care and rehabilitation, to advise about the proper utilisation of drugs and to assist in improving the record system of the hospital.

In the department of ophthalmology Philomena Guinan was joined by John Blake in 1970. The unit had close associations with the Royal Victoria Eye and Ear Hospital. As with other units in the hospital there was considerable referral of patients from outside the south-east catchment area.

In the department of orthopaedics, one of the busiest in the hospital, J.E. Gallagher (appointed in 1959) was joined by J.M. Sheehan (appointed in 1970). The department worked in close association with the joint replacement centre at St Mary's Hospital Cappagh. Sheehan was a pioneer and has gained international fame for his work in joint replacement. The priority of the unit was to expand in the area of joint replacement and for this purpose a clean air theatre was established in the hospital. At this time there were only fifteen beds available for orthopaedics and, in addition to the routine cases, the amount of bone work from trauma coming into the hospital daily placed great strain on the facilities of the department.

In otorhinolaryngology Brian O'Brien and Oliver McCullen were joined

219

by A.R. Dennis in 1972. In addition to the routine work of this busy speciality, sophisticated surgical techniques were available for the surgery of deafness. Associated with the otorhinolaryngology department an audiometry department was established.

Seamus O'Riain (appointed in 1969) conducted a small but very busy department in plastic surgery. With only eight beds available the turnover of cases was very considerable.

The respiratory unit, one of the most important in the hospital, was staffed by Philip Brennan and Muiris X. FitzGerald. There were forty beds available in this department. Plans were nearing completion for a fully-equipped respiratory laboratory which would help to keep up the traditional interest in respiratory medicine which was a feature of St Vincent's.

The department of rheumatology and physical medicine was under the care of Jack Molony. He had a unit of ten beds and worked in association with the nearby St Anthony's Rehabilitation Centre and also with St Joseph's Rehabilitation Centre at Our Lady's Hospice Harold's Cross. St Anthony's Rehabilitation Centre had come under the control of the hospital and was now an integral part of the hospital organisation.

Associated with respiratory medicine was the department of thoracic surgery. It was now hoped to expand this department, by the appointment in 1975 of Keith Shaw who was already consultant cardiac surgeon to the Royal City of Dublin Hospital, and Vincent Lynch who had just been appointed to St Vincent's as chest surgeon.

The department of vascular surgery was a very important unit in the hospital. Work in vascular surgery had been pioneered by Patrick FitzGerald in the 1940s and it was through his energy that a formal vascular surgery unit was established in the hospital before many of the other hospitals in the British Isles. He was responsible for the establishment of the vital link between the surgical department and the specialised radiological angiographic techniques which were an essential basis for vascular surgery. By now there was in Elm Park a unique angiographic theatre within the theatre suite and a blood flow laboratory within the department of surgery. By 1975 Professor FitzGerald and T.V. Keaveny headed a highly-trained vascular team.

The department of pathology consisted of microbiology, histopathology, biochemistry and haematology. In 1971, 328,599 tests were performed in the department of pathology; by 1974, 460,980 examinations were performed. The department of microbiology under P.N. Meenan was working in close liaison with the department of medical microbiology in UCD. Meenan was a pioneer in the development of virology in this country. The histopathology department was extremely busy also. R. Towers and Mary McCabe (appointed in 1974) provided a skilled and prompt service and were always ready and willing to shed light on a difficult diagnostic problem. John J. Dinn provided a specialist service in the histology of neurological tissue. Biochemistry was under the direction of Marian Doolin, a distinguished biochemist. Haematology, under the direction of Liam G. O'Connell, expanded considerably with the opening of the new hospital. He quickly proved the importance of such a department. It became one of the largest haematological departments in these islands. By 1974, routine laboratory tests were running at about 170,000 per annum. These tests included many specialist procedures not performed anywhere else in the country. O'Connell had four beds in this department.

The staff of the radiological department consisted of Dermot Cantwell, J.B. Hourihane (appointed in 1969) and D. MacErlaine (appointed in 1974). The department was divided into three sections:

1) the main department on the first floor of the hospital;
2) the angiographic suite in the theatre;
3) the casualty X-ray department.

Of major importance was the fact that the national school of radiography (diagnostic) was located on the hospital campus. As its name implies the school was and is responsible for the training of diagnostic radiographers in the country.

Besides the school for the training of radiographers, there were other para-medical schools which were associated with the medical school in providing practical training. These were schools of physiotherapy, occupational therapy, speech therapy, dietetics, medical social work and medical laboratory technology.

Summing up the report for 1974–75, the situation of specialisation in medicine in hospitals was clearly set out:

> Specialisation in medicine has occurred either because the equipment for the investigation and treatment of a particular disease is too expensive to be re-duplicated, or because the particular disease is seen too rarely because its incidence in the general population is so small that no one general unit sees enough of it to treat it well, or more usually, the evolution of a speciality is a combination of both. The logical, economical answer is to concentrate sophisticated diagnostic and therapeutic staff and equipment in one hospital, which must be large enough to accommodate the rest of the spectrum of general diseases. For if a specialised unit is separated from the general body of medicine and surgery, its perspective may be lost, its very autonomy proves its own undoing; we already have some examples of this in this country and in the rest of the British Isles . . .
>
> In summary then, we believe that St Vincent's is the natural hub or base hospital for the south-east, by virtue of its situation, its size, its staff and modernity. Its design and the size of its site area facilitates any expansion which may be required . . . The 550 beds at present available in the hospital are quite inadequate to sustain the service which we are presently providing, let alone to allow for any expansion. The matter of our immediate and long-term bed needs has been the

subject of some urgent discussions at Board of Management, Medical Board and executive council level for the past year. It is clear to us that the problem of bed needs must be examined from two points of view: firstly, our immediate bed needs to sustain our present services and to allow for limited expansion, and secondly, our long-term bed needs over the next ten to fifteen years.

Thus within five years of the opening of St Vincent's Hospital Elm Park, the hospital already found itself restricted as regards space for further expansion.

CHAPTER 23

CONSOLIDATION

As in the other departments of the hospital the Mary Aikenhead school of nursing developed rapidly after its move to Elm Park. At the time of the transfer to Elm Park Sr Frances Rose O'Flynn was appointed matron. The high regard in which she was held can be gauged from the award to her of the gold medal of the Institute of Hospital Administrators. Her tenure of the office of matron was to be a short one, as she was elected Mother General of the Congregation of the Irish Sisters of Charity in 1971.

The number of student nurses in training in 1974 was 324, this being the number sanctioned by the Department of Health. So high was the reputation of the school of nursing that demands for training reached a very high level and it became necessary to advertise in the public press that the waiting list was closed for two years. In 1976 the number of nurses who qualified was 102, the success rate in the examination being 98.04 per cent. During this period thirty-four qualified nurses undertook further training in specialised nursing care throughout the hospital: in theatre, accident and emergency department, coronary care and intensive care.

In July 1976 the first four of sixteen nurses from Bahrain came to the hospital to study nursing techniques and work administration. In 1979 the number of students in training was 329. Also in the summer of 1979 a group of nurses from Iraq attended the nursing school to gain medical experience. In the same year student nurse Betty Phelan won the competition in the nurses' year award sponsored by Lucozade.

All during the seventies the stream of new appointments to the consultant staff of the hospital continued. The appointment of Marian Rice in 1972 had strengthened the department of anaesthesia. Michael Moriarty became radiotherapist in 1975. In 1976 James J. Murphy was appointed consultant surgeon and Richard Assaf anaesthetist. 1978 was a particularly fruitful year: Mary Darby took up duty as psychiatrist, Michael Hutchinson as neurologist—he was consultant neurologist to the Adelaide Hospital. Other appointments in 1978: T.J. McKenna endocrinologist, B. Bresnihan rheumatologist, P. Brien radiologist, Geraldine Kelly ophthalmologist, D. O'Donoghue gastroenterologist and C. Pidgeon neurosurgeon. In 1979 F. Brady took up duty as oral surgeon, J.B. Masterson as radiologist, S. Rogers as dermatologist and M. Slazenger as anaesthetist. In 1980 W. Quinlan took up duty as orthopaedic surgeon and M. Fox as vascular surgeon.

The hospital bade farewell to several consultants who had given valuable service to St Vincent's. Denis O'Farrell died in 1974. In October 1975 many members of the hospital staff made a sad pilgrimage to Boherlahan in Co. Tipperary to say farewell to 'Jamsie' Maher, who had died too soon. He had been a friend and counsellor to everyone in the hospital. In 1976 the staff were saddened by the unexpected death of James O'Donnell, anaesthetist, who had been on the staff for only a few months. Not long after this loss, the anaesthetic department suffered a further blow through the death of Peter Tanham. Sister Borgia died in 1977. Patrick FitzGerald, Brian O'Brien and Harold Quinlan all died during 1978.

FitzGerald had retired from the chair of surgery in the hospital in 1976 and Francis A. Duff was appointed acting Professor of Surgery in the hospital. D.K. O'Donovan retired as Professor of Medicine in September 1975 but remained on as acting Professor until his successor was appointed. These retirements left the UCD chairs of medicine and surgery tenable in St Vincent's Hospital vacant. Declan Meagher, after his period of office as Master of the National Maternity Hospital, returned to the staff of the hospital in January 1977.

Niall O'Higgins was appointed Professor of Surgery in St Vincent's Hospital in September 1977 and took up duty in March 1978. He qualified M.B. NUI with first class honours in 1965. He had a distinguished postgraduate career. He was tutor in surgery in University College Dublin, senior registrar and tutor in surgery in the Royal Postgraduate medical school, Hammersmith Hospital London, and senior lecturer in surgery and honorary consultant surgeon, University College Hospital London.

Muiris Xavier FitzGerald was appointed Professor of Medicine in St Vincent's Hospital in 1977. He qualified M.B. NUI with first class honours in 1964. His postgraduate career was distinguished. He was research associate in the department of medicine and therapeutics in UCD and lecturer in medicine in the University of Birmingham. He was awarded a post-doctoral fellowship by the National Institute of Health in the USA and studied in the department of thoracic services at Boston University School of Medicine. He had been appointed to St Vincent's as consultant physician with a special interest in respiratory medicine in 1971.

The administration of such a large organisation as St Vincent's Hospital was becoming a formidable task and required the services of skilled administrators. Sean Fagan was appointed financial controller of the hospital in 1972. A qualified accountant, Sean Fagan began his career in industry. He moved to the Coombe Hospital as an accountant, and later worked in the Institute of Public Administration for five years before taking

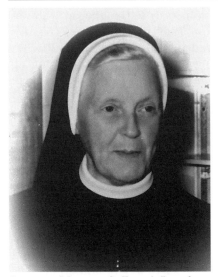

Secretary Manager Sr Francis Joseph
Lang, 1971–81

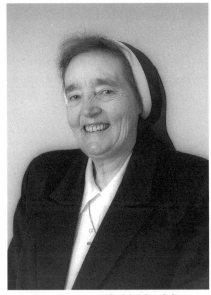

Secretary Manager Sr M. Magdalen
McParlan, 1981–93

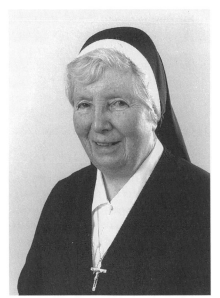

Rev. Mother Sr Joseph Cyril Fortune

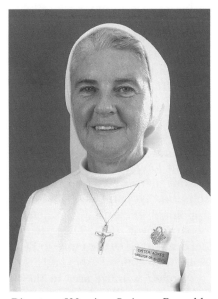

Director of Nursing, Sr Agnes Reynolds

up his position in St Vincent's. He was joined by F. Geoghegan who was purchasing officer in the hospital from 1969 to 1987; Noel Cassidy, personnel officer, who was appointed in 1973; and Kevin Roche, maintenance officer. The cost of running the hospital was also going up each year. In 1975 the total cost was £4,534,000. In 1977 this sum had crept up to £6,257,660. At the end of the decade the annual bill was £9,554,100.

In the old hospital 'the dog house'—as the accident and emergency department was inelegantly called—did not play a major role in the working of the hospital. On account of its location it was not readily accessible to ambulances, and the size of the hospital did not allow it to provide many beds for casualty patients. The situation improved when a new accident and emergency department was created in the new wing on Leeson Lane in 1961, but the relative shortage of beds was still a problem.

All this was to change rapidly after the move to Elm Park. The accident and emergency department was to become one of the most important areas in the hospital. Situated as it was in the southern suburbs of Dublin and near several major roads, an increasing number of ill and injured patients were brought to St Vincent's. An ageing population meant that many elderly people suffering from respiratory and cardiac disease had to be admitted as emergencies to medical wards particularly in the winter months. Excessive speed on the roads meant that the surgical wards had to make constant provision for the victims of road traffic accidents. There was also an unending stream of people requiring treatment for relatively minor conditions. Responding to these many needs meant a department working at full stretch all night and all day. People tend to judge a hospital by the performance of the staff that they first meet—and patients suffering from the effects of sudden illness or injury are not the easiest of people to deal with. Working in the accident and emergency department was becoming particularly onerous.

In 1979 the number of patients attending the department was 55,174. A certain percentage of these were emergencies and required urgent admission to the wards. This meant that vacant beds in the wards were occupied and the admission of patients on the waiting list for non-emergency surgery or investigations was blocked. Thus the waiting lists became longer and longer. In collaboration with the Department of Health various plans were tried but it is fair to say that this problem still awaits solution. To emphasise its increased importance Robert McQuillan was appointed whole-time consultant in charge of the accident and emergency department in 1983. The sisters in charge of the accident and emergency department since the move to Elm Park have been Sister Stephanie Murphy, Sister Conception Foskin and Sister Manus Daly.

Another sensitive area in the hospital was the out-patients' department. An extensive and well-equipped department had been built beside accident and emergency. The department consisted of six consulting rooms with five examination cubicles each, and specialised eye and dental rooms. There

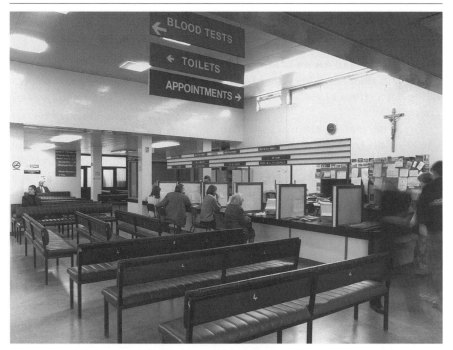

Out-patients' department, 1994

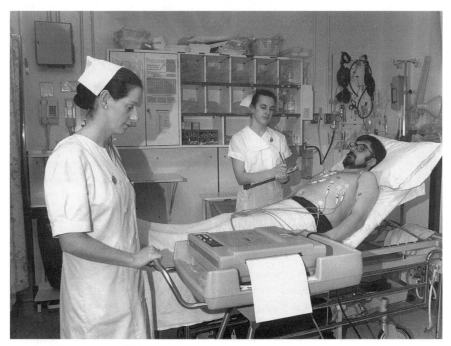

Casualty department, 1994

were two small operating theatres suitable for dealing with minor surgery, seven waiting areas near the consulting rooms and one main waiting area at the reception desk. There was a canteen which was especially useful for patients who had come a long way to be examined, a room for social workers, a dieticians' room and sisters' office and of course facilities for doing the various blood tests so that patients would not have to come back another day.

Over the years there was a swift increase in the number of conditions which could be dealt with on an out-patient basis. This in turn put great pressure on the department and the waiting lists for appointments grew. By 1979 the annual attendance was 57,665; in the same year in an average week there were fifty-two specialist clinics conducted by members of the staff. No matter how good the organisation in an out-patients' department might be, an element of waiting cannot be totally eliminated. In some specialities patients could be seen more rapidly than others. Furthermore the out-patients' department had to be geared so that patients from the country could get all their tests done in the same day. This demanded patience and there were inevitably some complaints—but such complaints were kept to a minimum. The out-patients' department has been under the skilled and tactful direction of the sister-in-charge, Sister Teresa McDermot, for many years.

In the hospital itself, the work in the wards was also increasing. In 1979 there were 17,111 admissions to the wards. In January 1978, a new day-care/five day unit consisting of twelve beds was opened in the hospital. This unit proved to be of enormous benefit to patients who came into hospital for short stay procedures and minor surgery. The day-patients came in for their investigation or procedures and went home again that evening. In a five day unit patients came into hospital at the beginning of the week and then went home the following Friday before the weekend. The unit has been under the efficient care of Sister Nuala Donnelly.

A recital of all the work done in the hospital, the number of attendances at casualty and out-patients', the amount of beds occupied during the year, the increasing numbers of specialist appointments and the rapid expansion of the hospital staff might give the impression that the new St Vincent's was a grim and earnest place to work in and that there was no time for social activities and relaxation. This was far from the truth. The atmosphere in the new hospital might have been earnest but it was by no means grim.

St Vincent's on the Green was a happy place in which to work. The staff were relatively few and specialities and departments were in constant contact with each other. Colleagues were readily available and consultations concerning difficult cases and other hospital problems were easily arranged. Everybody knew what was going on, and at times of crisis there could be immediate contact between community and staff. There was a pleasant custom in the Green that after Mass on a Sunday morning many members of the medical staff would drop into the Medical Boardroom to discuss current affairs and the weekly occurrences in the hospital. It would be fair to say that the staff were like one large happy family giving advice and support to one another when the need arose. There was an unspoken and indeed at times spoken fear that all these activities would cease in the rarefied atmosphere of Elm Park. Another fear was that everybody would be working in their own department with no knowledge of what was going on around them, and that the old Vincent's family spirit would be diluted. Fortunately this did not happen and the old spirit of loyalty to the traditions of the hospital survived the move to Elm Park.

From the beginning there was an active social life in the new hospital. The medical staff settled down quickly in their comfortable boardroom on the front corridor. Surrounded by the portraits and photographs of former members of staff, they continued to meet and discuss the matters of the day. There was another factor which helped to bring them together and which was absent in the Green: the new hospital had a large cafeteria on the ground floor. Members of the staff from the most senior and distinguished of physicians to the most junior lab boy could be seen taking their meals there, often at the same table, no doubt to their mutual benefit. The catering department of the hospital continued under the expert direction of Philip Fletcher.

An important building in the life of the new hospital was the assembly hall. This was constructed in the grounds beside the nurses' home and many major social and professional events took place in it. The building consisted of a large auditorium and stage. The annual prize-giving ceremony was held here. Happily revived in the 1950s by the then Reverend Mother, Mother Canisius, these ceremonies continued to take place annually. An especially noteworthy prize-giving ceremony was that of 1972 when the newly-appointed Archbishop of Dublin, Most Rev. Dr Dermot Ryan—the son of a Vincent's graduate—presided. Bishop James Kavanagh, Bishop Desmond Williams and Bishop Eamon Walsh have been welcome visitors also and have presented the prizes to the medal winners from the nursing school and the medical school.

The annual hospital concert took place at Christmas in the assembly hall and became a regular feature of the social life of the hospital. The amount of hidden talent revealed amongst the hospital staff, the many fine tenor voices and promising pianists and violinists were very impressive. Some of the 'nurses' who appeared on the stage never did or never would belong to any nursing school. Some of the jokes might be a bit 'near the bone' and there would be an accurate and merciless 'take off' of hospital consultants with their little foibles and habits. There was the occasional worry afterwards that they might have gone a little bit too far with this surgeon or that physician. They need not have worried—the consultants who took umbrage were those whose names were not mentioned. It was a matter of prestige to be mentioned in the concert. For a few years the annual hospital dance also took place on the campus, a special marquee being erected beside the assembly hall. These were particularly happy affairs.

A spirit of co-operation between members of the staff is not created by accident and once established it must be maintained. The hospital chaplains have been of great assistance in this respect. We remember especially Father Fox and Father Cloonan of the Holy Ghost Fathers and the Rev. Canon Bertram, Rector of Donnybrook and Sandymount. As well as their vital work on the wards they took a conscious interest in the welfare of all members of the staff. Fr Fox and Fr Cloonan retired in 1978 and were succeeded by Fr O'Brien and Fr Smith. In 1987 the chaplaincy department was formally established. The chaplains then were Fr Tom Cremin O.S.Cam., Fr Brendan Conway O.S.Cam., Canon Bertram, the Rev. Trevor Hipwell; Sister Marie Therese was appointed assistant chaplain and Fr Joe Cahill director of clinical pastoral education.

The old private nursing homes in Leeson Street and Pembroke Street carried on for a few years after the transfer to Elm Park.[1] However, they were now working in isolation from the main hospital and this naturally created enormous difficulties for the running of a modern nursing home. A committee comprising some of the senior members of the medical staff was set up to consider the feasibility of building a private nursing home at Elm Park to cater for the ever-increasing numbers of the population who were members of the VHI. The committee advised Mother General, Mother Frances Rose O'Flynn, that the most practical plan would be to build a new nursing home beside the main hospital. The recommendation of the committee was accepted by Mother General and on 6 June 1972, a wet windy day, Fr Fox turned the first sod for the new nursing home at Elm Park. Due to the efficiency of the architects Robinson Keefe and Devane and the builders John Sisk and Co., the building was completed in less than two years and the new nursing home opened for patients on 1 May 1974. The new building was entirely financed by the Sisters of Charity and remains totally independent of the general hospital.

The original building consisted of 140 beds, mostly four-bedded and five-bedded rooms, and twenty-four single rooms complete with bathrooms. A building project completed in the early eighties added another twenty single rooms, four with individual bathrooms and sixteen with bathrooms shared between two rooms. The completed extension also added much-needed space on three levels, basement, ground floor and first floor. In the basement extension there was a mortuary room, a staff changing room and a coffee shop. There was also a new medical records department and a computer room. On ground level there was a self-contained X-ray department and offices for the financial controller, personnel officer and clerical staff. Also off the ground floor there were consultant clinics where members of the consultant staff of the hospital conducted their private practices. The first floor extension comprised five extra single rooms as did the second, third and fourth floors. On the first floor there was a new twin theatre suite and a procedure room for minor surgery; a new conference room on the same floor was built. The private hospital has also under its roof a physiotherapy department and a pharmacy.

Over the years the work of the private hospital has been intensive and there is a huge turnover of patients, the bed occupancy being almost always 100 per cent. From January 1984 two resident house doctors were appointed to the private hospital.

The new private nursing home may lack the majesty and Georgian splendour of its predecessor in Leeson Street, but it is more efficient and more suitable for the practice of modern medicine. Most of those who worked in the old nursing home made the transition to the new modern nursing home without any difficulty. It was always a source of pleasure to see such stalwarts of 96 as Lil Fleming and Lil Tuohy working happily in the new building. There were many other nurses also who came from 96 in the early days. On the first floor Mary Hoban, on the second floor Maureen Smith, on the third Mary O'Neill and on the fourth Maura Smart. The night sisters in the mid-1980s were Gretta Colbert and Mary Sullivan and the theatre sister was Deirdre Campbell.

The private nursing home is under the efficient care of Sister Baptist Somers. Helping her over the years have been Sister Margaret Cecilia Curley, Sister Rosaleen Foley in charge of nursing administration and pastoral care, Sister Marie Joan McNamara, director of the radiological department, and Sister Joseph Rosario O'Brien, in charge of that most necessary department in any nursing home or hospital, the catering service.

In the 1980s the nursing home installed an MRI scanner (magnetic resonance imaging), a sophisticated X-ray diagnostic machine. In the 1990s the private nursing home was planning the establishment of a comprehensive radiotherapy service. It has also concentrated on a number of specialities for day-care patients. Out of a total of 163 beds, thirteen have been designated for day-care in the areas dealing with gastroenterology, chest investigations, minor surgery, urology and gynaecology, among other specialities. Oncology—chemotherapy treatment—is a very large speciality at both day-care and in-patient levels. In 1993 the private hospital has over two hundred and fifty full-time staff as well as consultants who have practising privileges. There is also a chaplain and a pastoral care worker. The average ward has a ward sister, two junior ward sisters, a team of staff nurses, a porter and a floor secretary.

CHAPTER 24

THE DIFFICULT EIGHTIES

In the 1980s the country as a whole faced another series of financial and economic crises. In simple terms the country was living beyond its means and serious remedies had to be introduced to correct the worsening situation. Retrenchment, cut-backs in government subsidies and grants and higher taxes were the order of the day. The Department of Health was by its very nature a big spender. A substantial amount of the funds allocated to the health services went to finance the general voluntary teaching hospitals. These hospitals were expensive to run and were particularly vulnerable to economic and financial pressures.

The administrators in St Vincent's, as in other hospitals, waged a constant battle to maintain essential standards in the hospital and to provide for the necessary increase in new and expensive medical equipment and also for the employment of trained personnel. The annual reports of the financial controller during these years make for rather gloomy reading. In his report for 1982 he offered a pessimistic forecast which unfortunately proved to be all too true: 'The acceleration of the recession is noticeable particularly in the reducing percentage increases in pay between 1980, 1981 and 1982. It would appear that in the present climate the input of resources to this and other acute hospitals and the health sector in general would be reduced in real terms for some years to come.' The total expenditure for 1981 was £16,072,210.

In the report for 1983 it was stated that: 'The final revenue allocation for 1982 was £16,867,000', and it was pointed out that while this was 9 per cent more than the previous year it was 'below the rate of general inflation of 12.50 per cent recorded in 1982. The total expenditure for 1982 was £17,682,470.' Apart from a new vital form of radiological diagnosis, a CAT scanner (computerised axial tomography), which became operational in 1984, only nominal capital grants had been received towards new and replacement equipment in 1984.

The financial constraints in 1987 resulted in closures of in excess of one hundred and thirty-five beds and a reduction of 130 in staff. The financial difficulties eased slightly in 1988, although it was not possible to open closed beds and the hospital was under severe pressure to meet its commitments to patients seeking its services. In 1989 the hospital strove to live within its financial allocation. It nearly succeeded but at the cost of closing beds in the summer period. By 1990 there was some slight evidence that the harsh financial problems facing the hospital were beginning to ease. The total expenditure for 1989 was £26,598,592. Much credit is due to Mr Sean Fagan, financial controller, and his colleagues for steering the hospital safely through such stormy financial times.

In spite of the clouds on the economic front there was much activity during the 1980s amongst the medical and administrative staff. Several important appointments were made to the staff and on the other side were the inevitable resignations and farewells. Sister Joseph Cyril Fortune was appointed principal nursing officer (formerly matron) in 1980 and Sister Ann Riordan was appointed theatre superintendent. Michael Fox, vascular surgeon, resigned in 1981.

In June 1981 everyone in the hospital was shocked to hear of the sudden and unexpected death of Gussie Mehigan. He was a man of many talents which he used selflessly in the service of his hospital and his colleagues. He was a pioneer in cardio-thoracic surgery and an accomplished administrator. He played a large part in the successful transfer of the hospital from St Stephen's Green to Elm Park, and in the new hospital he contributed much to the organisation and administration of the Medical Board. The enormous number of mourners at his funeral was eloquent testimony to the great respect in which he was held by his colleagues and many friends both inside and outside the profession.

Sister Francis Joseph Lang who held the post of Secretary Manager from 1971 retired in 1981. She did not live long to enjoy her retirement as she died in 1983. Her role was a most difficult and exacting one to perform —she had to deal with all aspects of hospital life and activity. 'She was a woman of the highest integrity and refused to compromise in matters related to truth or justice no matter what pressure was brought to bear on her. Her steadfast trust in God sustained her in all trials and there was about her an air of serenity and calm that nothing could disturb . . . She never imposed on others her expectations of herself. In particular the constancy of her concern and the gentleness of her care for the sick and the old was outstanding.'[1] In any history of St Vincent's Hospital Sister Francis Joseph Lang must have an honoured place. The hospital was happy to welcome as the new Secretary Manager Sister Mary Magdalen McParlan in 1981. A graduate of the nursing school, Sister Magdalen had been administrator in a home for the elderly in Culver City, California.

In 1982 Sister Catherina O'Brien, who was staff nurse and subsequently sister on the staff of the hospital, died. She had spent many years as sister-in-charge of 96. Emma McDonnell died in May 1982. Miss McDonnell was a dedicated member of the staff of St Vincent's Hospital for almost half a

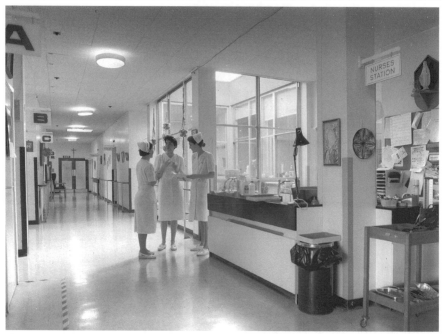

Our Lady's ward

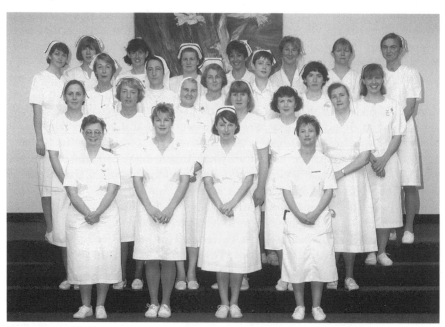

Ward Sisters 1994

century. After being seconded as matron to Clongowes Wood College, Naas for several years she returned to take the position of sister-in-charge of the out-patients' department; six years later that post was combined with the assistant matron's post. She was assistant matron for fifteen years and for two years 1968–70 she held the position of matron in the hospital on the Green.

In 1982 a new oratory was opened on the concourse, where people passing through the hospital could stop for a short period of prayer and recollection. The oratory was dedicated to the memory of the deceased consultants and staff of the hospital.

In 1982 Noel Gibney (radiologist), D. Molyneux (anaesthetist), T. Healy (anaesthetist) and A. Cunningham (anaesthetist) were appointed to the staff and in the same year two former stalwarts of the hospital, Professor John F. Cunningham (gynaecologist) and Frank McLaughlin, the first psychiatrist to the hospital, died.

In 1983 Bob O'Connell, Philomena Guinan, Oliver FitzGerald, Kevin Feeney, Frank Duff, Fergus Donovan and Raymond Davys, staff members who had contributed much to the life and welfare of the hospital, retired. In the same year the hospital welcomed John Hyland (surgeon), and Brian Keogh (nephrologist) to the staff. Richard Nolan died after a short illness in the same year.

Another group of highly-qualified consultants were added to the staff in 1984. They were G. Dorrian (anaesthetist), P. Barry (ophthalmologist), J. Hegarty (gastroenterologist), A. Owens (radiologist), A. Heaney (urologist), J. Griffin (radiologist), N. Duignan (gynaecologist), W. McNicholas (physician in respiratory medicine) and D. Mehigan (vascular surgeon) who was also appointed to St Michael's Hospital.

During these years that most necessary of services in a teaching hospital, the library service, continued to expand rapidly under the direction of Hylda Beckett. Mrs Hylda J. Beckett M.A., Dip.Ed., Dip.L.I.S., A.L.A.I. was appointed Librarian to St Vincent's Hospital in July 1980. She was the first professional medical librarian to hold such a post. She was instrumental in setting up and organising the medical library, making it a model for other hospitals. She was also a founding member of the health sciences libraries section of the Library Association of Ireland. She was awarded the A.L.A.I. for her work in the medical library of St Vincent's Hospital. In spite of constriction in space and staff she continued to provide a first class service for all members of the staff. There were constant requests for manual searches for which the Cumulated Index Medicus was invaluable. Computer searches in the literature were also carried out in increasing numbers. Finance for the library caused a certain amount of anxiety—donations to it from firms and drug companies had fallen off dramatically. Many members of the staff contributed text books and specialist medical journals.

The approach of the year 1984 conjured up different sentiments in different people. It reminded many of the dire events foretold by George Orwell in his famous novel *Nineteen eighty-four*. Many were relieved when

1984 passed without anything too untoward or drastic happening. For staff of St Vincent's Hospital 1984 had much more pleasant connotations. It was the year in which the hospital celebrated the one-hundred-and-fiftieth anniversary of its foundation. This anniversary was officially described as the sesquicentenary of St Vincent's Hospital. It also had further significance as it was the first major anniversary of the hospital to be celebrated at Elm Park. It was therefore an event of special importance in the life of the hospital. In a message for the hospital's sesquicentenary booklet the Archbishop of Dublin, Dr Dermot Ryan, stated:

> The celebration of the sesquicentenary of St Vincent's Hospital gives us an opportunity to inform ourselves of the achievements of the Irish Sisters of Charity, to be proud of them, to support them and to imitate them. St Vincent's Hospital in spite of its size represents but a fraction of the apostolates and institutions in Ireland and abroad which owe their origin to the Irish Sisters of Charity and continue to flourish under their inspiring care.

A special committee was set up under the chairmanship of Professor Oliver FitzGerald to organise the celebrations. The opening celebration took place on Sunday 22 January 1984 with a Mass of thanksgiving in the hospital chapel. Archbishop Ryan was the principal celebrant. Concelebrants included priests associated with the Sisters of Charity and former hospital chaplains. The hospital was honoured by the presence of the President of Ireland, Dr Patrick Hillery, the Minister for Health, Mr Barry Desmond, and many distinguished representatives of Church, State, university and medical bodies.

Mass was followed by a formal lunch in the hospital presided over by Mr Justice Brian Walsh, chairman of the Board of Management. Speeches were made by the Minister for Health, the chairman of the Medical Board, Mr J. McMullin, and Mother Francis Ignatius, Mother General. That evening a celebrity concert 'An Evening of the Stars' was held in the National Concert Hall to celebrate the achievements of the hospital. Taking part were Geraldine O'Grady, Bernadette Greevy, Maureen Potter, Frank Patterson and Joan Merrigan; also the RTE Symphony Orchestra and Our Lady's Choral Society. Compères were Des Keogh and Charles Mitchell and the producer was Fred O'Donovan. On 4 February a very special function was held in the hospital, where former members of the staff from the Green were invited to lunch. Many old friendships were renewed and happy memories of the old hospital revived.

During the period 17 May to 19 May a well-attended scientific programme was organised. It was opened by An Taoiseach Dr Garret FitzGerald. Recent advances in medicine and surgery were discussed in a series of presentations. The final session was taken up by a symposium on the future of nursing. Twenty-minute communications detailing current research in the hospital were also presented. J.J. Fennelly was chairman of the scientific exhibition committee which organised the symposium. He was ably helped by Mary Monaghan, secretary of the postgraduate department. Associated with the scientific exhibition a historical programme was arranged by F.O.C. Meenan, depicting life in the hospital over the previous 150 years.

A formal sesquicentenary banquet was held in the Shelbourne Hotel on 18 May. Mrs Gemma Hussey, Minister for Education proposed the health of the hospital. Professor M.X. FitzGerald, Professor N. O'Higgins, Mr T.C.J. O'Connell and Professor Courtney Bartholomew, a distinguished graduate of the hospital, replied to the toast. There were also many sporting fixtures during the week, including a very successful night at the races in the Phoenix Park arranged by Dr Tony Healy. Other sporting events included a week of sports at St Michael's College, Ailesbury Road and a well-attended golf outing in Elm Park.

A specially happy and successful function was a garden party for the present and past graduates of the nursing school. Many nurses travelled long distances to be present. Another notable event during the year was when a 26p stamp with a picture of Mother Mary Aikenhead was issued by An Post to celebrate the sesquicentenary. The stamp was formally presented to the hospital by the Minister for Posts and Telegraphs, Mr Jim Mitchell.

The National University of Ireland honoured the achievements of the hospital by conferring the honorary degree of Doctor of Laws on Mother Canisius O'Keeffe, a distinguished former Reverend Mother of the hospital. The Fellowship in Nursing, Faculty of Nursing, Royal College of Surgeons in Ireland was conferred on Sister Pauline Campbell, Sister Marie John Sexton, Miss Josephine Bartley, Sister Joseph Cyril Fortune, Sister Margaret Vincent Dockery, Miss Geraldine McSweeney, Sister M. Canisius O'Keeffe and Miss Petronilla Martin.

In 1985 Bob O'Connell, Kevin Feeney and Sister Mary Conception Foskin died. All of them in their various ways had given generously to the welfare and development of the hospital. P. Brennan, N. Martin and K. Shaw retired during the same year. Marian Rice retired in 1986. Appointed to the staff in 1985 were Ann O'Brien histopathologist to St Vincent's and also to St Michael's, D.A. Luke cardio-thoracic surgeon, John F. Murphy gynaecologist, J.F. Keane anaesthetist and B. Ferris anaesthetist. In 1987 Risteard Mulcahy retired from the department of cardiology where he did much pioneer work in the prevention of heart disease.

The second half of the 1980s saw no slackening in the pace of change and in the arrival of new talent to the hospital. Peter Lenehan was appointed gynaecologist and Oscar Traynor surgeon in 1987. Oliver FitzGerald died in the same year. Mr Justice Brian Walsh resigned from his position as chairman of the Board of Management in December 1988. He was succeeded by Professor Michael McCormac, former Professor of Business Administration and dean of the faculty of commerce at University

College Dublin. The department of anaesthesia was particularly active during these years and was greatly strengthened by the appointment in 1989 of Edward Gallagher, Niall McDonald, Kevin Keating, Declan O'Keeffe and Vincent Hannon. Considerable new facilities were required for the intensive care unit which was under the direction of G. Dorrian. David Quinlan was appointed consultant in urology, and Kieran O'Rourke and Eamon Kelly consultants in orthopaedics. Peter Quigley became consultant cardiologist. There was also a major development in pain control and palliative care with the collaboration of the department of anaesthesia and Our Lady's Hospice in Harold's Cross. Michael Kearney joined the staff as consultant in palliative medicine and Lynda Fenelon was appointed clinical microbiologist to the hospital.

St Vincent's was disappointed when during 1989 the Department of Health decided to re-locate neurosurgery at Beaumont Hospital. The hospital owes a great debt of gratitude to Fergus Donovan, Christopher Pidgeon and the neurologists Edward A. Martin and Michael Hutchinson for their pioneer work in the speciality. The Department of Health agreed that certain speciality areas would be developed in St Vincent's Hospital, particularly cardiology, oncology and liver transplantation.

In spite of difficulties the various departments which go to make up the essential framework of the hospital continued to work in a highly efficient manner. Pharmacy continued to play its vital role. Mary Fitzpatrick who had been chief pharmacist since the move out to Elm Park retired at the end of 1987, her successor being Mrs June O'Shea. The increase in the price of drugs had been a major factor in the accelerating cost of running the hospital, and it required constant vigilance on the part of the pharmacist and the members of the medical staff to keep drug expenditure down to a minimum.

The department of nutrition and dietetics under June Ruigrok dealt successfully with the increasing calls on its expertise and skill. The medical social work department continued to be one of the most essential departments in the hospital under the senior medical social worker, Miss K. Hennigan. The goal of the department was the timely and effective re-integration of the patient into the community following a stay in hospital. Modern social trends tended to make the work of the medical social department increasingly complex. Another important commitment of this department was the training of student medical social workers in association with University College Dublin and Trinity College.

The department of physiotherapy was very active. It had been highly organised on the Green by successive physiotherapists: Dan Moloney, Helen Lowry, Gerry Brereton, Bertha Howard and Joy O'Farrell. Joy O'Farrell started the department in Elm Park and enhanced its already high reputation. She was succeeded by Bridie Barrett. The present senior physiotherapist is Pauline Leahy.

The department of speech therapy worked in close collaboration with the ear nose and throat surgeons.

The medical records department, without whose constant skill and care no department could function adequately, was under the direction of Tricia McDonagh. The latter part of 1989 was spent in preparing for the computerisation of the admissions department. The main benefit to the hospital and the medical records department was the availability of more detailed information on admissions—necessary for planning and reporting purposes.

St Anthony's rehabilitation centre under the direction of Jack Molony and Barry Bresnihan continued its active course in spite of financial cut-backs. Oliver FitzGerald (junior) joined the staff as rheumatologist in 1990. Football injuries were a speciality of the department—both Bresnihan and Molony had represented Ireland in rugby football. A feature in St Anthony's has been the juvenile arthritis clinic conducted by Dr Bresnihan; it provides a unique service of its kind in Ireland.

The department of occupational therapy also passed through difficult times. 'The object of occupational therapy is to bring back to normal the persons whose occupational performance has been impaired by illness or injury, emotional disorders, development disorders, social disadvantages or the ageing process.' The department has been working in close co-operation with St Anthony's rehabilitation centre. The department co-operated with Trinity College Dublin in its course for occupational therapy and it plays a role in training students of occupational therapy.

It is difficult to mention and pay just tribute to all the various departments and committees who labour to make St Vincent's an efficient unit. So many committees were established that it is impossible to mention them all or to give adequate recognition for their contribution to the life of the hospital. However, there is one small committee which surely merits special attention. Judging from its name one would be pardoned for thinking that the lands on which the new hospital was built were richly endowed with elm and other trees. Nothing could be further from the truth, for the ground between the various buildings and the hospital complex was bleak and infertile. To improve the appearance and increase the amenities a landscaping committee was established under the chairmanship of Mr Arthur Ganly, a member of the Board of Management. The committee also received considerable help from Risteard Mulcahy.

A tree-planting programme as well as the planting of flower beds and the paving of unsightly areas was organised in the early 1970s. A number of trees and shrubs were ordered and planted under the direction of Risteard Mulcahy. In the autumn of 1978 the landscaping programme was reviewed and about twenty-five new trees were planted. Some of these were to replace young trees which had failed to thrive. These were planted as additions along the Merrion Road front or amongst the old trees on the right hand side of the carriageway leading from the Merrion Road entrance. The old trees to the right of the Merrion Road entrance were beginning to fail but it was hoped that young beech, oak and chestnut trees set amongst the old trees would grow quickly to replace them.

Attention was paid to the mature trees between the south façade of the hospital and the Elm Park golf course which are a very considerable amenity. Some of these had been damaged by crows; an anti-crow campaign was organised but according to the report of the landscape committee it was relatively unsuccessful. The programme was reviewed in 1982. Some new trees were planted, many to replace previous plantings which had succumbed to drought and to the generally hostile environment created by the poor soil and a lack of day-to-day attention. The losses through drought occurred during the summers of 1981 and 1982. A plantation between the hospital cafeteria and the nursing home parking lot was completed: five silver birch, five variegated maples, four wild crab and four oak trees had been planted but some were lost. Mr Ganly and Dr Mulcahy received much help and co-operation from the head porter Larry Quinn and from Val Brady, Alistair Roche and Mr Hickey of the maintenance department. It will take many years before the labours of the landscaping committee produce fruitful results.

It is to be hoped that the pioneer work of the landscaping committee will be carried on by other members of the staff and that future generations will work in green and pleasant surroundings.

In a hospital above all other places it is important to welcome patients and visitors in an agreeable and courteous manner. This was achieved by Michael Hanly, who retired in 1972 after many years service as hall porter. He was well known to generations of medical students and nurses in the hospital on the Green. Larry Quinn continued to maintain the same tradition in the possibly more austere surroundings of Elm Park. He in turn has worthy successors in Paddy O'Neill and John O'Grady and Eddie Griffin, who keep the communications open between the hospitals.

CHAPTER 25

TOWARDS THE MILLENNIUM

A s the eighties sped on and merged with the nineties many new projects matured. Indeed there were so many exciting developments in the hospital that it was difficult for the historian to keep pace with all its activities. Situated as it was in the south of Dublin, and drawing the majority of its patients from the south-east, the hospital had several sister hospitals in close proximity. Over the years St Vincent's and the other hospitals in the area have developed a close relationship, particularly in the areas of joint appointments.

St Vincent's has joint appointments with St Columcille's Hospital Loughlinstown. In geriatrics, they are Denis Keating and Morgan Crowe (who was appointed geriatrician to St Vincent's in 1988). Other joint appointments are John Hyland in general surgery, Kieran O'Rourke and Eamon Kelly in orthopaedics and Niamh Nolan in pathology. Joint appointments with St Michael's Hospital Dun Laoghaire are W. Quinlan in orthopaedics, Ann O'Brien in pathology and Denis Mehigan in vascular surgery. There are also many areas of co-operation with St Luke's/St Anne's Hospital, the Skin and Cancer Hospital Hume Street and the National Maternity Hospital.

A particularly useful relationship has grown up between the hospital and the Royal Hospital in Donnybrook. This is basically due to the fact that in the area of south-east Dublin there is a very large percentage of the population who are over sixty-five years of age and make special demands on the health services. In 1983 a meeting took place between representatives of St Vincent's, the Royal Hospital and the Eastern Health Board to devise a suitable scheme of collaboration. A plan was drawn up defining the role of both hospitals. The acute assessment geriatric unit in St Vincent's would have access to long stay beds in the Royal Hospital; on the other hand the Royal Hospital would have access to beds in St Vincent's for acute medical and surgical emergencies. The Royal Hospital would be given an increased complement of junior hospital doctors from St Vincent's. Also the various rehabilitation units so necessary in the treatment of the elderly patient, such as physiotherapy and speech therapy, would be available to the Royal Hospital. Equally important, by the terms of the agreement the Royal Hospital was to maintain its independence and autonomy. This scheme has been working extremely well to the benefit of patients in both hospitals. The scheme started in 1987.[1]

In 1985 without warning the Department of Health announced a scheme by which the otorhinolaryngological services of the Royal Victoria Eye and Ear Hospital would be transferred to St James's Hospital; and the ophthalmological services to St Vincent's Hospital.[2] Representatives of the Royal Victoria Hospital, with whom the hospital has had a happy relationship over many years, and representatives of St Vincent's had discussions on the proposal. They concluded that if the eye department was to be transferred to the Elm Park site new buildings would have to be provided. At this time money to fund the buildings was simply not available. The matter still rests.

In 1992 a full-time post of consultant intensivist was established in the hospital. The function of the consultant intensivist is to give dedicated and exclusive care to patients with critical care illness. Dr Kieran Crowley was appointed to the post which was unique in St Vincent's Hospital and indeed in intensive care in Ireland.

Another development in the early nineties has been the expansion of the department of oncology and cancer services. This department is under the care of Professor James Fennelly who is the first person to occupy a chair of medical oncology in Ireland—at University College Dublin. The department works in close co-operation with the palliative and terminal care services located in Our Lady's Hospice Harold's Cross. John Crown from the Sloan Kettering Cancer Institute New York has been appointed oncologist in St Vincent's.

Three members of the staff who had given most valuable service to the hospital retired. P.N. Meenan (first chairman of the Medical Board in Elm Park) and J. Molony retired in 1989. E.A. Martin (neurologist) also retired. He was also a distinguished medical historian and had made many significant contributions to the history of medicine in Ireland. Marion Doolin had given much skill and valuable service to the hospital and her death in October 1992 was a cause of grief amongst all her colleagues on the staff. Professor M. McCormac resigned as chairman of the Board of Management in September 1991 and was succeeded by Professor N. Whelan, Vice-President of the University of Limerick.

T. Joseph McKenna writes about education and research in St Vincent's:

When the plans for the development of a new St Vincent's Hospital on the Elm Park site were developed in the 1950s there was little appreciation of the need for specialised educational and research facilities. However, by the time the building was finally commissioned it was apparent that major deficiencies existed in this area.

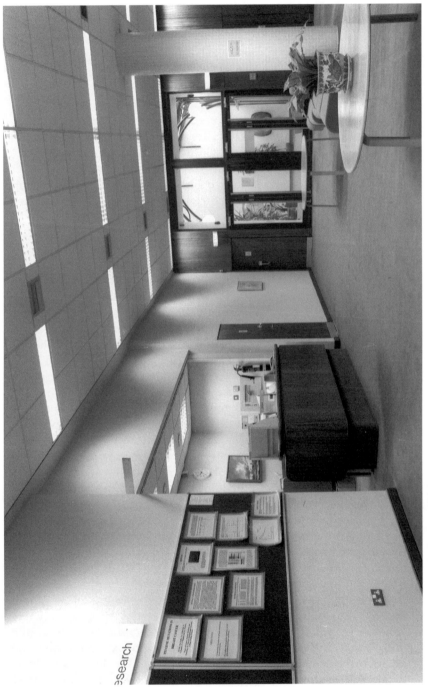

Education and Research Centre, 1994

Representations were made to the hospital administration and to the Sisters of Charity, by the consultant staff, to undertake a development which would repair these deficiencies. The Sisters of Charity recognised that in order to maintain St Vincent's Hospital's standing as a creditable teaching hospital, improved research and education facilities were necessary. Initially, discussion focused on the need for laboratories and medical research space. Subsequently the new development was seen as providing an opportunity to improve other components in the broad area of education and research. Thus the final plan for the Education and Research Centre included a lecture hall with a seating capacity of 200, a seminar room with a seating capacity of fifty and a conference room with capacity approximately twenty-five. In addition, plans were agreed for a greatly expanded and improved medical library to be re-located in the Education and Research Centre.

The centre was to be located on the south side of the existing hospital complex between what used to be known as the students' hostel and the golf course. Access to the centre would be by way of a new entrance between the two-storey pathology and teaching building and the reading room, through what used to be a kitchen and thence under a new 'covered way' through the courtyard which at this time contained the lecture theatre. It was planned that the new centre would be built in two stages: stage one, east block containing library, graphics, seminar room and laboratories and stage two west block containing lecture theatre. Considerable emphasis was to be placed upon flexibility of use, pleasing environment and comfort. The financial projection for the complete building and site works was £2,700,000. It was planned that the building would be completed in March 1988. On 11 November 1987 the laying of the corner stone of the Education and Research Centre was performed by the President of Ireland Dr Patrick Hillery. The Education and Research Centre was completed in 1989 and the building was handed over to the hospital authorities early in February 1989. The official blessing and opening of the building took place on 26 May 1989.

Gradually a number of departments transferred to the centre from the hospital, such as the postgraduate department, the library and medical professorial staff, the development and fund-raising office and finally the department of preventive medicine, and one laboratory floor was equipped. It had been hoped that University College Dublin department of medicine and department of surgery research laboratories would be moved from the university site to the Education and Research Centre. With this in mind approximately twice the laboratory space initially planned was approved for the final building. As a result of this the third floor laboratories were not immediately assigned, with the exception of that area designed for the department of epidemiology under the direction of Noel Hickey. It was on the second floor that the initial research projects approved for the Education and Research Centre were activated.

The first floor of the centre houses the library which is supported by a subvention from University College Dublin and this floor also is the location for the offices of the department of medicine and department of surgery. The ground floor is the location for the lecture hall, seminar room and conference room. The department of postgraduate medicine is also sited at this level.

Around 1990 the decision was taken in University College Dublin not to transfer activities of the professorial laboratories to the centre.

While the activities within the Education and Research Centre contributed immensely to the academic well-being of the hospital and thus to patient care, a significant economic impact was also appreciated. The Sisters of Charity had not only great foresight in meeting a need which would not be met at the time by the Department of Health or the Department of Education; the order also had great courage in underwriting the entire project. The plan was that privately-generated funding would repay the financial commitment made by the sisters.

Initial fund-raising under the effective direction of Mrs Margaret Heffernan was highly successful and provided support for the belief that payment for the centre would be completed over a relatively short period. However, the second half of the 1980s proved more resistant to the fund-raising forces. By the early 1990s it became clear that a funding crisis existed. A debt for the original building and furnishing costs of £1.2 million existed, on which considerable annual interest accrued. To this could be added the ongoing running costs.

Among the strategies employed to meet the debts on the centre it was agreed to locate the immunology and bacteriology laboratories of St Vincent's Hospital on the third floor of the Education and Research Centre. In recognition of this move the Department of Health took over responsibility for the five salaried members of staff who previously had been on the payroll of the Education and Research Centre Trust. In addition, University College Dublin initiated an annual grant to the Education and Research Centre. In recognition of the services provided, including housing several activities previously conducted in the hospital proper, St Vincent's Hospital assumed the responsibility to make an ongoing contribution. However, at the time of writing the funding of the Education and Research Centre continues to pose a major problem.

It is hoped that when the financial problems of the centre have been solved it will play a major part in the future development of St Vincent's Hospital. When it becomes a fully-integrated part of the hospital, the wisdom of taking the bold step to support the building and equipping of the centre will be recognised to the immense credit of the Sisters of Charity.[3]

According to the chairman of the Medical Board: by 1993 the Education and Research Centre has become the centre point of the scientific and intellectual life of the hospital.[4] T.J. McKenna, the first director, has been succeeded by Barry Bresnihan. There are indications that the financial problems are easing. A considerable debt of gratitude is owed to Dr McKenna for initiating such a major contribution to the work of the hospital.

It is not to be suggested that all medical research requires expensive facilities and funding, as judging from a report by John Blake of the department of ophthalmology:

> Front seat car occupants have always been at risk of serious injury to face and eyes, often resulting in blindness, from shattering of toughened glass windscreens. With the enactment of seat belt legislation in Ireland (1979) some amelioration was expected; in the event, this law was so poorly complied with that it effected no change in the high incidence of eye perforation.
>
> We therefore published the result of a twenty-year study of eye injuries on the roads (including a national survey), and submitted these findings to the government. We then campaigned to secure legislation in favour of high penetration resistant laminated windscreens, which protect the individual from both eye and general injuries. In time, appropriate legislation was passed through the Dáil making these windscreens mandatory in all new cars from 1 January 1986. Since then, against a background of a rising trend in the number of deaths and general casualties on the roads, there has been a dramatic fall by 77 per cent in the number of eye perforations from traffic accidents seen at the Eye and Ear Hospital and St Vincent's Hospital, Dublin.

During this period a major development in the department of surgery was the establishment of the liver transplant programme in the hospital. Some years earlier St Vincent's, in association with Our Lady's Hospital for Sick Children Crumlin, had been designated the national liver transplant centre. Funding for such a programme was made available during the previous three years and the Department of Health made arrangements for specialised training of staff at King's College Hospital London. Intensive training of medical staff was undertaken there. Surgeons, hepatologists and anaesthetists spent time with the liver unit at King's College and members of the nursing staff spent periods of up to six months in London. Medical staff from other disciplines and also members of the paramedical disciplines spent varying lengths of time in London.

246

A broad range of medical nursing and laboratory expertise was available now to St Vincent's. Gerry McEntee was appointed surgeon and in association with Oscar Traynor provided the consultant surgical service to the transplant programme. John Boylan, who has a special expertise in liver transplant anaesthesia care, was appointed to the unit. John Hegarty provided the back-up medical skill for the unit. During 1992 the new purpose-designed liver unit in St Brigid's ward was commissioned, and received its first patients in November 1992. This is an eleven bed medical and surgical unit which includes two high dependency beds with facilities for full ventilation of patients with liver disease. By 1993 the unit could report 'a very high rate of success in its programme'.[5]

The nursing school was no less active than the medical school. In June 1992 the Mary Aikenhead school of nursing organised a seminar on the evolution of nursing to celebrate the centenary of the foundation of the nursing school. The seminar was opened by Sister Agnes Reynolds, director of nursing. The first session was devoted to the history of nursing in St Vincent's Hospital, with contributions from Pauline Doyle, deputy director of nursing, and Loreto Browne, nurse tutor. The theme of the second session was specialities in nursing and the chairperson was Geraldine McSweeney, nurse tutor. In the third session the future of nurse education was discussed, the principal speaker being Judith Chavasse, director of nursing in University College Dublin.

A magnificent exhibition of historical photographs vividly depicting the history of nursing in the hospital over the last one hundred years was put on display in the nurses' home. On the social side there was a very successful garden party which many present and former members of the nursing staff of the hospital attended. In 1993, the school of nursing continued to shed lustre on the hospital. Geraldine McSweeney was elected national president of the Irish Guild of Catholic Nurses. Maureen Ashe, nurse tutor, retired from the school in the same year. She made history by being the first member of the nursing school to deliver the address at the prize-giving ceremony. Her paper, 'Forty-Five Years in Nursing: Some Reflections', was received with much interest.

In the latter part of 1993 the hospital lost two of its most respected and valuable members. Sister Marie John Sexton spent most of her professional life as a ward sister in the hospital and was devoted to its service. The death of Noel Hickey was keenly felt in all departments in the hospital. In his speciality of preventive medicine he contributed much to all aspects of hospital affairs. On a personal note he was a wise and loyal friend. Professor Frank Lavery who also died during the year had built up a very efficient ophthalmological department in the hospital.

In 1984 the hospital welcomed as one of its chaplains Fr Ambrose O'Farrell O.P., a member of a family who played an important role in the development of the hospital.

The chaplaincy continued its work for the spiritual care of the patients in the hospital. Fr Ciaran O'Mathuna was transferred from St Vincent's to Blanchardstown Hospital in July and Fr William King was appointed in his place. The full chaplaincy team is Fr Donal Sullivan, Fr Joseph Cahill, Fr Matthew Gaffney, Fr William King, Sister Marie Therese Claire and Rev. Canon Richard Bertram (Church of Ireland).

Sister M. Magdalen retired from the post of Secretary Manager in April 1993 after more than ten years of service to St Vincent's. Her period of office was particularly arduous as it coincided with recurrent financial crises and difficulties. In spite of the many problems that she had to deal with on a daily basis, her office door was always open to members of the staff seeking advice and encouragement. Mr Nicholas Jermyn was appointed Chief Executive Officer of the hospital in 1994.

In the early nineties the hospital was working to full capacity. There was an ever-increasing demand on its services. Apart from carrying out their routine duties many consultants were engaged in their own medical specialist interests and research. This was becoming more and more difficult as facilities were not matching requirements. Apart from the liver unit the department of surgery under the direction of Niall O'Higgins had a special interest in breast cancer. John Hyland, Oscar Traynor and James Murphy had particular expertise in gastroenterological surgery. In vascular surgery T.V. Keaveny and Denis Mehigan continued their research. William Quinlan and Brian Hurson travelled widely and attended many meetings in the field of orthopaedic surgery.

Peter Lenehan, Niall Duignan and John F. Murphy organised a meeting of the British Society for Colposcopy and Cervical Pathology in Dublin in April 1992. In the department of urology 1992 was a progressive year for Daniel Kelly and David Quinlan and it was marked by the introduction of the laser to urology. The number of patients attending the plastic surgery department continued to increase and Seamus O'Riain had a very busy year, helped by Michael Early who has now left to take up an appointment in another Dublin hospital. The department of anaesthesia in addition to its normal duties was expanding pain services in the hospital. The appointment in 1992 of Kieran Crowley as an intensivist working in the intensive care unit has already been noted. As well as his many other commitments in the hospital, especially as director of the Education and Research Centre, T.J. McKenna, assisted by his colleague M.J. McKenna, who was appointed in 1992, was in charge of the department of endocrinology and diabetes mellitus. Valuable publications came from the department and its work was featured in medical journals throughout the world.

Many advances in the treatment of renal disease have come from the department of renal and metabolic medicine under the direction of F.P. Muldowney. In association with the liver unit, gastroenterology continues to be extremely busy and the number of patients presenting for special investigations is continually rising. In 1992 D.P. O'Donoghue and his colleague in the gastroenterology unit presented fifteen papers at

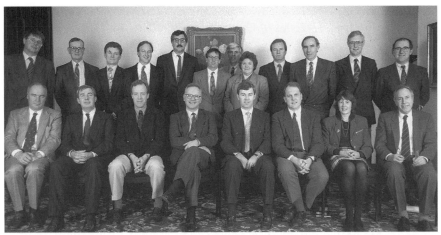

Consultant medical staff, 1994. (Back row, left to right) Dr T. McDonnell, Prof. G. Bourke, Dr D. O'Donoghue, Dr A. Watson, Dr J. Crown, Dr M. McKenna, Dr M. Hutchinson, Dr S. Rogers, Dr J. Hegarty, Prof. T.J. McKenna, Dr M. Crowe, Dr P. Quigley; (front row, left to right) Dr B. Maurer, Prof. B. Keogh, Prof. B. Bresnihan, Prof. M.X. FitzGerald, Dr W. McNicholas, Dr O. FitzGerald, Dr L. Fenelon, Dr. D. Keating

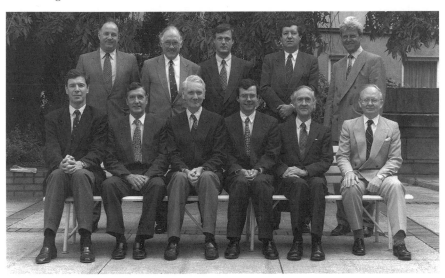

Consultant surgical staff, 1994. (Back row, left to right) Mr W.R. Quinlan, Dr J. Murphy, Mr O. Traynor, Mr J. Hyland, Mr P. Barry; (front row, left to right) Mr D. Quinlan, Mr T.V. Keaveny, Mr V. Lynch, Mr E. McDermott, Mr J. Blake, Prof. N. O'Higgins

international and national meetings including the American, British, European and Irish Societies of Gastroenterology. Dermot O'Donoghue has also been a highly active and successful director of the postgraduate education department in the hospital.

Cardiology under the direction of Brian Maurer and Peter Quigley maintained its high reputation. A new investigative laboratory was opened and patients no longer had to be transferred from St Vincent's Hospital to another institution for a full range of cardiac services. The departments of cardiology, preventive medicine, physiotherapy and dietetics co-operated to produce a comprehensive rehabilitation programme for patients who had sustained myocardial infarction and were undergoing cardiac surgery.

Janice Redmond was appointed consultant neurologist to St James's Hospital with sessions also in St Vincent's. She has a particular interest in neuromuscular disorders. Michael Hutchinson has continued to publish the fruits of his neurological research in major medical journals. In the department of respiratory medicine Walter McNicholas is carrying out major research into the problems of sleep and has a unique department in the shape of a respiratory sleep laboratory. In addition to his considerable administrative duties Professor M.X. FitzGerald has a particular interest and skill in thoracic medicine, especially in the problems of cystic fibrosis and sarcoidosis.

The department of psychiatry under the direction of Noel Walsh and Mary Darby runs an active programme on the problems of stress and also has developed a specialised biofeedback clinic. The rheumatology department under Barry Bresnihan and Oliver FitzGerald is one of the busiest departments in the hospital. The juvenile arthritis clinic has already been mentioned, and the department has also initiated research programmes with the departments of orthopaedics and dermatology. Barry Bresnihan has been appointed to a chair of rheumatology established by UCD in 1991.

The department of medical oncology under the direction of James Fennelly located in St Anne's ward has been referred to. In addition to its work in the hospital this department has links with the Children's Hospital Temple Street and special studies are in progress on child leukaemia. The department of dermatology under the direction of F.O.C. Meenan and S. Rogers has continued to publish a series of valuable papers on many aspects of diseases of the skin. The department is taking part in a multi-centre European study on psoriasis.

There has also been necessary expansion in the field of pathology. Medical microbiology and immunology have moved to new quarters in the research centre, and haematology and histopathology have taken over the space vacated in the main hospital. In the haematology department Liam O'Connell has been joined by Donal McCarthy. Conferences in the various specialities are held routinely once weekly and are under the direction of N. Parfrey, M. McCabe, D.K. Sheehan, S. Kennedy and A. O'Brien. The school

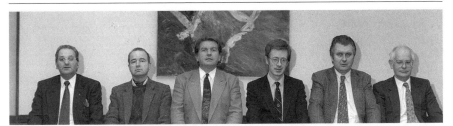

Consultant anaesthetists, 1994. (Left to right) Dr R. Assaf, Dr B. Ferris, Dr V. Hannon, Dr J. Boylan, Dr D. O'Keeffe, Dr T. Healy

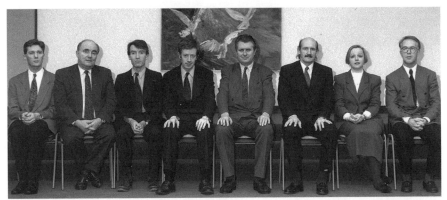

Consultant anaesthetists, 1994. (Left to right) Dr K. McKeating, Dr E. Gallagher, Dr K. Crowley, Dr J. Boylan, Dr D. O'Keeffe, Dr A. McShane, Dr B. O'Kelly, Dr J. Keane

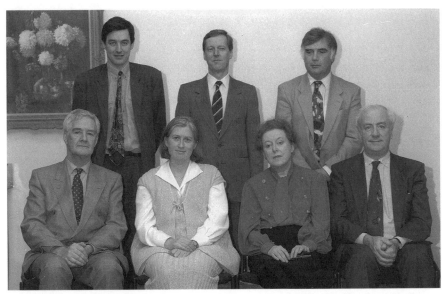

Diagnostic committee, 1994. (Back row, left to right) Dr Kieran Sheahan, Dr James Griffin, Dr Anthony Owens; (front row, left to right) Dr George Duffy, Dr Niamh Nolan, Dr Mary McCabe, Dr James Masterson

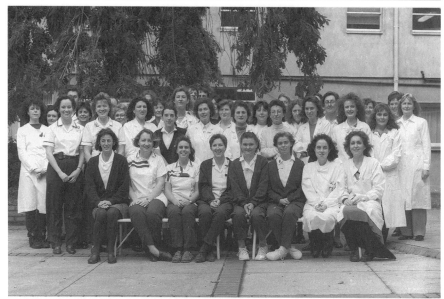

Paramedical staff, 1994

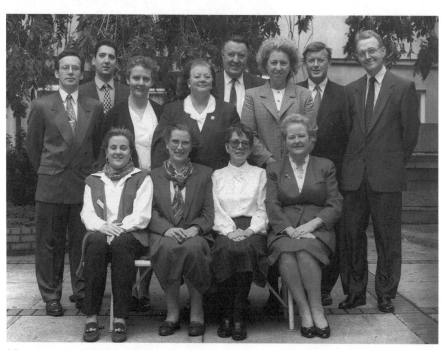

Management/Administration staff, 1994. (Back row, left to right) Mr N.C. Jermyn, Mr G. Russell, Ms K. Gill, Mrs P. Cuddihy, Mr K. Roche, Ms T. McDonough, Mr A. Moriarty, Mr P. Fletcher; (front row, left to right) Ms E. Couse, Mrs A. Greenan, Ms M. Bellew, Ms E. Carroll

of diagnostic imaging has organised a four year degree programme for radiography students and is being currently validated by the senate of the NUI. The department of nuclear medicine, as well as providing routine services to St Vincent's, also provides services for many other hospitals in Dublin. A total of thirty-three hospitals, fourteen in Dublin and nineteen outside Dublin, availed of these services for their patients in 1992.

In addition to healing and research the other great task of a voluntary hospital is to teach, and the high priority given to education has been one of the major characteristics of St Vincent's Hospital. From its earliest days the foundress Mary Aikenhead laid stress on the importance of producing trained personnel. This tradition has been maintained and enhanced over one hundred years of the hospital's existence. By their fruits you shall know them, and the number of members of the St Vincent's staff who have achieved professorial rank in their speciality is impressive.

In 1995 apart from the Professors of Medicine and Surgery, current professors include:

B. Keogh, Professor of Renal Medicine;

J.J. Fennelly, Research Professor of Oncology;

G. Bourke, Professor of Community Medicine and Epidemiology;

T.J. McKenna, Professor of Investigative Endocrinology;

B. Bresnihan, Professor of Rheumatology;

D.P. MacErlaine, Professor of Radiology;

N. Walsh, Professor of Clinical Psychiatry;

N. Duignan, Professor of Obstetrics and Gynaecology;

N. Parfrey, Professor of Pathology.

All these chairs are held in University College Dublin except for that of B. Keogh which is held in Trinity College Dublin.

The names of previous professors on the staff of the hospital are listed in an appendix.

The number of former students of the hospital who have been appointed professor in other institutions in this country is remarkable. The current list includes:

M. Cullen, Associate Professor of Endocrinology, St James's Hospital, TCD;

S. McCann, Professor of Haematology, St James's Hospital, TCD;

David Bouchier-Hayes, Professor of Surgery, Beaumont Hospital, RCSI;

Michael Brady, Professor of Surgery, UCC;

John FitzPatrick, Professor of Surgery, Mater Hospital, UCD;

Garret Fitzgerald, Professor of Medicine, Mater Hospital, UCD;

J. Stephen Doyle, Professor of Medicine, Beaumont Hospital, RCSI and President of the Royal College of Physicians of Ireland;

Anthony Clare, Professor of Psychiatry, St Bartholomew's Hospital London, and TCD;

A. (Conal) Hooper, Associate Professor of Anatomy, UCD;

L. Collum, Professor of Ophthalmology, Royal Victoria Eye and Ear Hospital, RCSI;

John H. Horgan, Associate Professor of Cardiology, Department of Medicine, Beaumont Hospital, RCSI;

Professor Brendan O'Donnell, Medical Officer of Health, Dublin, RCSI;

E.J. Guiney, Professor of Paediatric Research, Our Lady's Hospital for Sick Children, UCD;

Francis V. O'Brien, Professor of Oral Pathology, Queen's University Belfast;

It may be permissible to pick out one former student of the hospital who influenced the destiny of kings. Peter Kerley was born in Louth and graduated M.B., UCD in 1923. He was a house officer in St Vincent's in the years 1923–24. He was a pioneer in the speciality of radiology and achieved eminence in his field. He was called into consultation in the diagnosis of the illness of King George VI. It was Kerley who diagnosed the 'bronchial neoplasm which claimed the King's life'. His career has been described by Davis Coakley. 'During the 1950s and 1960s in addition to his hospital appointments Kerley had a flourishing practice, numbering Winston Churchill among his patients. He also continued to act as radiologist to the British Royal Family. In 1939 Kerley was one of the founder members of the Faculty of Radiology in London, and he was elected president in 1952, serving in the post for three years.'[6]

His photograph with colleagues can be seen hanging in the corridor of the hospital.

Such a busy programme of healing and teaching ensured that every available space in the main corridor of the hospital would be utilised and with new developments and projects more and more space was required. M.X. FitzGerald has pointed out that 'a high increase in activity has been generated by the highly-efficient organisation of the day-care and five-day investigation units in both medicine and surgery'. The accident and emergency department and the out-patients' department also have increasing demands on their services and urgently need more space and facilities. FitzGerald emphasised the fact that 'St Vincent's Hospital was now a quarter-century old and was designed at a time which preceded the vast expansion in diagnostic technology.'[7] This is an ever-present modern problem.

The torrent of new medical and scientific knowledge has been pouring out from centres all over the world at such speed that it outstrips the rate at which hospitals can be built. No one can foretell with accuracy what the twenty-first century will bring, but it is safe to assume that this torrent of scientific discoveries will continue unabated. In its day, St Vincent's on the Green faced similar problems and overcame them. Although a relatively small hospital the old St Vincent's made a major contribution to Irish medicine. Shortage of space was never allowed to hamper its progress. It was realised then that human ingenuity and perseverance were as important as bricks and mortar. St Vincent's Hospital Elm Park with its proud tradition can surely face the challenge of a new century with a firm heart and great confidence.

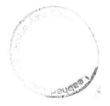

EPILOGUE

If Mr Inglis could make a return visit to Stephen's Green, he would witness the inevitable change of nearly two hundred years. However, some buildings would appear familiar. Number 56 still stands tall and elegant. Through its windows one can get a glimpse of the plasterwork on the walls and ceilings which was one of the glories of Georgian Dublin. On the front of the house above the entrance the crest of Archbishop Murray is displayed; recently added is a plaque proudly proclaiming that 'This building was the site of St Vincent's Hospital, founded by Mary Aikenhead and the Sisters of Charity, which has served the people of Dublin for over 130 years'.

At the corner, no. 60 has been extensively renovated and incorporated into the Building Society offices which occupy the block. Through the trees on the Green one can discern the austere outline of 86 St Stephen's Green where John Henry Newman dreamed of establishing a Catholic University which would be the pride of European civilisation—that same John Henry Newman who frequently said Mass in the hospital chapel and whose name is inscribed in its visiting book. Beside no. 86 is an equally significant symbol, Iveagh House, now the Department of Foreign Affairs of an independent Ireland. The park itself consists of pleasant tree-shaded walks, and a feast of flower beds reflecting the changing seasons. Also in the park there are monuments commemorating—among others—Countess Markievicz, James Joyce and Tom Kettle 'who died not for King nor Flag nor Emperor but for a dream born in a herdsman's shed and the secret scripture of the poor'.

Nos. 65 and 66 St Stephen's Green have fallen victim to the voracious appetite of the inevitable office block. Up the way in Earlsfort Terrace there is the National Concert Hall, where previously there was University College Dublin—built on the site of the Royal University of Ireland (1879–1909), which incorporated some of the buildings constructed for the Dublin International Exhibition of 1865.

Around the corner in Lower Leeson Street there have been changes also. The Department of the Marine has taken over most of Leeson Lane. A large

256

new office block has been built behind the old private nursing home. The out-patients' department and St Mary's nurses' home have also been taken over by the Department of the Marine. No longer do immaculately-starched figures emerge from St Mary's and proceed in stately manner across the bridge to nursing home or hospital to care for their patients. The residency stands empty and forlorn, but there still is a familiar face in the lane—John Fitzpatrick like his father before him continues to practise his art of shoemaking.

Over the years many shops had sprung up to serve the student population. A walk around Lower Leeson Street where it merges with the Green brings back memories of days gone by—Miss O'Connor watching over the magazine counter in the Post Office, the Misses McCarthy with their infinite supply of 'smokes'. Even during the grim days of war they could always find enough cigarettes under the counter to satisfy the most addicted smoker. Gone is Mr Hall who presided for many years over his grocer's shop, succeeded by Mr Fitzpatrick. No longer is there Mr Louis Hatch's Dairy, where one could drink vast quantities of milk for a penny in the company of distinguished professors from University College; on more affluent days a cream bun could be consumed. Mr McGuirk who provided the hospital's supply of meat is also gone.

Still happily present is the pharmacy of Joseph O'Reilly, whose voice inspired a generation of worshippers in University Church on a Sunday morning. His niece Christine Leahy succeeded him in the business and for many years provided unrivalled service to doctors and patients alike. And what about the oases of peace and tranquillity where one could discuss affairs of State, and of the hospital?—perhaps not so tranquil on the nights that the final results came out. They are all flourishing, but under different names: Mulligan's which succeeded Dwyer's and before Dwyer's was Grogan's; Lynch's which begat Hartigan's; and Hourican's whose ancestors were the Green Bar and John Ryan the Wake.

The tide of history has now swept out to Elm Park. Under the proud care of Mary Aikenhead and Daniel Murray, the sons and daughters of the new St Vincent's will make their own history and create their own traditions as a new century unfolds.

APPENDIXES

Appendix 1

MOTHERS GENERAL

Mother Mary Aikenhead 1843–58

Mother M. Francis Magdalene McCarthy 1858–76

Mother M. Scholastica Margison 1876–1905

Mother M. Canisius Cullen 1905–09

Mother Agnes Gertrude Chamberlaine 1909–28

Mother M. de Ricci O'Connor 1929–35

Mother M. Bernard Carew 1935–53

Mother Teresa Anthony Heskin 1953–71

Mother Frances Rose O'Flynn 1971–83

Sister Francis Ignatius Fahy 1983–

Appendix 2

SUPERIORS OF ST VINCENT'S HOSPITAL 1834–1993

Mother Mary Augustine Aikenhead 1834–36

Mother Francis Magdalene McCarthy 1836–58

Mother Mary Scholastica Margison 1858–76

Mother Mary Loyola Seagrave 1876–82

Mother Mary Canisius Cullen 1882–1905

Mother Mary Bernard Carew 1905–18

Mother Joseph Theckla Maunsell 1918–24

Mother Mary Bernard Carew 1924–30

Mother Mary Fidelis Butler 1930–31

Mother Mary Bernard Carew 1931–35

Mother Joseph Theckla Maunsell 1935–41

Mother Joseph Ignatius Austin 1941– (became ill)

Mother Mary Baptist Magan (temporary) 1942–43

Mother Joseph Ignatius Austin 1943–48

Mother Mary Baptist Magan 1948–54

Mother Mary Canisius O'Keeffe 1954–60

Mother Mary Paula Gleeson 1960–72

Mother Mary Catherina O'Brien (94 Lower Leeson Street) 1972

Mother Mary Canisius O'Keeffe (Elm Park) 1968–74

Mother Mary Teresita Stewart 1974–80

Sister Francis Mary Lawn 1980–86

Sister Teresa Avila Osborne 1986–92

Sister Joseph Cyril Fortune 1992–

Appendix 3

MEMBERS OF THE BOARD OF MANAGEMENT 1972

The Hon. Mr Justice Brian Walsh—chairman

Reverend Mother M. Canisius—Superioress

Mother Mary Baptist

Sister Joseph Ignatius

Mr Denis C. Crowley

Mr Sean Galvin

Mr Arthur Ganly

Senator John Kelly

District Justice Eileen Kennedy

Mr Thomas Lenehan

Mr Cathal McAllister

Professor Patrick Meenan

Professor Patrick Masterson

Mr J.A. Mehigan

Mr J.J. Nolan

Mr T.C.J. O'Connell

Mr John Ryan

Mr Kyran P. Tanham

MEMBERS OF THE BOARD OF MANAGEMENT 1989

Professor Michael McCormac—chairman

Mr C. McAllister—secretary

Sr Frances Rose O'Flynn

Professor John Kelly

Mr J.J. Nolan

Sister Agnes Reynolds

Sister Teresa Avila Osborne

Professor M.X. FitzGerald

Mr B. Quinlan

Dr T.J. McKenna

Miss M. Doolin

Mrs Patricia Maguire

Mr B. Kilcoyne

Mr Denis J. Bergin

Mr Gerald B. Scanlan

Dr Noel Whelan

Mrs Joyce Andrews

Mr Patrick Meade

MEMBERS OF THE BOARD OF MANAGEMENT 1993

Professor Noel Whelan—chairman

Mr C. McAllister—secretary

Mr Patrick Meade

Professor M.X. FitzGerald

Mr Gerald B. Scanlan

Dr T.J. McKenna

Mrs Joyce Andrews

Mr William Quinlan

Professor John Kelly

Sister Joseph Cyril Fortune

Sister Agnes Reynolds

Mrs Pat Maguire

Mr Stewart Harrington

Mr Denis Bergin

Appendix 4

MEMBERS OF THE EXECUTIVE OF THE MEDICAL BOARD 1993

Professor Muiris X. FitzGerald—chairman

Mr William R. Quinlan—hon. secretary

Dr Vincent Hannon

Mr John Hyland

Dr James Masterson

Dr Mary McCabe

Dr Terence J. McKenna

Dr Walter McNicholas

Dr Brian Maurer

Mr Denis Mehigan

Dr James Griffin

Appendix 5

SECRETARY MANAGERS

Sister Francis Joseph Lang 1971–81

Sister Mary Magdalen McParlan 1981–93

Mr Nicholas Jermyn—Chief Executive Officer 1994

Appendix 6

CHAIRMEN OF THE MEDICAL BOARD

P.N. Meenan 1969–73

F. Duff 1973–75

F.O.C. Meenan 1975–78

D. Cantwell 1978–83

J. McMullin 1983–84

D. Kelly 1985–89

M. FitzGerald 1989–

SECRETARIES OF THE MEDICAL BOARD

J.A. Mehigan 1970–72

F.O.C. Meenan 1972–74

D. Cantwell 1974–76

D. Kelly 1976–80

N. Walsh 1980–81

B. Maurer 1981–82

V. Keaveny 1982–84

D.A. MacErlaine 1984–86

B. Bresnihan 1986–88

J. Masterson 1988–90

J. Hegarty 1990–92

W. Quinlan 1992

Appendix 7

CONSULTANT MEDICAL STAFF

Notes

1. A.P. = Assistant Physician

    P. = Physician

    A.S. = Assistant Surgeon

    S. = Surgeon

    A.G. = Assistant Gynaecologist

    G. = Gynaecologist

2. Up to 1910 professorial chairs were held in the Catholic University School of Medicine (Cecilia Street), except for those of E.D. Mapother, whose chairs were held in the Royal College of Surgeons in Ireland. After 1910 the chairs were held in University College Dublin, except for B. Keogh, whose chair is held in Trinity College Dublin.

3. Dates are based on official hospital records.

PHYSICIANS

Joseph M. O'Ferrall First Medical Advisor in Ordinary 1835–68

O'Bryen Bellingham Second Medical Advisor in Ordinary 1836–57

Sir Henry Marsh Honorary Consulting Physician

Francis B. Quinlan P. 1864–89 Professor of Materia Medica

Robert Cryan P. 1868–81 Professor of Anatomy and Physiology

Michael F. Cox P. 1881–1925

Michael McHugh A.P. 1885–89 P. 1889–1915

Paul Dillon A.P. 1889–90

William Thompson A.P. 1890

Matthew B. Savage A.P. 1890–92

F.G. Adye-Curran A.P. 1892

Alexander Blayney A.P. 1895–96

William J. Dargan A.P. 1897 P. 1906–43

James N. Meenan A.P. 1906 P. 1915–50 Professor of Hygiene & Medical

Jurisprudence Professor of Medicine (Systemic)

James B. Magennis A.P. 1915 P. 1924–40

Patrick T. O'Farrell A.P. 1924 P. 1940–60

Harold Quinlan A.P. 1924 P. 1940–75

Denis K. O'Donovan A.P. 1934 P. 1943–76 Professor of Medicine

Oliver FitzGerald A.P. 1940 P. 1950–83 Professor of Therapeutics

Edward L. Murphy A.P. 1941 P. 1960–62

Phillip Brennan A.P. 1944 P. 1963–84

Francis McLaughlin Psychiatrist 1945–73

F.O.C. Meenan Dermatologist 1949

Risteard Mulcahy Physician 1950–88 Professor of Preventive Cardiology

Francis P. Muldowney Physician 1960–93 Research Professor of Medicine

Jack Molony Rheumatologist 1961–89

Ann Goff A.P. 1963–65

Alexander McDonald Paediatric Cardiologist 1955

James J. Fennelly Oncologist 1963 Research Professor of Oncology

Noel Walsh Psychiatrist 1970 Professor of Psychiatry

George J. Duffy Nuclear Medicine 1970

Edward A. Martin Neurologist 1971–89

Denis Keating Geriatrician 1971

Muiris X. FitzGerald Respiratory 1971 Professor of Medicine & Therapeutics

Andrew Heffernan Physician 1972

Brian Maurer Cardiologist 1974

Michael Moriarty Radiotherapist 1975

Geoffrey Bourke Preventive Medicine and Epidemiology 1975 Professor of Preventive Medicine & Epidemiology

Noel Hickey Preventive Medicine 1975–93 Professor of Preventive Cardiology

Mary Darby Psychiatrist 1978

Michael Hutchinson Neurologist 1978

Barry Bresnihan Rheumatologist 1978 Ciba-Geigy Professor of Rheumatology

Dermot O'Donoghue Gastroenterologist 1978

T.J. McKenna Endocrinologist 1978 Professor of Investigative Endocrinology

Sarah Rogers Dermatologist 1979

Brian Keogh Nephrologist 1983 Associate Professor of Renal Medicine

Robert McQuillan Accident and Emergency 1983

Walter McNicholas Respiratory 1984

John Hegarty Gastroenterologist 1984

Morgan Crowe Geriatrician 1987

P. Quigley Cardiologist 1989

M. Kearney Palliative Medicine 1989

Oliver FitzGerald Rheumatologist 1990

T. McDonnell Respiratory Physician 1991

M.J. McKenna Endocrinologist 1992

Kieran Crowley Intensivist 1992

Janice Redmond Neurologist 1992

John Crown Oncologist 1993

P. McCormick Gastroenterologist 1994

A. Watson Physician 1993

SURGEONS

Sir Philip Crampton Honorary Consulting Surgeon

Kevin Izud O'Doherty S. 1857–59

Edward D. Mapother S. 1859–89 Professor of Political Medicine Professor of Anatomy & Physiology

William H. O'Leary S. 1865–80

Matthew J. Keogh S. 1880–82

John S. McArdle S. 1882–1928 Professor of Surgery

F.G. Adye-Curran A.S. 1883–93

Richard F. Tobin A.S. 1885–86 S. 1886–1917

C. Burke Gaffney A.S. 1886–89

Glasgow Patterson A.S. 1889–93

Patrick J. Fagan A.S. 1896–1905 S. 1905–10 Professor of Natural Philosophy

Robert McDonnell A.S. 1905–08

Denis Kennedy A.S. 1908–10 S. 1910–45

Henry S. Meade A.S. 1910 S. 1917–52 Professor of Surgery (Systemic)

William Doolin A.S. 1914 S. 1928–57 Professor of History of Medicine

Francis J. Morrin A.S. 1924 S. 1940–68

Christopher Shortall A.S. *c.* 1927–35

T.C.J. O'Connell A.S. 1934 S. 1945–85

Patrick FitzGerald A.S. 1940 S. 1952–78 Professor of Surgery

Francis A. Duff A.S. (and urological) 1941–57

James Maher A.S. 1946–69 S. 1969–75

J.A. Mehigan A.S. 1954–69 S. 1969–81

J.P. McMullin A.S. 1955–69 S. 1969–84

James J. Murphy Surgeon 1976

Niall O'Higgins Surgeon 1977 Professor of Surgery

John Hyland Surgeon 1982

Denis Mehigan Surgeon 1985

Oscar Traynor Surgeon 1987

Gerry McEntee Surgeon 1991

E. McDermott Surgeon 1993

VASCULAR SURGEONS
T. Vincent Keaveny 1971

M.J. Fox 1979–81

UROLOGICAL SURGEONS
Francis A. Duff 1957–83

Daniel Kelly 1968

A. Heaney 1984–86

David Quinlan 1990

NEUROLOGICAL SURGEONS
Fergus Donovan 1958

Christopher Pidgeon 1978–89

CARDIO-THORACIC SURGEONS
Keith Shaw 1975–85

D.A. Luke 1985

ORTHOPAEDIC SURGEONS
Joseph Gallagher 1959–90

James Sheehan 1970–86

William Quinlan 1979

Kieran O'Rourke 1989

Eamon Kelly 1990

Brian Hurson 1991

THORACIC SURGEON
Vincent Lynch 1975

PLASTIC SURGEONS
Seamus O'Riain 1969

Michael Earley 1989–92

T. O'Reilly 1992

ORAL SURGEONS
Nicholas Martin 1949–86

F. Brady 1979

GYNAECOLOGISTS

John A. Byrne G. 1876–91 Professor of Midwifery

Alfred Smith G. 1891–1922 Professor of Obstetrics & Gynaecology

Arthur P. Barry A.G. 1919–22

John F. Cunningham A.G. 1922–31 G. 1942–60 Professor of Obstetrics & Gynaecology

Reginald White G. 1924–42

Gerald Tierney A.G. 1931–37

J.K. Feeney A.G. 1937–49 G. 1956–83 Associate Professor of Obstetrics & Gynaecology

Charles Coyle G. 1949–63

Declan Meagher G. 1964–70 1977–85

Brendan Murphy G. 1970–77

Anthony Keane G. 1970–77

Niall Duignan G. 1984 Associate Professor of Obstetrics & Gynaecology

John F. Murphy G. 1984

Peter Lenehan G. 1987

OPHTHALMOLOGISTS

Denis Redmond 1880–92 Professor of Ophthalmology

Ferdinand Odevaine 1892–1908

Herbert Mooney 1908–40

Joseph B. McArevey 1924–51

Philomena Guinan 1945–83

Francis Lavery 1953–71 Professor of Ophthalmology

John Blake 1970

Geraldine Kelly 1978

Peter Barry 1984

ANAESTHETISTS

Richard Shaw 1895–1922

Oswald J. Murphy 1927–67

Michael Mullen (O.P.D.) 1930

G.R. Davys 1947–83

M. Nash 1947–74

Denis O'Leary 1953–92

Richard Nolan 1965–83

Marian Rice 1971–86

James O'Donnell 1975–76

Richard Assaf 1976

Michael Slazenger 1978–84

D. Molyneaux 1982

P.A. Healy 1982

A. Cunningham 1982–86

G. Dorrian 1984–91

B. Ferris 1984

J.F. Keane 1985

A. McShane 1987

W. Casey 1988

V. Hannon 1988

N. McDonald 1989

E. Gallagher 1989

D. O'Keeffe 1989

K. McKeating 1989

J. Boylan 1992

B. O'Kelly 1992

P. Benson 1994

OTORHINOLARYNGOLOGISTS

Michael Curran 1903–04

William L. Murphy 1908–19

P.J. Keogh 1924–44

Albert Fagan 1924–66

Brian O'Brien 1944–78

O. McCullen 1951–88

A.R. Dennis 1972

PATHOLOGISTS

Thomas T. O'Farrell 1906–55 Professor of Pathology and Bacteriology

John McGrath 1927–57 Professor of Pathology, Bacteriology & Medical
   Jurisprudence

Patrick N. Meenan 1947–89 Microbiologist Professor of Medical Microbiology

Robert P. Towers 1955–92 Histopathologist

John Harman 1958–82 Pathologist Professor of Pathology

James J. Dinn 1973–90 Histopathologist

Mary McCabe 1974 Histopathologist

Anne O'Brien 1985 Histopathologist

Lynda Fenelon 1991 Microbiologist

Nollaig Parfrey 1991 Immunologist Professor of Pathology

Niamh Nolan 1992 Histopathologist

K. Sheahan 1992 Histopathologist

S. Kennedy 1993 Histopathologist

HAEMATOLOGISTS

Liam O'Connell 1954

D. McCarthy 1993

PHARMACISTS

Richard Shaw 1895–1922

Richard Shaw (Jr) 1922–26

John Shiel 1926–50

RADIOLOGISTS

M.F. O'Hea 1913–58

W.J. Murphy 1928–34

T.D. O'Farrell 1938–69

S.J. Boland 1938–74

Dermot Cantwell 1959–90

J.B. Hourihane 1969

D.A. MacErlaine 1974 Professor of Radiology

P.Bryan 1978–79

J.B. Masterson 1979

A. Owens 1984

J. Griffin 1984

R. Gibney 1990

J. Lorrigan 1993

SURGEON DENTISTS

Edward Corbett 1884–90

Marcus Bloom 1890–98

Kevin O'Duffy 1898–1903

John I. Potter 1903–06

J.J. Murphy 1924–49

Leo Smyth 1924–57

BIOCHEMISTS

Daniel Hingerty 1973–90 Associate Professor of Biochemistry Honorary Consultant
    in Biochemistry

Peter Smyth 1974– Honorary Consultant in Laboratory Endocrinology

M. Doolin 1956–92 Biochemist

Appendix 8

MARY AIKENHEAD SCHOOL OF NURSING
PRINCIPAL NURSING OFFICERS

MATRONS

1892–1906 Miss Campbell

1906–18 Miss Sutton

1918–46 Miss Angela Halbert

1946–68 Miss Annie Kelly

1968–70 Miss Emma McDonnell

1970–71 Sister Frances Rose O'Flynn

1971–76 Sister Mary Ignatius Killeen

1976–80 Sister Mary Stephanie Murphy

1980–85 Sister Joseph Cyril Fortune

1985–87 Sister Marie Peter McEneaney

1987–present Sister Agnes Reynolds

TUTORS

1947–49 Miss Loretta Pillon

1949–52 Miss Brigid Barlow

1952–55 Miss Rosanna Cunningham

1955–70 Sister Frances Rose O'Flynn

1970–90 Sister Margaret Vincent

1990–91 Miss Maureen Ashe

1991–present Sister Anne Curry

Appendix 9

LADY PRESIDENTS OF FINANCIAL AID COMMITTEE SINCE 1957

Mrs Kay Quinlan

Miss Nora Green

Mrs T.C.J. O'Connell

Mrs McCall

Mrs Kathleen Fagan

Miss Annie Kelly

Mrs William Doolin

Mrs Mgt Feeney

Mrs Kathleen Murphy

Miss Emma McDonnell

Mrs Maura Martin

Mrs F. Lavery

Miss Nora Maher

Dr Livina Meenan

Miss Eileen Kennedy

Mrs Nancy Coyle

First hon. sec. Mrs P.N. Meenan

Appendix 10

PAST STUDENTS OF ST VINCENT'S HOSPITAL
1834–1909

Adye–Curran, Francis G., Lieut–Colonel, A.M.S. Dublin, F.R.C.S.I., 42 Upper Rathmines

Adye–Curran, S., L.A.H. Dublin 1900, R.A.M.C.

Ahern, John Maurice, L. & L.M., R.C.P. & S.I., M.B., Bac.Surg., R.U.I. (Bellingham Gold Medallist in Medicine 1889), H.M. Prison, Liverpool

Ambrose, John Michael, L.R.C.P. & S. Edin., Newcastle West, Co. Limerick

Ambrose, Michael, L. & L.M., R.C.P. & S.I. 1904, Mayo County Infirmary, Castlebar

Ambrose, Thomas, L. & L.M., R.C.P.I., L.A.H., 10 Park Road, Dewsbury, Yorkshire

Anderson, Walter H., L.R.C.P. & S. Edin., L.F.P.S. Glasg., Sandhill, Boyle, Co. Roscommon

Anglim, William Joseph, L. & L.M., R.C.P. & S.I. 1900, Riverview, Arthurstown, Co. Wexford

Ballesty Michael J., L. & L.M., R.C.P. & S.I. 1900 (Bellingham Gold Medallist in Medicine 1900), Harbour Street, Mullingar, Co. Westmeath

Barrett, J. Francis, M.B., Bac.Surg., R.U.I. (Bellingham Gold Medallist in Medicine 1892), Ebburga House, The Bank, Highgate, London

Barry, Arthur Patrick, M.B., Bac.Surg., R.U.I. 1904 (O'Ferrall Gold Medallist in Surgery 1903), 50 Lower Baggot Street, Dublin

Barry, Harte Lionel Aloysius, L. & L.M., R.C.P. & S.I. 1901 (O'Ferrall Gold Medallist in Surgery 1901), Egmont Place, Kanturk, Co. Cork

Barry, James, L.R.C.P. & S. Edin., L.F.P. & S. Glasg., Rathcormac, Fermoy, Co. Cork

Bayer, Henry Michael, L.R.C.P. & S. Edin., L.F.P.S. Glasg., 243 Boundary Street, Liverpool

Bell, Hamilton Joseph, L.R.C.P. & S. Edin. 1899, 63 Sheen Lane, East Sheen, Surrey

Benson, Francis A., L.R.C.P.I., 7 West Terrace, Ormsby, Middlesborough, Yorks.

Beveridge, William John, L. & L.M., R.C.P. & S.I., Kalgoorlie, W. Australia

Born, Edward Turner, M.B., Univ. Durham 1900, Fox Bay, West Falkland Islands, South America

Bourke, Ulick Joseph, L.R.C.S.I., L.S.A., London Army Medical Staff

Boyd James, F.R.C.S.I., Ebor, Clonbur, Co. Galway

Boyd–Barrett, J., M.B., B.Ch., R.U.I. 1907 (O'Ferrall Gold Medallist in Surgery 1907), Asst Surgeon, Children's Hospital Temple Street, Fitzwilliam Street, Dublin

Brannan, Francis, M.B., B.Ch., R.U.I. 1892, Castledermot, Co. Kildare

Broderick, Simon, L.R.C.P. & S.I. 1908, Resident Medical Officer, St Vincent's Hospital

Brogan, John Francis, L. & L.M., R.C.P. & S.I. 1901, Castlepollard, Co. Meath

Bulfin, John F.A., L. & L.M., R.C.P. & S.I., Sierra Leone

Burke, John, L.R.C.P. & S.I. 1906, 26 Leeson Park, Dublin

Burke, Patrick Hannan, L. & L.M., R.C.P. & S. Edin., Coalview House, New Birmingham, Thurles

Burke, T.A., L.R.C.P. & S.I. 1906

Butler, John Joseph, L.R.C.P. & S. Edin., Ormonde House, Carnforth, Lancs.

Butler, Padget O'Brien, L. & L.M., R.C.P. & S.I. 1905, R.A.M.C.

Byrne, Benjamin, L. & L.M., R.C.S.I., L.A.H. Dublin, 79 East India Road E

Byrne, George, M.R.C.S. & P. London, Sunwick, Wilbraham Road, Chorlton–cum– Hardy, Manchester

Byrne, Herbert Unsworth, M.B., B.Ch. Dublin Univ., 1 Upper Merrion Street, Dublin

Byrne, John V., L.R.C.S.I., L.A.H. Dublin, 33 Laurence Street, Drogheda

Byrne, Peter K., M.R.C.S.E., L.R.C.P. London, 40 York Place, Portman Square, London W

Cahill, Francis Joseph, L. & L.M., R.C.P. & S.I. 1901, 24 Harcourt Street, Dublin

Cahill, Mark F., L. & L.M., R.C.P. & S.I., 93 Shankill Road, Belfast

Caithness, Geo. Edgar, L. & L.M., R.C.P. & S.I., 16 Tritonville Road, Sandymount, Co. Dublin

Calnan, R., L.R., C.P. & S.I. 1905, Main Street, Bandon, Co. Cork

Cane, Richard James, L. & L.M., R.C.P. & S.I. 1900, Highland Lodge, Kilkelly, Co. Mayo

Carrigan, Edward, M.D., 204 Southwark Park Road, London SE

Carroll, Denis J., L. & L.M., R.C.P. & S.I. 1894, Ballynattin, Clonmel, Co. Tipperary

Carroll, William Stanislaus, M.B., Bac.Surg., R.U.I. 1895, Trehafod, Pontypridd, Glamorganshire

Casey, Joseph, L. & L.M., R.C.P. & S.I. 1903, 39 Dockhead, Bermondsey, SE

Clarke, Denis Francis, L. & L.M., R.C.P. & S.I. 1897, Easkey, Co. Sligo

Clarke, J., M.B., York House, Castleblayney, Co. Monaghan

Clarke, John, L.R.C.S. & P.I., Farlhadreen, Bailieboro', Co. Cavan

Cleary, Martin, L.R.C.P. & S. Edin, L.F.P. & S. Glasg., Ballycroy, Co. Mayo

Clendinuing, James H., L. & L.M., R.C.P. & S., L.A.H., 152 Rathgar Road, Dublin

Clutterbuck, Lewis Augustus, I.R.C.P. & S. Edin., L.F.P. & S. Glasg., 43 Welbeck Street, London

Coen, John Augustus, L.R.C.P. & S.I. 1886, Frenchpark, Co. Roscommon

Coen, Patrick Joseph Dowell, L. & L.M., R.C.P. & S.I. 1894, The Lodge, Croghan, Boyle, Co. Roscommon

Coghlan, Michael Patrick, L.R.C.P. & S. Edin., L.F.P. & S. Glasg. 1893, Newrath Lodge, Waterford

Coghlan, Thomas, L. & L.M., R.C.P. & S.I., L.A.H. 1889 Dublin, Clare Castle, Ennis, Co. Clare

Conlon, Thomas Peter, L. & L.M., R.C.P. & S.I. 1894, District Asylum, Monaghan

Connolly, Capt. Edward Patrick, L. & L.M., R.C.P. & S.I. 1898 (O'Ferrall Gold Medallist in Surgery 1898), Army Medical Service

Conry, Charles William, L. & L.M., R.C.P. & S.I. 1901, Howth, Co. Dublin

Considine, Patrick Oswald, M.D., Q.U.I., L.R.C.S.I. 1877, Port Elizabeth, South Africa

Considine, Thomas Ivory, L. & L.M., R.C.P. & S.I. 1894, The Central Asylum, Dundrum, Co. Dublin

Conway, Thomas, L.R.C.P. & S.I. 1905, Asst Master Coombe Hospital

Cooke, Robert Philip, L.R.C.P. & S. Edin., L.F.P. & S. Glasg. 1891, Unity Place, Oldbury, Birmingham

Cooper, Charles, L.R.C.P. & S.I. 1905, Wygram House, Wexford

Corbet, Edward, L. & L.M., R.C.P. & S.I., Fairfield House, Alpington Road, Exeter

Cormac, Charles Henry, L. & L.M., R.C.P. & S.I. 1899, Sydney, Australia

Cormack, Thomas Patrick, L. & L.M., R.C.P. & S.I. 1902, Urlingford, Thurles, Co. Tipperary

Cormack, William Petrie, M.B. B.S. Edin. 1900, 16 Sinclair Terrace, Wick, N.B.

Cosgrove, Edward, L. & L.M., R.C.P. & S.I., Kilcock, Co. Kildare (Bellingham Gold Medallist in Medicine 1890)

Costello, Francis Xavier, L. & L.M., R.C.P. & S.I., L.D.S.I. 1904, Hong Kong

Costello, Joseph, L. & L.M., R.C.S.I., L.A.H. Dublin 1887, Doon Lodge, Ballybunion, Co. Kerry

Cotton, Edward J., L.R.C.P. & S.I. 1885, Buenos Aires

Cowell, William I., L. & L.M., R.C.P. & S.I. (O'Ferrall Gold Medallist in Surgery 1904)

Cox, Michael F., B.A., C.U.I., F.R.C.P., M.D., Hon. Causa., R.U.I., 26 Merrion Square

Coyne, Michael, L.R.C.P. & S.I. 1906, Crossmaglen, Co. Armagh

Craig, Barry Alexander, L. & L.M., R.C.P. & S.I. 1899, Army Medical Service

Crean, Thomas Joseph, V.C., L. & L.M., R.C.P. & S.I. 1896, Army Medical Service

Crean, William, L.R.C.P. & S. Edin., L.F.P. & S. Glasg., Fethard Dispensary, Co. Tipperary

Cremin, John, L. & L.M., R.C.P. & S.I. 1870, Charleville, Co. Cork

Cremin, William, L. & L.M., R.C.P. & S.I. 1903 (O'Ferrall Gold Medallist in Surgery 1902), 13 South Circular Road, Dublin

Cuffe, Joseph, L. & L.M., R.C.P. & S.I. 1904, 5 Usher's Island, Dublin

Cullen, Vincent J., L.R.C.P. & S.I. 1905 (O'Ferrall Gold Medallist in Surgery 1905), R.M.O., South Dublin Union

Cummins, Thomas C., L. & L.M., R.C.P. & S.I., Silverleigh, Cole Park, Twickenham

Curran, John James, L.R.C.P. & S.I. 1879, Mount Belle, Killeagh, Co. Cork

Curtin, Patrick Joseph, L.R.C.S.I. 1885, Grove Villa House, Crumlin, Co. Dublin

Cusack, Christopher Albert, L. & L.M., P.C.P. & S.I. 1904 (Bellingham Gold Medallist in Medicine 1904), 6 Nth Gt George's St, Dublin

Daly, Charles Francis, M.D., M.A.O., R.U.I., L.R.C.S.E., Silverdale, Staffordshire

Davies, Naunton W., L.R.C.P. & S. Edin., F.R.C.S. Edin., Penllwyn Park, Carmarthen

Davys, John J., L. & L.M., R.C.P. & S.I. 1895, 26 Westland Row, Dublin

Delany, Julius Barry, L. & L.M., R.C.R. & S.I., L.A.H., 103 Church Place, Runcorn, Cheshire

Delany, Thomas H., M.B., Bac.Surg., R.U.I. 1893, Indian Medical Service

Delany, William Francis, L. & L.M., R.C.P. & S.I. 1902, 6 Gardener's Place, Dublin

Delany, William, L. & L.M., R.C.P. & S.I. 1889, Bagnalstown, Co. Carlow

Dempsey, Alexander, M.D., Q.U.I., L.R.C.S.I., 36 Clifton Street, Belfast

Dempsey, Patrick Joseph, L. & L.M., R.C.P. & S.I. 1881, Kingscourt, Co. Cavan

Devlin, Hugh Patrick, M.B., Bac.Surg., R.U.I. 1904, Irish Street, Downpatrick, Co. Down

Dickenson, R.F., L.R.C.P. & S.I., R.A.M.C.

Dillon, Thomas Augustus, L. & L.M., R.C.P. & S.I. 1902 (Bellingham Gold Medallist in Medicine 1902), Croydon Union Infirmary, Mayday Road, Thornton Heath, Croydon, Surrey

Dolphin, Michael O'Farrell, L.R.C.P. & S.I. 1882, 19 South Third Street, Neward, USA

Donnellan, Robert Vincent, L.R.C.P. & S. Edin., L.F.P. & S. 1897, Glasg., 2 Lewisham Park, London SE

Dooley, M.B., L.R.C.P. & S.I. 1908

Dooley, Patrick Francis, L.R.C.P. & S. Edin., L.F.P. & S. Glasg. 1903, Carrick–on–Shannon

Dowling, Francis T., M.B., B.Ch., R.U.I. 1906, R.A.M.C.

Dowser, John Joseph Michael, L. & L.M., R.C.P. & S.I., Green Bank, Patricroft, Manchester

Duigenan, Patrick Samuel, L.R.C.S.I., 35 Manchester Road, Denton, Manchester

Dundon, Michael, M.D., M.Ch., Q.U.I., Army Medical Staff

Dunne, Thomas E., M.B., B.Ch., B.A.O., Edenfield, Castletown, Mountrath, Queen's Co.

Esmonde, John, L.R.C.P. & S.I., Thurgsland, Sheffield

Eyre, Robert Smyth, L.R.C.P. & S.I., Ohilly, Woodford, Loughrea, Co. Galway

Falvey, Charles Hebbert, L.R.C.P. & S.I. 1901, Wood House, Ardara, Co. Donegal

Fanning, James Joseph, L.R.C.P. & S. Edin., L.F.P. & S., Birr, King's Co.

Farrell, Louis Joseph, L.A.H. 1904, 195 Brunswick Street, Dublin

Fennelly, Martin, L.R.C.S.I., L.R.C.P.I., Richmond, Templemore, Co. Tipperary

Fetherston, Richard Herbert, M.B., M.Ch. Edin., L. & L.M., R.C.P. & S.I., Prabran, Melbourne, Australia

Finegan, Laurence, L. & L.M., R.C.P. & S.I. 1876, Navan, Co. Meath

Finnegan, Arthur D., L. & L.M., R.C.P. & S.I. 1877, Medical Superintendent District Asylum, Mullingar, Co. Westmeath

Fitzgerald, Daniel Aloysius, L. & L.M., R.C.P. & S.I., F.R.C.S. 1899, Cardiff

Fitzgerald, Edward, L. & L.M., R.C.P. & S.E., 5 Castlehill Avenue, Folkestone

Fitzgerald, Joseph, L.R.P. & S.E. 1884, Ballyneety, Pallasgreen, Queensland

Fitzgerald, Michael, L. & L.M., R.C.P. & S.I. 1880, Isisford, Queensland

Fitzmaurice, Thomas, L.R.C.S.I., L.R.C.P.E. 1879, Moate, Co. Westmeath

Flanigan, E.H., M.B., B.Ch., R.U.I. 1908, R.M.O. St Vincent's Hospital

Flood, Charles, L. & L.M., R.C.S.I., L.A.H. 1887 Dublin, Dewanan House, Northfleet, Kent

Flood, Edward Fitzgerald, L.R.C.S.I., L.A.H. Dublin, 89 Clanbrassil Street, Dundalk

Flood, Philip, L. & L.M., R.C.I., L.A.H., 318 Stapleton Road, Bristol

Foley, Cornelius, L. & L.M., R.C.P. & S.I. 1902, Ruardean, Gloucester

Foley, J.M.G., L.R.C.P. & S.I. 1907, Australia

Foley, John, L. & L.M., R.C.P. & S.I. 1899, Ballynoran, Charleville, Co. Cork

Forde, Bernard, M.B., M.Ch., Royal Univ., Army Medical Staff

Fottrell, Wm Joseph, L. & L.M., R.C.P. & S.I., 2 Rutland Square, Dublin

Freeman, Denis W., M.B. Dublin, L.M. Rotunda, 67 Eccles Street, Dublin

Gallagher, Gerald, H.L. & L.M., R.C.P. & S.I. 1905, Apollo, Bunder, Bombay

Gardiner, Charles E. Roche, L. & L.M., R.C.P. & S.I. 1888, Dungloe, Co. Donegal

Geoghegan, Charles Edward, L. & L.M., R.C.P. & S.I., Fleet Surgeon, Royal Navy

Gerrard, J.J., M.B. Dublin, Major, A.M.S. Brighton

Gibbons, James Barry, L. & L.M., R.C.P. & S.I., Indian Medical Department, Bengal

Gibbs, Andrew A., L. & L.M., R.C.P. & S.I., Indian Medical Department

Gilbert, John, L. & L.M., R.C.P. & S.I. 1891, Ennis, Co. Clare

Gill, James Geoffrey, L. & L.M., R.C.P. & S.I., Army Medical Service

Gilleran, Edward Joseph, L.R.C.P. & S. Edin., L.F.R. & S. Glasg., 120 Central Park West, New York, USA

Godfrey, William, M.B., B.Ch., B.A.O., R.U.I. 1905, Cork

Gordon, C., L.R.C.P. & S.I. 1906, Sheepwalk House, Frenchpark, Co. Roscommon

Gordon, James, L. & L.M., R.C.P. & S.I. 1898, Ballyshannon, Co. Donegal

Gordon, William, L.R.C.P. & S.E., L.F.P. & S., Glasg., 6 Marlborough Road, Salisbury

Grant, Hugh, M.B., B.Ch., R.U.I. 1908, R.M.A., St Vincent's Hospital

Gray, James, M.B., Mast.Surg., F.R.C.S.E., 9 South Jay Street, Dundee

Gray, Thomas, L.R.C.P. Edin., L.F.P. & S. Glasg., St Mary's, Ontario, Canada

Greehy, Wm Joseph, L. & L.M., R.C.P. & S.E., L.F.P. & S. Glasg. 1902, Main Street, Tallow, Co. Waterford

Green, James S., M.B., B.Ch. Dublin, L. & L.M., R.C.P. & S.I., Army Medical Staff

Griffin, John, L.R.C.S.I., Denton, Lancs.

Griffin, Reginald Edward J., St John, L. & L.M., R.C.P. & S.I., 5 Patrick Street, Kilkenny

Griffin, Thomas Francis, L.R.C.P. & S.I. 1885, St Denis, Edge Hill, Wimbledon, London SW

Griffith, Albert Edward, L.R.C.P. & S.E., L.F.P. & S. Glasg., Edinburgh

Hackett, Bartholomew James, M.B., Bac.Surg. R.U.I. 1899, Mountjoy Prison, Dublin

Hall, George Joseph, L. & L.M., R.C.P. & S.I., Kimbolton, Fielding, New Zealand

Hall, Helena Adelaide, L. & L.M., R.C.P. & S.I. 1902, Isolation Hospital, Chingford

Hamilton, Richard Moorhead, L. & L.M., R.C.P. & S.I., Annesley, Woodhouse, Notts.

Hannan, Mary Josephine, L. & L.M., R.C.P. & S.I., Glengadiffe, Pietermaritzburgh, Natal

Hanrahan, James A., L. & L.M., R.C.P. & S.I., Pollymount, Co. Mayo

Harding, James Joseph, L. & L.M., R.C.P. & S.I., Ballincollig, Co. Cork

Hardwicke, William Wright, L. & L.M., R.C.P. & S.I., Argyil Mansions, Chelsea, London SW

Harold, James T., L. & L.M., R.C.P. & S.I., 20 Brunswick Square, London WC

Hart, Patrick Joseph, L.R.C.P. & S.I., 11 Grantham Street, South Circular Road

Hartigan, William, L. & L.M., R.C.P. & S.I., 4 Bond Court, Walbrook, London EC

Hayes, Edwin Charles, L.R.C.P. & S.E., L.F.P. & S. (O'Ferrall Gold Medallist in Surgery 1894), Glasgow Army Medical Staff

Hayes, J.M., L. & L.M., R.C.P. & S.I. (Bellingham Gold Medallist in Medicine 1905), Limerick

Hayes, William J., L.R.C.P. & S.E., L.F.P. & S., Glasg., 288 Liverpool Road, Patricroft, near Manchester

Hearn, William Edward, L. & L.M., R.C.S.I., L.A.H., Wentworth House, Oldham, Lancs.

Heatly, Robert John, L. & L.M., R.C.P. & S.I., 138 Stockwell Street, Brixton, London SW

Heffernan, James, L.R.C.P. & S.I., 619 Green Lanes, Harringay

Henegan, Patrick J., L. & L.M., R.C.S.I., L.A.H. 1891, Glen Heather Lodge, Mulranny

Henry, John Patrick, M.D., B.Ch. Dublin, L. & L.M., R C.P. & S.I., 32 Lower Leeson Street, Dublin

Hickey, Garret Aloysius, L. & L.M., R.C.S.I., L.A.H. 1890 Dublin (O'Ferrall Gold Medallist in Surgery 1890), New Ross, Co. Wexford

Hickey, Gerald, M.B., B.Ch., R.U.I., 7 Park Terrace, Sunderland

Hogan, Edward James Kirby, L. & L.M., R.C.P. & S.I. 1895, 145 Albert Road, Southsea, Hants

Holms, John, F.R.C.S.I., L.R.C.P.E., 7 The Crescent, Limerick

Hopkins, James John, L. & L.M., R.C.P. & S.I. 1891, Castlebar, Co. Mayo

Horne, Andrew J., F. & L.M., R.C.P. & S.I., 94 Merrion Square, Dublin

Hosty, H., L. & L.M., R.C.P. & S.I. 1905, Ballyglunin, Co. Galway

Hourigan, William P., L.R.C.S.I., L.R.C.P.E., Freshford, Co. Kilkenny

Howley, Edward Joseph, L.R.C.P. & S.E., L.F.P. & S. Glasg., 78 Dundas Street, Sunderland

Howley, Henry Edward, L. & L.M., R.C.P. & S.I. 1899, Rich Hill, Lisnagry, Co. Limerick

Hughes, Christopher J., L.R.C.S.I., L.A.H. Dublin, 18 Trafalgar Square, Peckham, London SE

Hughes, Richard Lawlor, L. & L.M., R.C.P. & S.I., 101 Endlesham Road, Balham, London SW

Hughes, William, L.R.C.P. & S.E., L.F.P. & S. Glasg. 1903, Tokyo, Japan

Hutch, William, L.R.C.P. & S.E., L.F.P. & S. 1901, Conna, Co. Cork

Hynes, Edward Charles, L.R.C.S.I., L.R.C.P.E., 54 Shakespeare Street, Nottingham

Irwin, Peter Joseph, L. & L.M., R.C.P. & S.I. 1903, Pallas Cottage, Kilmeedy, Co. Limerick

Jennings, E.C., L. & L.M., R.C.P. & S.I. 1904, Broadmoor Asylum, Crowthorne, Berks.

Jones, John Langdale, L. & L.M., R.C.P. & S.I. 1899, 6 Burlington Road, Dublin

Jones, William Midwinter, L. & L.M., R.C.P. & S.I. 1899, Brownlow Hill Infirmary, Liverpool

Jordon, Thomas Joseph, L. & L.M., R.C.P. & S.I. 1895, Mortomley Hall, High Green, near Sheffield

Joyce, Garret W., L. & L.M., R.C.P. & S.I., 26 Rathmines Road, Dublin

Kearney, Anthony Joseph, L. & L.M., R.C.P. & S.I. 1894, Bishop Gate Street, Mullingar, Co. Westmeath

Kearney, James, L. & L.M., R.C.P. & S.I., George's Street, Panamatta, New South Wales

Keary, Patrick, M.B., B.A.O., R.U.I. 1890, Woodford, Co. Galway

Keays, William, L. & L.M., R.C.P. & S.I., F.R.C.S.I., Army Medical Staff

Keegan, Denis F., Surgeon-Major, M.D. Dublin, M.R.C.S. England, Indian Medical Department, Bengal Army, Bengal

Keegan, John Francis Leo, L. & L.M., R.C.P. & S.I., F.R.C.S. (Bellingham Gold Medallist in Medicine 1901, O'Ferrall Gold Medallist in Surgery 1900), Lower Baggot Street, Dublin

Kelly, George, M.B., Bac.Surg., R.U.I., Army Medical Staff

Kelly, Thomas, L. & L.M., R.C.P. & S.I. 1904, Donahill, Co. Tipperary

Kelly, William A., L.R.C.P. & S.I. 1886, 87 Pitt Street, Sydney, New South Wales

Kennedy, Denis, L. & L.M., R.C.P. & S.I., F.R.C.S.I. (O'Ferrall Gold Medallist in Surgery also Bellingham Gold Medallist in Medicine 1896), 20 Harcourt Street, Dublin

Kennedy, Edward, L. & L.M., R.C.P. & S.I. 1898, 4 Leeson Park Avenue, Dublin

Kennedy, Patrick, L. & L.M., R.C.P. & S.I., Albury, New South Wales

Kenny, Charles Aloysius, L. & L.M., R.C.P. & S.I. 1898, Ballymahon, Co. Longford

Kenny, Denis P., L. & L.M., R.C.P & S.I., Baltinglass, Co. Wicklow

Kenny, Michael Joseph, L.R.C.P.E., L.R.C.S.I. & L.M., Bridge House, Tallow, Co. Waterford

Keogh, Stephen, L. & L.M., R.C.P. & S.I., L.A.H. 1891, Dundrum Villa, Cashel, Co. Tipperary

Kerr, William, M.B., B.Ch., R.U.I., J.P. Armagh

Killeen, Timothy Robert, L.R.C.P. & S.I. 1885, Clonfeigh, Ennis, Co. Clare

Kinsella, Harmon Eugene Waters, L. & L.M., R.C.P. & S.I. 1896, Kilronan, Aran Islands

Kinsella, John Ignatius, L. & L.M., R.C.P. & S.I., Maryboro', Queen's Co.

Kinsella, John Jerome, M.B., Bac.Surg., R.U.I. 1897, Edenderry, King's Co.

Kinsella, Patrick, L. & L.M., R.C.P. & S.I. 1904, Crosstown, Castlebridge, Co. Wexford

Kirwin, James St, M.B., Bac.Surg., R.U.I. 1896, District Lunatic Asylum, Ballinasloe, Co. Galway

Kirwin, Richard R., M.B., B.Ch, B.A.O., R.U.I. 1907, District Lunatic Asylum, Ballinasloe, Co. Galway

Lawlor, Purcell N. O'Gorman, M.B., Bac.Surg., R.U.I. 1894, Indian Medical Service, Bombay

Lee, William Patrick, L. & L.M., R.C.P. & S.I., Kilfinane, Co. Limerick

Lee, William Stephen Ignatius, L. & L.M., R.C.P. & S.I., 34 Beaufort Street, King's Road, Chelsea, London SW

Lemass, Peter Edward, L.R.C.S.I., 4 Leeson Park, Dublin

Lennan, Francis Joseph, L. & L.M., R.C.P. & S.I. 1904, 32 Milnrow Road, Shaw, Oldham, Lancs.

Leybourne, Edward Smyth, L.R.C.P. & S. Edin., L.F.P. & S. Glasg., 151 Rathgar Road, Dublin

Little, Thomas Joseph, M.B., Bac.Surg., R.U.I. 1900, 125 Stephen's Green West

Longford, John M., L. & L.M., R.C.P. & S.I., Stoke Union Hospital, Newcastle–under–Lyne

Loughrey, Thomas Francis, L. & L.M., R.C.P. & S.I. 1890, 250 Upper Parliament Street, Liverpool

Lovett, William L., L.R.C.P. & S. Edin., L.F.P. & S. Glasg., 2 Keighey Road, Colne, Lancs.

Lowrey, John, L.R.C.P. & S.I., Naval Medical Service

Lynch, Edmund William, L. & L.M., R.C.P. & S.I., Royal Infirmary, Phoenix Park, Dublin

Lynch, Edward J., L.R.C.S.I., Newtownmountkennedy, Co. Wicklow

McArdle, John S., F.R.U.I., F.R.C.S.I., etc., etc., 72 Merrion Square, Dublin

McArdle, Robert F., L.R.C.S.I., L.R.C.S.E., 30 Bristol Road, Bournbrook, Birmingham

MacAulay, Roger, M.D., Q.U.I., L.R.C.S.I., L.M., L.A.H. Dublin, Ballina, Co. Mayo

McCann, William Francis Augustus, L. & L.M., R.C.P. & S.I. 1895, 4 Park Place, Liverpool

McCartan, Michael Joseph, L. & L.M., R.C.P. & S.I., J.P., Rostrevor, Co. Down

MacCarthy, Brendan, M.B., Bac.Surg., M.D., R.U. Dublin, Londonderry

McCarthy, Denis T., M.B., B.Ch., B.A.O., R.U.I. 1906, R.A.M.C.

McCarthy, Henry, L.M. & L.R.C.S.I., L.A.H. Dublin, Tastura, Victoria, Australia

McCarthy, James, L. & L.M., R.C.P. & S.I., Milford, Charleville, Co. Cork

McCarthy, William, M.B., Bac.Surg., R.U.I. 1900, Abbeyfeale, Co. Limerick

McCaul, Bernard, L. & L.M., R.C.P. & S.I. 1896, Carrickmacross, Co. Monaghan

McClancy, J.B., L.R.C.P. & S.I. 1907, Infirmary, Ennis, Co. Clare

McCleland, Hugh A., M.R.C.S.E., L.R.C.P. London, 9 Burlington Road, Bayswater, London

McConnell, John Joseph, L. & L.M., R.C.P. & S.I. 1903, Main Street, Moville, Co. Donegal

McCormack, Wm, L.R.C.P. & S.I. 1906, Nenagh, Co. Tipperary

McDermott, Thomas, M.B., B.Ch., B.A.O. Royal Univ., Army Medical Service

McDonald, Peter, Surgeon–Major, M.D., M.Ch., Q.U.I., L.R.C.S.I., Indian Medical Department, Bengal

McDonnell, Robert Percy, L. & L.M., R.C.P. & S.I., F.R.C.S.I., Extern Surgeon to the Hospital, 20 Lower Leeson Street, Dublin

McDonogh, Francis Joseph, J.P., L.R.C.P. & S.I., L.M., L.A.H., Newpark House, Kilmeague, Co. Kildare

McDonogh, Vincent E.J., L. & L.M., R.C.P. & S.I., Navarino, Surrey Road, Bournemouth

McElligott, Patrick Edward, L.R.C.P. & S.E., L.F.P. & S. Glasg., Andover House, Sheffield

McEvoy, Thomas Michael, L. & L.M., R.C.P. & S.I., 1 Lower Prince Edward Terrace, Blackrock, Co. Dublin

McGann, James, Surgeon–Major, L.R.C.P. & S.I., Army Medical Staff

McGann, Michael, L.R.C.P. & S.E.L.F.P. & S. Glasg., 113 Old Woolwich Road, East Greenwich, London SE

McGauran, Arthur, L.R.C.S.I., Newtowngore, Carrick–on–Shannon

McGuinness, Luke, L. & L.M., R.C.P. & S.I. 1905, Ardnaree House, Ballina, Co. Mayo

McHugh, Michael, M.A., M.B. Dublin, L.R.C.S.I., 25 Harcourt Street, Dublin

McHugh, Patrick William, L. & L.M., R.C.P. & S.I., Palmfield House, Crook, Co. Durham

McInerney, James Joseph, L. & L.M., R.C.P. & S.I. 1902, Corraclare, Ennis, Co. Clare

McKenna, Peter, M.B., M.Ch., Royal View, Carrickmacross, Co. Monaghan

McLoughlin, Ed. P., M.B., B.Ch., B.A.O., R.U.I., Medical School, Cecilia Street, Dublin

McNaboe, John Joseph, L. & L.M, R.C.P. & S.I., 2 Church Road, Kingsland, London N

McNamara, Matthew, L. & L.M, R.C.P. & S.I., Brisbane, Queensland

McQuaid, E.W., L. & L.M., R.C.S.I., L.A.H. Dublin, Cootehill, Co. Cavan

McQuillan, J., L.R.C.P. & S.I. 1906, Ardee, Co. Louth

McSwiney, Myles O'Connell, L. & L.M., R.C.P. & S.I., Naval Medical Service

Madden, M.J., L. & L.M., R.C.P. & S.I., Thomastown, Golden, Co. Tipperary

Madden, Thomas, L.R.C.P. & S.I. 1906, Kiltimagh, Co. Mayo

Magee, William J., L.R.C.P. & S.I., 88 Hampden Street, Bolton, Lancs.

Magner, James, M.D., M.Ch., M.A.O. Royal Univ., L.A.H. Dublin, Timoleague, Co. Cork

Magner, Thomas, L. & L.M., R.C.P. & S.I., Rathkeale, Co. Limerick

Maguire, James Henry, L.R.C.P. & S.I., Chesterton, Newcastle, Staffordshire

Maher, James, L.R.C.P. & S.E., L.F.P. & S. Glasg., Gawler, South Australia

Mahon, Ralph Bodkin, M.D., M.Ch. Royal Univ., Ballinrobe, Co. Mayo

Malone, Michael Joseph, M.D., Q.U.I., F.R.C.S.I., 5 Percy Square, Limerick

Mandel, Frederick P., L.R.C.P. & S.E., L.F.P. & S. Glasg., 53 Bromham Road, Bedford

Manning, James Michael Aloysius, L.R.C.P. & S.E. 1899, 45 Bell Street, Edgeworth Road, London

Marnell, James Patrick, L. & L.M., R.C.P. & S.I. (O'Ferrall Gold Medallist in Surgery 1892), Kilmaganny, Co. Kilkenny

Martin, George, L. & L.M., R.C.P.I., 4 Park Terrace, Silloth, Cumberland

Mason, Henry William, L.A.H. 1902, 35 Pembroke Road, Dublin

Meagher, William, L. & L.M., R.C.P. & S.I. 1898, Ferbane, King's Co.

Meenan, James N., M.B., B.Ch., D.P.H., R.U.I. (Bellingham Gold Medallist in Medicine 1903)

Meldon, James Bernard, M.B., Bac.Surg., Royal Univ. 1901, Army Medical Service

Meredith, Richard Graves, L.A.H. 1903, M.B., B.Ch., R.U.I. 1904, Army Medical Service

Moloney, Michael Charles, L.R.C.S.I., L.A.H., Tulla, Co. Clare

Moloney, Patrick Joseph, L.R.C.P.I., Brisbane, Queensland

Monahan, Patrick Francis, L. & L.M., R.C.P. & S.I., Mount Bellew, Ballinasloe, Co. Galway

Monks, Charles, L. & L.M., R.C.P. & S.I., Indian Medical Department, Bombay

Moore, Charles John, M.B., Bac.Surg., R.U.I. (O'Ferrall Gold Medallist in Surgery 1897), 77 Markhouse Road, Walthamstow, London NE

Moore, Edward Joseph, L. & L.M., R.C.P. & S.I. 1894 (Bellingham Gold Medallist in Medicine 1894), District Medical Office, Southern Nigeria

Moore, Henry Joseph, M.B., Bac.Surg., R.U.I. 1893, Ivy House, Ardee, Co. Louth

Moore, Henry, L. & L.M., R.C.P. & S.I., 40 Lower Baggot Street, Dublin

Moore, Joseph Henry, L.R.C.P. & S.E., Army Medical Staff

Moore, Louis Thomas, M.B., Bac.Surg., R.U.I. 1902, Kilgarvan, Co. Kerry

Moore, Stanley, L. & L.M.R., C.P. & S.I. (Bellingham Gold Medallist in Medicine 1889), Maynooth, Co. Kildare

Moran, Austin Joseph, L. & L.M., R.C.P. & S.I., 12 Cambridge Gardens, Kilburn, London NW

Moran, James Joseph, M.D., M.Ch. Dublin, Indian Medical Department, Madras

Moriarty, John Michael, L.R.C.P. & S.E. & L.F.P. & S. Glasg. 1904, Strand Street, Dingle, Co. Kerry

Morris, Michael A., M.B., Bac.Surg., M.D. Dublin, Clonmore, Piltown, Co. Kilkenny

Morris, William Richard, M.B., B.Ch., B.A.O. Royal Univ., 37 Lady Lane, Waterford

Morrissey, Martin Rowland, L.R.C.P. & S.E. & L.F.P. & S. Glasg. 1898, Hill House, Coalbrook, Thurles, Co. Tipperary

Morrissey, Patrick Joseph, L. & L.M., R.C.P. & S. 1891, Knockane House, Dungarvan, Co. Waterford

Mulcahy, Patrick, L.R.C.S.I., L.R.C.S.E., Ballinamore, Co. Leitrim

Mulcahy, Thomas K., L. & L.M., R.C.P. & S.I., 2 Upper Hartstronge Street, Limerick

Murphy, John, L. & L.M., R.C.P. & S.I. 1902, Castleview, Macroom, Co. Cork

Murphy, M.D. & M.S., Q.U.I., 13 New Church Road, Hove, Brighton

Murphy, Philip John, L. & L.M., R.C.P. & S.I., L.A.H. 1898, Main Street, Carrick–on–Suir, Co. Tipperary

Murphy, Richard, L.R.C.P. & S.I., Cork Street Fever Hospital

Murray, P.J., L.R.C.P. & S.I. 1907, Drogheda

Nangle, James Joseph, M.D. & Mast.Surg., R.U.I., 24 Woburn Place, London WC

Nash, William H., L.R.C.P. & S.E., L.F.P. & S. Glasg., 8 Rathdown Terrace, North Circular Road

Neilan, John Alexander, L. & L.M., R.C.P. & S.I. 1899 (Bellingham Gold Medallist in Medicine 1899), Seatonview, Seaham, Durham

Nicholls, John William, M.D., M.Ch., R.U.I. Dublin, Carlow

Nolan, Cornelius Joseph, L. & L.M., R.C.P. & S.I., Elm View, Shanagolden, Co. Limerick

Nolan, Francis Joseph, L. & L.M., R.C.P. & S.E., L.F.P. & S. Glasg.

Nolan, Michael James, L. & L.M., R.C.P. & S.I., District Asylum, Downpatrick

Nowlan, John Patrick, L.A.H. Dublin, 59 Amiens Street, Dublin

O'Brien, Christopher, M., M.D., L. & L.M., R.C.P. & S.I., 29 Merrion Square, Dublin

O'Brien, Daniel Patrick, L. & L.M., R.C.P. & S.I., F.R.C.S.I., 'Avonsleigh', Rockhampton, Queensland

O'Brien, John Robert, L. & L.M., R.C.P. & S.I. 1898, 282 Portobello Road, N. Kensington, London

O'Brien, Michael Patrick, L.R.C.P. & S.E., L.F.P. & S. Glasg. 1898, King's Square, Mitchelstown, Co. Cork

O'Brien, Richard F., L. & L.M., R.C.P. & S.I., Army Medical Staff

O'Carroll, Joseph Francis, M.D., M.Ch., R.U.I., F.R.C.P. & S.I., 43 Merrion Square, Dublin

O'Connell, John Henry, L. & L.M., R.C.P. & S.I. 1900, 38 Healthfield Road, Wavertree, Liverpool

O'Connell, Morgan D., L. & L., R.C.P. & S.I., Army Medical Staff

O'Connor, Arthur P., L. & L.M., R.C.P. & S.I., F.R.C.S.I., Army Medical Staff

O'Connor, John Edward, M.B., Bac.Surg., R.U.I., White Lodge, Kirby, Muxloc, Leicester

O'Connor, John Francis, L. & L.M. R.C.P. & S.I., Rockforest Lodge, Mallow, Co. Cork

O'Connor, John, L.M., L. Surg. Dublin Univ., British Hospital, Buenos Aires

O'Connor, S.V., L.A.H. Dublin 1907, Wexford

O'Doherty, Michael Joseph, L. & L.M., R.C.P. & S.I., Newtown Hall, Middleswick, Cheshire, 696 Oldham Road, Newton Health, Manchester

O'Doherty, William Joseph, L. & L.M., R.C.P. & S.I. 1902, Carndonagh, Co. Donegal

O'Donnell, James Joseph, L. & L.M., R.C.P. & S.I., 65 Jude Street, Brunswick Square, London WC

O'Donnell, John D., L.R.C.P. & S.E., L.F.P. & S. Glasg., Ooorgaum, Mysore State, India

O'Donnell, Thomas Moore, L.R.C.P. & S.I., 20 Bucklersbury, London EC

O'Donnell, William, L. & L.M., R.C.P. & S.I., Castlehill, Fishguard, Pembrokeshire

O'Donoghue, John, L. & L.M., R.C.P. & S.I. 1891, Clontarf, Co. Dublin

O'Donohoe, Hugh Tyrell, L.R.C.P. & S. Edin, L.F.P. & S. Glasg. 1897, 26 Mill Street, Leeds

O'Donovan, Robert Arthur, L. & L.M., R.C.P. & S.I. 1900, Mount Haigh, Kingstown, Co. Dublin

O'Dwyer, D., L.R.C.P. & S.I.

O'Dwyer, Peter, L. & L.M., R.C.P. & S.I., The Cottage, Ennistymon, Co. Clare

O'Farrell, Thomas T., L.R.C.P. & S.I., 44 Waterloo Road, Dublin

O'Farrell, William R., L.R.C.P. & S.I. 1907, R.A.M.C.

O'Ferrall, Lewis Richard More, L. & L.M., R.C.P. & S.I. 1899 (O'Ferrall Gold Medallist in Surgery 1899), Finsbury H., Stackport Road, Bristol

O'Flaherty, Richard, L. & L.M., R.C.P. & S.I. 1904, Leenane, Co. Galway

O'Gorman, Michael C., L. & L.M., L.R.C.P. & S.I., Aughrim, Co. Wicklow

O'Gorman, William, L. & L.M., R.C.P. & S.I., L.A.H. Dublin, Ballyragget, Co. Kilkenny

O'Kane, M., L.R.C.P. & S.I. 1907, Londonderry

O'Keeffe, Arthur Lanigan, L. & L.M., R.C.P. & S.I. 1904, Navan, Co. Meath

O'Keeffe, M., L.R.C.P. & S.I., Avoca, Co. Wicklow

O'Keeffe, Thomas F., M.B., Bac.Surg., R.U.I. 1900, Royal Navy

O'Kelly, Robert, L.R.C.P. & S.I. 1907, R.A.M.C.

O'Loughlin, William, F.W., L.R.C.P. & S.I., 30 James's Street, Liverpool

O'Malley, David Joseph, M.D., M.Ch., Q.U.I., Glenamaddy, Co. Roscommon

O'Mara, Joseph E., L.R.C.P. & S.I., 14 Dudley Road, Wolverhampton

O'Meara, Patrick Michael, M.B., Bac.Surg., R.U.I., Francis Street, Kilrush, Co. Clare

O'Reilly, A., L. & L.M., R.C.P. & S. 1905, Portarlington, Co. Laois

O'Sullivan, Carol Naish, L. & L.M., R.C.P. & S.I. 1899, 1 Queen's Parade, Barking Road, E. Ham., Essex

O'Sullivan, Daniel, L.R.C.S. & P.E., Rathmore, Killarney, Co. Kerry

O'Sullivan, Michael, L.R.C.P. & S.E., L.F.P. & S. Glasg., Alexandra Road, Swansea

Palmer, Francis Joseph, L.R.C.P. & S.I. 1898 (Bellingham Gold Medallist in Medicine 1897), Army Medical Service

Peart, Joseph Frederick, L. & L.M, R.C.P. & S.I. 1901, 65 Elgin Mansions, London W

Pierce, M.J., L.R.C.P. & S.I. 1908, 24 Drummond Place, Harold's Cross, Dublin

Pierse, Thomas, L.R.C.P. & S.I., 1 Upper George Street, Wexford

Pigott, John George Glynn, L. & L.M., R.C.P. & S.I. 1896, Belmont, Shrewsbury

Poett, Patrick M., M.K., Q.C.P.I. & L.M.R.C.S.E., Dispensary House, Tallaght, Co. Dublin

Potter, Thomas James, L. & L.M., R.C.P. & S.I. 1897, Army Medical Service

Power, J.H., L. & L.M., R.C.P. & S.I. (O'Ferrall Gold Medallist in Surgery 1893), Army Medical Service

Power, Edward Francis, L. & L.M, R.C.P. & S.I. 1894, Naval Medical Service

Power, Patrick William, L. & L.M., R.C.P. & S.I. 1902, Rathmore, Croom, Co. Limerick

Power, William Moroney, L. & L.M., R.C.P. & S.I., Army Medical Service

Purcell, Edward Alphonsus, L.R.C.P. & S.E., 44 Queen's Road, Wimbledon, Surrey

Quigley, Luke Joseph, L.R.C.P. & S.E., L.F.P. & S. Glasg., Cloughjordan, Co. Tipperary

Quirk, John Joseph, M.R.C.S.E., L.R.C.P. London, Oakland House, Hunters Road, Hansworth, Birmingham

Raye, Daniel O'Connor, Surgeon–Major, M.D., R.U.I., F.R.C.S.I., Indian Medical Department, Calcutta

Rearden, J., L.R.C.P. & S.I. 1907, Cork

Redahan, Thomas, L. & L.M., R.C.P. & S.I., Mohill, Co. Leitrim

Redmond, Gabriel O'Connell, L. & L.M., R.C.P. & S.I., Cappoquin, Co. Waterford

Redmond, Henry O'Connell, L. & L.M., R.C.P. & S.I., 15 Talbot Street, Dublin

Roberts, James, L. & L.M., R.C.P. & S.I. 1904, Limerick

Roche, Jas D., M.B. Univ. Dublin 1907

Roche, Wm, L.R.C.P. & S.I. 1906, West Africa

Ronayne, James Francis, L. & L.M., R.C.P. & S.I., 90 Salisbury Road, Wavertree, Liverpool

Rowan, Edward A., L.R.C.P. & S.E., L.F.P. & S. Glasg., Rondebosch, Cape Colony

Ryan, David Joseph, M.B., Bac.Surg., R.U.I., Monasterevan, Co. Kildare

Ryan, James Dwyer, L. & L.M., R.C.P. & S., Rathdrum, Co. Wicklow

Ryan, John Coffey, L. & L.M., R C.P. & S.I., Brookville, Broadford, Co. Clare

Ryan, Martin Joseph, L. & L.M., R.C.P. & S. 1903, Station House, Bamber Bridge, Preston, Lancs.

Ryan, Michael Joseph, L. & L.M., R.C.P. & S.I., 207 Derby Street, Bolton, Lancs.

Ryan, Patrick J., L.S.A. London, 15a Gower Street, London WC

Ryan, Richard, M.D., M.Ch., R.U.I., J.P., The Villa, Bailieboro', Co. Cavan

Ryan, Thomas John, L. & L.M., R.C.P. & S. 1904, 126 George Street, Limerick

Ryan, Walter Henry, L. & L.M., R.C.P. & S.I., Roade, Northamptonshire

Ryan, William, L. & L.M., R.C.P. & S.I., Albury, New South Wales

Sage, Michael Christopher, L. & L.M., R.C.P. & S.I. 1904, Wakefield, Grosvenor Road, Rathgar, Dublin

Sampson, Francis Cornelius, M.B., Bac.Surg., R.U.I. 1903, Army Medical Service

Sampson, William, M.B., B.Ch., B.A.O., R.U.I., Moyne House, Scarriff, Co. Clare

Sellers, John C., L. & L.M., R.C.P. & S.I., Roden Place, Dundalk, Co. Louth

Sexton, George Joseph, L. & L.M., R.C.P. & S.I. 1902, Tinahely, Co. Wicklow

Sexton, Joseph P., L. & L.M., R.C.P. & S.I., Tamworth, New South Wales

Shanahan, John Francis, L.R.C.P. & S.I., 2 The Crescent, Limerick

Shaw, Hugh, L.R.C.P. & S. Edin., L.F.P. & S. Glasg., 146 Upper Parliament Street, Liverpool

Shaw, Richard F., L.R.C.P. & S.E., L.F.P. & S. Glasg., The Lymes, Audlem, Cheshire

Shaw, Richard, L. & L.M., R.C.S.I., L.A.H., 86 Ranelagh Road, Dublin

Sheedy, Patrick J., L.R.C.S. & P.I., L.F.P. & S. Glasg., Oaks House, Evenwood

Sheedy, Thomas, L.R.C.S.I., L.R.C.P.E.

Sheppard, John, L.R.C.P. & S. Edin., L.F.P. & S. Glasg. 1898, 1 Rostrevor Terrace, Clontarf, Co. Dublin

Sinton, Joseph Richard, M.B., Bac.Surg., R.U.I., Kenhard, Cape Colony

Slattery, James Beary, M.B., Bac.Surg., R.U.I. 1898, Seaverden Asylum, King's Langley, Herts.

Slevin, Laurence C., L. & L.M., R.C.P. & S.I., 48 Lower Mount Street, Dublin

Smith, Alfred J., M.D., M.Ch., M.A.O., R.U.I., F.R.C.S.I., 30 Merrion Square, Dublin

Smith, Michael Joseph, L.M., L.Surg., M.B., Bac.Surg. Dublin, Naval Medical Service

Smith, Robert, L.R.C.S.I., L.A.H. Dublin, Ormiston, Cremadyna, Hobart, Tasmania

Smyth, John Francis, L. & L.M., R.C.P. & S.I. 1900, 22 Stockport Road, Ardwick, Manchester

Smyth, Patrick J., L.R.C.S.I., Stedalt, Stamullen, Balbriggan, Dublin

Sparrow, Thomas Francis, M.L., Q.U.I., L.R.C.P. & S.E., Kells, Co. Meath

Starkey, William, M.B., Bac.Surg., R.U.I. 1900, County Asylum, Prestwick, Manchester

Stephenson, Alexander Berchmans, L. & L.M., L.R.C.P. & S.I., Gorey, Co. Wexford

Stephenson, Edward A., L.M., T.C.D., M. & L.M.R.C.P. & S.I., Clareville, Tramore, Co. Waterford

Stoker, Sir William Thornley, Fellow and Examiner, R.C.S.I., M.D., Ely Place, Dublin

Stone, Henry E., L. & L.M., R.C.P. & S.I., 78 The Green, Bloxwick, Staffordshire

Sutcliffe, John Forest, L.R.C.P. & S.E., L.F.P. & S. Glasg., Harbury, Warwickshire

Sweeney, Terence Humphrey, L. & L.M., R.C.P. & S.I., F.R.C.S.I., Indian Medical Department, Surgeon–Major, Bengal Army

Talbot, Thomas Joseph, L.R.C.P. & S.E., L.F.P. & S. Glasg., 21 Poulton Road, Seacombe, Cheshire

Teahan, Timothy T., L.R.C.P. & S.I., Castlegregory, Co. Kerry

Teevan, Francis J., L. & L.M., R.C.P. & S.I., Bawnboy, Co. Cavan

Tench, Charles G., M.B., Bac.Surg. Dublin, Alverston House, Bagshot, Surrey

Thompson, Sir William J., F.R.C.P.I., M.D., 59 Fitzwilliam Square N

Tiernan, John, L.R.C.P. & S.E., L.F.P. & S. Glasg., 35 Heathurst Road, Hampstead, London NW

Tobin, J.R., L.R.C.P. & S.I., Kapunda, S. Australia

Tobin, Richard Francis, Fellow and Member of Council, R.C.S.I., M.R.C.P.I., 60 Stephen's Green, Dublin

Tobin, William, F.R.C.S.I., Late Army Medical Staff, Halifax, Nova Scotia

Trant, James, J.P., L. & L.M., R.C.P. & S.I., Waterville, Co. Kerry

Treston, John Francis, L. & L.M., R.C.P. & S.I. 1899, 13 Merrion Square, Dublin

Tynan, Edward Joseph, L. & L.M., R.C.P. & S.I. 1894, Ballyconky, Rathowen, Co. Westmeath

Vasquez, J., L. & L.M., R.C.P. & S.I. 1905, Gibraltar

Verdon, John, L. & L.M., R.C.P. & S.I. 1900, Royal Navy

Vereker, C.V., L. & L.M., R.C.P. & S.I. 1890, Holly House, Walton, near Liverpool

Walsh, Edmund, L. & L.M., R.C.P. & S.I. 1904, Cresswell, Mansfield, Notts.

Walsh, James A., L.R.C.P. & S.E., L.F.P. & S. Glasg. 1892, 30 Westmoreland Street, Dublin

Walsh, John Joseph, L.R.C.P.E., L.R.C.S.I. 1898, Main Street, Mallow, Co. Cork

Walsh, John Thomas, L.R.C.P. & S.I., Balrath, Liscard, Cheshire

Walsh, Michael, L.R.C.P. & S.I., Airmount, New Ross, Co. Wexford

Walsh, P.D., L.R.C.P. & S.I. 1907, Kinlough, Co. Donegal

Walsh, Patrick Francis, L. & L.M., R.C.P. & S.I., Callan, Co. Kilkenny

Walsh, Thos John, L.R.C.P. & S.I. 1903, Brooklyn Terrace, South Circular Road, Dublin

Walsh, Wm, L.R.C.P. & S.I. 1906

Watts, Vincent Leonard, L. & L.M., R.C.S.I., L.A.H. Dublin, Bankeera, Bengal

Westwood, Samuel Constantine, M.B., B.Ch., B.A.O. Dublin, L.M., Belgravia, Kiida, Melbourne, Australia

White, George, M.B., B.Ch., R.U.I. 1908, R.M.O, St Vincent's Hospital

White, Matthew L.F., Brigade Surgeon, L.R.C.S.I., Army Medical Service

White, Reginald J., L. & L.M., R.C.P. & S.I. 1899, 39 Lower Baggot Street, Dublin

Wilkin, Richard McKim, L.R.C.P., S.E., L.F.P. & S. Glasg. 1900, 2 Ardskeagh Villas, St Luke's, Cork

Wilson, George O'Keeffe, L. & L.M., R.C.P. & S.I., F.R.C.S.I., 34 North Frederick Street, Dublin

Wilson, J.W., L. & L.M., R.C.P. & S.I., The Square, Portaferry, Co. Down

Woods, Thomas Arthur, M.B. Dublin, L.R.C.S.I. & L.M., Rose Lodge, Brada Mt., Douglas, Isle of Man

Wright, Douglas, M.D., L.R.C.P. & S.E., 229 Camden Road, London NW

Wright, Edward, L.R.C.P. & S. Edin. 1898, Medical Mission, 123 Moncar Street, Glasgow

Yarr, Michael Thomas, L. & L.M., R.C.P. & S.I., Army Medical Staff

Yourelle, Michael J., L.M. & R.C.P. & S.I. 1875, 10 Ailesbury Road, Dublin

Appendix 11

MEDICAL EXAMINATIONS MEDAL AND PRIZEWINNERS

THE BELLINGHAM GOLD MEDAL IN MEDICINE

1888 F.B. Nolan B.A.

1889 Stanley Moore

1890 Edward Cosgrave

1891 Not Awarded

1892 J.P. Marnell

1893 Not Awarded

1894 E.J. Moore

1895 Joseph McArdle

1896 D. Kennedy

1897 Francis J. Palmer

1898 John M. Ahern

1899 John A. Neilan

1900 M. Ballesty

1901 J.L. Keegan

1902 A. Dillon

1903 J.N. Meenan

1904 C.A. Cusack

1905 J. Hayes

1906 F.T. Dowling

1907 W.R. O'Farrell

1908 A.P. O'Connor

1909 H.S. Meade

1910 M.F. O'Hea

1911 P.J. Ryan

1912 N. Atken

1913 J.G. Green

1914 J. Pierce

1915 M. Moriarty

1916 T.J. Canton

1917 M. Carboy

1918 J.W. Healy

1919 O. Morphy

1920 A. Scully

1921 W. Magauran

1922 T. McWeeney

1923 Miss A. Brereton

1924 J.A. McGrath

1925 John Mowbray

1926 Timothy Ryan

1927 Not Awarded

1928 C. Shortall

1929 W. Callaghan

1930 T.C. O'Connell

M.J. Mullen Ex-Aequo

1931 F.P. Ryan

1932 Not Awarded

1933 D.K. O'Donovan

1934 Not Awarded

Silver Replica

E. O'Shaughnessy

C.F. Stanford

1935 O.P. FitzGerald

1936 J. Martin

1937 Miss K.A. Roche

Special Prize

Miss N. McNally

1938 J. Hallissey

1939 J.T. O'Reilly

1940 J.W. Magner

1941 P. Moroney

1942 P.C. Brennan

1943 Not Awarded

1944 P. Twomey

1945 P.J. O'Dwyer

1946 P. McGill

1947 O. McCullen

1948 Miss P. Phelan

Silver Replica

J. Considine

1949 Miss M. Dardis

1950 Miss M. Fitzgerald

1951 B. Lemass

1952 M.J.T. Fitzgerald

Silver Replica

B. O'Hanlon

1953 T. Poon King

1954 Miss E. Bastible

P. Morrin Ex-Aequo

1955 M.P. Brady

1956 Not Awarded

Silver Replica

R.J. Mansfield

P. Whelan

1957 A. Heffernan

1958 Miss M. McCabe

1959 J.A. Carney

1960 Miss E. Keane

1961 G. Duffy

1962 M. Carey

1963 J. Sheehan

1964 M.X. FitzGerald

Silver Replica

D.J. Murnaghan

1965 M.J. Cullen

Silver Replica

Miss O'Brien

1966 Sr M.H. Hester

1967 J.F. Donohoe

Silver Replica

N. Behan

1968 T. O'Gorman

1969 Dr E. Griffen

1970 Dr A. Gorman

1971 Dr F. Sheridan

1972 Dr K. McGarry

1973 Dr J. Hegarty

1974 Dr P. Broe

1975 Dr D.C. Costigan

1976 Dr B. Sheehy

1977 Dr R. Finn

1978 Dr W.P. Roche

1979 Dr W. Powderly

Second Prize

Dr D. Lynch

1980 Not Awarded

Silver Replica

Dr J. Redmond

1981 Dr S. O'Reilly

Silver Replica

Dr E. McFadden

1982 Dr N. Keenan

1983 Dr H. Enright

1984 Dr Patricia Holland

1985 Dr Marie Therese Keogan

1986 Dr D. Mulherin

1987 Dr P. Blake

1988 Dr A. O'Callaghan

1989 Dr D. McGowan

1990 Dr Richard Farrell

THE O'FERRALL GOLD MEDAL IN SURGERY

1890 Garret A. Hickey

1891 Patrick J. Henehan

1892 J.F. Barrett

1893 John H. Power

1894 E.C. Hayes

1895 J. Roughan

1896 D. Kennedy

1897 Chas. J. Moore

1898 Edward P. Connolly

1899 Louis More O'Farrell

1900 J.L. Keegan

1901 H.L. Barry

1902 W. Cremin

1903 A.P. Barry

1904 C. Cowell

1905 V.J. Cullen

1906 W. Walsh

1907 J. Boyd Barrett

1908 C. Tierney

1909 E. Kirwan

1910 P.T. O'Farrell

1911 T.F. O'Donnell

1912 G. Sheil

1913 Not Awarded

1914 E. De C. Keogh

1915 F. Morrin

1916 L. O'Mahony

1917 M. Lawler

1918 T. McKinney

1919 J. Bookey

1920 H. Quinlan

1921 A. Fagan

1922 O.C. Blanc

1923 W. Prendergast

1924 J.D. Hourihane

1925 P.A. Hanratty

1926 M.L. Kennedy

1927 Not Awarded

1928 P. Keane

1929 Sean Lavin

1930 J.F. Ferguson

1931 D. Kennedy

1932 J.K. Feeney

1933 D.K. O'Donovan

1934 T.M. Kavanagh

Silver Replica

B. O'Brien

1935 P.A. Fitzgerald

Silver Replica

A.P. Barry

1936 T.M. Hennebry

1937 Miss K.A. Roche

Silver Replica

S. McHale

1938 S. McHale

Silver Replica

F.A. Duff

1939 E.P. Campbell

1940 Miss P.M. Guinan

Silver Replica

D.J. Leahy

1941 S.D. Daly

1942 F. Donovan

1943 B. McMahon

1944 M. Lochrin

1945 R. Mulcahy

1946 B. Daly

1947 E. O'Dwyer

1948 Miss P. Phelan

Silver Replica

S. Malone

1949 Not Awarded

1950 Miss M. Fitzgerald

1951 L. McElearney

1952 M.J.T. Fitzgerald

1953 T. Poon King

1954 P. Morrin

1955 V. Hughes

1956 R.J. Mansfield

Silver Replica

B. Flanagan

1957 B. Hannan

1958 T. Waldron

1959 Miss A. Sharrett

1960 C. McCarthy

Silver Replica

C. Bartholomew

1961 V. Keaveny

1962 L.O. Tuama

1963 J. Sheehan

1964 Miss M. O'Keefe

Silver Replica

T.B. Conlon

1965 L.M T. Collum

Silver Replica

J. Horgan

1966 M. Meagher

1967 D. Duff

Silver Replica

G. O'Malley

1968 J. Harman

Silver Replica

D.K. McDowell

1969 Dr B. Stuart

1970 Dr S. McCann

1971 Dr T.J. Keane

Special Prizes

Dr D. O'Reilly

Dr T. Hutchinson

1972 Dr D. Doyle

1973 Dr B. Silke

1974 Dr O. Traynor

1975 Dr P. Lenehan

1976 Dr D. de la Harpe

1977 Dr J. Kirby

Dr S. O'Donnell Ex-Aequo

1978 Dr W.P. Roche

1979 Dr P.A. McCormick

2nd Prize

Dr D. Lynch

1980 Dr D. Quinlan

1981 Dr E McFadden

1982 Dr N. Kennan

1983 Dr F. Stafford

1984 Dr Alice Stanton

1985 Not Awarded

Special Prize

Dr Patrick Hartly

1986 Dr S. O'Gorman

1987 Dr P. Blake

Special Prize

Dr J. Harty

1988 Dr P. Deegan

1989 Niall Mulligan

THE MCARDLE PRIZE IN SURGERY

1923 Sean O'Dea

Annie Brereton Ex-Aequo

1924 J.D. Hourihane

1925 Kathleen Kennedy

1926 M.L. Kennedy

1927 J.A. Timony

1928 C. Shortall

1929 W. Callaghan

1930 T.C. O'Connell

1931 Not Awarded

1932 J.K. Feeney

1933 D.K. O'Donovan

E.L. Murphy, Residual 1931

1934 T.M. Kavanagh

1935 A.P. Barry

P.A. Fitzgerald Ex-Aequo

1936 T.M. Hennebry

1937 Not Awarded

1938 F.A. Duff

Special Prize

J.T. O'Reilly

1939 Not Awarded

1940 D.F. O'Connor

S.D. Daly, Residual 1939

1941 P.L. Brennan

1942 F. Donovan

1943 E. Shanahan

M.O.P. Mansfield

1944 Half McArdle. P.R.

F.O.C. Meenan

1945 *Special Prize*

B.J. O'Sullivan

1946 Miss D. Donovan

1947 Miss J. McCarthy

1948 J. Considine

Special 2nd Prize

E. O'Kelly

1949 D. Donovan

1950 J.B. Healy

1951 M.J.T. Fitzgerald

L.D. O'Carroll Ex-Aequo

1952 C.B. McGann

1953 P. Morrin

J.G. Devlin

Additional McArdle

1954 M.P. Brady

Special 2nd Prize

S. Doyle

1955 Not Awarded

Supplementary Prize

E.J. Guiney

1956 ——

1957 J. Fennelly

1958 Miss M. Murnane

1959 Miss A. Sharrett

1960 C. McCarthy

1961 V. Keaveny

1962 M. Carey

1965 L.M T. Collum

Junior Prize

Sr M. Hilda Hester

2nd Prize

F. Brady

B. St J. Canning Ex-Aequo

1966 J. Murphy

1967 J.F. Donohoe

1968 Miss M. Fogarty

2nd Prize

C. Ryan

1969 J. O'Callaghan

1970 Dr R. Healy

1971 Dr C. O'Donoghue

1972 Dr D. Doyle

1973 Dr F. Sheehan

1974 Dr O. Traynor

Dr G. Fitzgerald Ex-Aequo

1975 Dr R.N. Gibney

1976 Dr B. Sheehy

1977 Dr R. Finn

1978 Dr K. Butler

1979 Dr P.A. McCormick

2nd Prize

Dr D. Lynch

1980 Dr D. Quinlan

1981 Dr E. McFadden

1982 Dr N. Kennan

1983 Dr. R. Gray

1984 Dr Eoin Mooney

1985 Not Awarded

Special Prize

Dr Shaun O'Keeffe

1986 Dr D. Mulherin

1987 Dr M. Keane

1988 Dr G. O'Neill

Dr L. McKenna Ex-Aequo

1989 Dr Margaret James

Dr Peter Hogan Ex-Aequo

THE MAGENNIS GOLD MEDAL IN CLINICAL MEDICINE

1942 B. O'Donnell

1943 E. Nugent

1944 F.O.C. Meenan—*Silver Replica*

1945 Not Awarded

1946 Not Awarded

1947 Miss J. McCarthy

1948 Not Awarded

1949 D. Donovan

1950 B. Lemass

1951 L.D. O'Kelly

1952 T. Poon King

1953 P. Morrin

1954 M.P. Brady—Silver Replica

1955 Not Awarded

Silver Replica

E.J. Brady

1956 Not Awarded

1957 Miss D. Tomey

1958 Miss M. Murnane

1959 Miss A. Sharrett

1960 C. McCarthy

1961 J. Woods

1962 M. Carey

1966 B. St J. Canning

Junior Prize

D. Duff

2nd Prize

N. Keaney

J. O'Driscoll Ex-Aequo

1967 J.F. Donohoe

Junior Prize

J. Harman

1968 Miss M. Fogarty

Silver Replica

D.K. McDowell

1969 Dr E. Griffen

1970 Dr A. Gorman

1971 Dr J.M. Fitzpatrick

1972 Dr D. McCarthy

1973 Dr J. Waterhouse

1974 Dr G. Fitzgerald

1975 Dr C.D. Costigan

Dr R.N. Gibney Ex-Aequo

1976 Dr B. Sheehy

1977 Dr R.Finn

Special Prize

Dr S. O'Donnell

1978 Dr W.P. Roche

1979 Dr W. Powderly

Dr D. Lynch

1980 Dr J. Redmond

1981 *Silver Replica*

Dr E. McFadden

1982 Dr H. Brady

1983 Dr F. Stafford

1984 Dr Patricia Holland

1985 Dr Brian Kavanagh

1986 Dr G. McMahon

1987 Dr M. Keane

1988 Dr F. Hayes

1989 Dr D. MacGowan

1990 Dr Aisling Denihan

THE TOBIN PRIZE IN SURGERY FOR JUNIOR STUDENTS

1952 P. Morrin

1953 M.P. Brady

2nd Prize

E.J. Guiney

1954 Miss Z. Betowska

1955 J.P. O'Sullivan

2nd Prize

J.J. Fennelly

1956 R. Reilly

1957 Miss A. Sharratt

1958 *1st Place*

Miss S. McNamara

2nd Place

C. McCarthy

1959 *1st Place*

A. Dennis

2nd Place

V. Keaveny

1960 D. Dunne

1961 J. Sheehan

1962 J.J. Walsh

Miss M. Collins

1963 J. Horgan

2nd Prize

G. Foyle

M. Cullen Ex-Aequo

1964 Miss G. Hester

2nd Prize

D. Johnston

1965 *1st Place*

M. Behan

M. Keaney

2nd Place

H. McLoughlin

1966 D.K. McDowell

1967 Miss C. Corcoran

2nd Prize

J. O'Callaghan

1968 Miss R. Healy

Miss E. Lawlor Ex-Aequo

2nd Place

Miss A. Gorman

1970 Miss C. O'Donoghue

2nd Prize

T. Hutchinson

1971 Miss P. Gorman

D. Mehigan Ex-Aequo

1972 H. Durkin

1973 P. Broe

1974 R.N. Gibney

2nd Prize

P. Lenehan

1975 Miss J. Power

1976 Miss P. O'Donnell

293

1977 Miss C. O'Reilly

Special Prize

W.P. Roche

1978 D. Lynch

2nd Prize

Miss M. Judge

1979 Miss J. Redmond

1980 Miss K. Reilly

1981 H. Brady

1982 Miss F. Stafford

1983 Miss P. Holland

1984 Ms Margaret Dolan

1985 Miss Bridget Byrne

1986 Mr Maccon Keane

Replicas

Miss Patricia Blake

Miss Ailis Ni Riain

1987 Miss Anne Burke

1988 Miss Margaret James

Silver Replica

Mr John Lyne

1989 Miss Catherine Fleming

1990 Miss Ethna Mannion

THE DARGAN PRIZE IN MEDICINE FOR JUNIOR STUDENTS

1968 J. O'Callaghan

2nd Prize

Miss L. Groarke

1969 Miss R. Healy

2nd Prize

Miss E. Lawlor

1970 F. Sheridan

2nd Prize

K. Martin

1971 D. McCarthy

1972 B. Silke

1973 Miss U. O'Callaghan

1974 P. Lenehan

2nd Prize

Miss H. Daly

1975 Miss H. Dillon

1976 Miss S. O'Donnell

1977 W.P. Roche

Special Prize

B. O'Kelly

1978 D. Lynch

2nd Prize

W. Powderly

1979 Miss K. Lyons

Miss J. Redmond Ex-Aequo

1980 Miss S.O'Reilly

1981 H. Brady

1982 Miss F. Stafford

1983 Not Awarded

Silver Replica

Miss S. O'Brien

1984 Not Awarded

Silver Replica

Ms Margaret Dolan

1985 Dermot Mulherin

1986 Mr Maccon Keane

1987 Miss Ann O'Callaghan

1988 Not Awarded

Special Prize

Miss Aideen O'Hara

1989 Mr Andrew Keaveny

1990 Mr Fergal Malone

THE MCGRATH PRIZE IN PATHOLOGY

1968 J. O'Callaghan
1969 Miss A. Gorman
1970 Miss C. O'Donoghue
1971 Miss P. Gorman

Special Prize

N.J. Brennan
1972 Not Awarded
1973 A. Landy
1974 R.N. Gibney
1975 Not Awarded
1976 H. O'Conor
1977 K. Butler
1978 Not Awarded
1979 Dr D. Lynch
1980 Not Awarded
1981 Not Awarded
1982 Miss H. Enright
1983 Not Awarded
1984 Ms Imelda Lambert

2nd Award

Mr Brian Kavanagh
1985 Miss Patricia Blake
Mr Maccon Keane Ex-Aequo
1986 Mr Patrick Deegan
Mr Gilmore O'Neill Ex-Aequo
1987 Mr D. MacGowen
1988 Mr Michael Stewart
Mr Alan O'Connor Ex-Aequo
1989 Mr Aidan Moran

THE J.N. MEENAN PRIZE
Awarded for original research by young graduates of the Hospital

Winners of the prize included:

Fergus O'Rourke
Francis Muldowney
Robert Towers
Robert Carroll
Vincent Keaveny
Turlough FitzGerald

In 1978 the prize was changed to a biennial lecture on a suitable topic in medicine given by a former student of the hospital, who was not a member of the hospital staff.

1978 John F. Fleetwood
1980 William F. O'Dwyer
1982 Arthur Barry
1984 Anthony Clare
1986 J. Stephen Doyle
1988 Michael Brady
1990 Michael Boland
1992 Shaun McCann
1994 Peter Boylan

Appendix 12

NURSING EXAMINATIONS MEDAL AND PRIZEWINNERS

GOLD BADGE (SENIOR NURSES)
Awarded by the community for loyalty and long service to the hospital

1972 Sr Marie John Sexton

1974 Miss Eleanor Taylor

1982 Miss Pauline Doyle

1984 Sr Marie Therese

1987 Miss Mary Mulcahy

1989 Miss Maureen Ashe

1991 Miss Patricia Hennessy

1994 Miss Teresa McDermott

MOTHER MARY AIKENHEAD MEDAL
Loyalty and devotion to duty (senior staff)

1971 Ms Pauline Doyle

1972 Ms Sheila O'Byrne

1973 Ms Josephine Bartley

1974 Ms Eileen Monaghan

1975 Ms Mary Mulcahy

1976 Ms Ann Riordan

1977 Ms Patricia Hennessy

1978 Ms Teresa McDermott

1979 Ms Geraldine McSweeney

1980 Ms Louise Hederman

1981 Ms Mary Frost

1982 Sr Philomena

1984 Ms Maureen Ashe

1985 Ms Nuala Donnelly

1986 Ms Mary McCormack

1987 Ms Geraldine O'Leary

1988 Ms Una Leydon

1989 Ms Mairead McDonnell

1990 Ms Petronilla Martin

1991 Ms Marie Maume

1992 Ms Valerie Feehan

1993 Ms Loretto Browne

1994 Ms Colette Kingston

MOTHER MARY BERNARD MEDAL

Loyalty and devotion to duty (junior staff)

1975 Ms Gabrielle Kenny

1976 Ms Petronilla Martin

1977 Ms Patricia Goodwillie

1978 Ms Mary Killeen

1979 Ms Patricia Kavanagh

1980 Ms Helen Delahunty

1981 Ms Anne Kiely

1982 Ms Irene Gordon

1982 Ms Mary Marnane

1985 Ms Monica Hurson

1986 Ms Dolores O'Neill

1987 Ms Vera Rogers

1988 Ms Angela Moriarty

1989 Ms Philomena Shovlin

1990 Ms Clare Maddock

1991 Ms Maureen Flynn

1992 Ms Delia Carr

1993 Mrs Bridget Corkery

1994 Miss Geraldine Carey

MAGENNIS MEDAL

Best student nurse over three years training

1984 —	1985 Catherine Meyler
1986 Anne Marie Cullinane	1987 Una Molloy
1988 Marguerite Doyle	1989 Brenda Sheridan
1990 —	1991 Deirdre Murphy
1992 Sally Anne McGroarty	1993 Eileen Cusack
1994 Therese Furlong	

Appendix 13

SOME CURRENT RESEARCH PROJECTS IN THE HOSPITAL

RESEARCH PROJECT
Name of consultant: Peter Barry

PHACOEMULSIFICATION AND BIFOCAL INTRAOCULAR LENS IMPLANTATION

This is part of an international multi-centre study to determine the place of the above procedure.

RESEARCH PROJECT
Name of consultant: John Blake

In glaucoma high intraocular pressure contributes to erosion of visual fields leading, if uncontrolled, to eventual blindness.

Our research has discovered that focusing on a near object, e.g. reading, reduces eye pressures in young adults; our continuing studies are designed to determine whether pressure falls also in older people who are more at risk of developing glaucoma.

RESEARCH PROJECT
Name of consultant: Barry Bresnihan

RHEUMATOID ARTHRITIS RESEARCH PROJECT 1990–93

Because the cause of rheumatoid arthritis is not known, there is no definitive treatment or cure. The damage is caused by the arrival in the joints of cells called lymphocytes, and specialised proteins called antibodies. In our studies we have focused on the particularly important arthritis-associated antibody called rheumatoid factor. Our experiments demonstrated that the source of rheumatoid factor is a particular type of lymphocyte which appears to proliferate in the bloodstream of patients with RA. These lymphocytes are called CD5+ B-lymphocytes. In our experiments we have studied factors which regulate the synthesis of rheumatoid factors and other antibodies by CD5+ B-lymphocytes. We have learned that the regulation of rheumatoid factor synthesis is quite specific and independent of all the other protective antibodies. This finding is particularly encouraging, as it suggests that rheumatoid factor formation could be suppressed therapeutically without having to suppress the entire immune system and creating the risk of unwanted side effects.

RESEARCH PROJECT
Name of consultant: Oliver FitzGerald

IMMUNOHISTOCHEMICAL ANALYSIS OF THE SYNOVIAL MEMBRANE IN PSORIATIC ARTHRITIS

Psoriatic arthritis is an unusual form of arthritis which affects 5 to 10 per cent of patients with psoriasis. The arthritis has been poorly studied and the changes within the joint tissues in patients suffering from psoriatic arthritis have not been well characterised. In this project tiny amounts of tissue are obtained from within the joint using a biopsy needle. These tissue samples are studied in detail and the changes observed are then compared with those seen in other forms of arthritis such as rheumatoid arthritis. It is hoped that with these studies we will be able to learn more about the nature of the disease in psoriatic arthritis and be in a better position therefore to influence it. This study is a combined study with Dr Sarah Rogers, consultant dermatologist from Hume Street and St Vincent's Hospital.

RESEARCH PROJECTS
Name of consultant: T.J. McKenna

THE CONTROL OF ADRENAL ANDROGENS

Polycystic ovary syndrome is the commonest cause of infertility in women. This condition may be related to excess production of androgens by the adrenals. However, the mechanism whereby androgens are controlled is unknown. Two Ph.D. students are pursuing closely related projects to shed light on this phenomenon. After a year of the necessary preparatory work with animal adrenals, Dara Clarke B.Sc. and Ursula Fearon B.Sc. have now moved on to working with human adrenal cell suspensions. Dara Clarke is using known fragments of the ACTH precursor POMC, and other potentially novel peptides e.g. Activin, to examine their ability to stimulate androgens and cortisol. In patients with what is essentially an experiment of nature, ectopic ACTH production, POMC fragments are present in very unusual ratios. This is associated with marked variability in the ratio of cortisol to androgens and this observation has led to the hypothesis that it may be possible to relate one or more of the non-ACTH POMC fragments directly to adrenal androgen biosynthesis. We are now using a sephidex column to separate POMC fragments in the serum of patients with ectopic ACTH with the intention of applying these to the human adrenal cell suspension and then measuring the relative cortisol to androgen responses. These exciting experiments are being carried out in collaboration with the Transplant Centre, Beaumont Hospital.

PITUITARY DYSFUNCTION IN POLYCYSTIC OVARY SYNDROME (PCOS)

Abnormalities of the pituitary hormones, LH and FSH, that control the functions of the ovaries have been identified in PCOS. LH is secreted in pulses about every sixty to ninety minutes in normal subjects. LH secretion is increased in PCOS. This may be due to excess oestrogen or deficient progesterone secretion by the ovary. Dr Tarek Fiad, Clinical Research Fellow, and Ms Jenny Dunbar, Research Nurse, are undertaking a very careful study of LH pulse frequency and quantity in normal subjects and subjects with PCOS in response to the addition of a progestagen and an oestrogen antagonist. These studies have already suggested explanations for the hormonal derangements which take place in PCOS.

EFFECTS OF BLOOD PRESSURE DRUGS ON SALT AND WATER METABOLISM

We are examining the clinical importance of an observation made by a previous Ph.D. graduate, Stephen Fitzpatrick, that calcium channel blockers in the treatment of coronary artery disease and hypertension impair aldosterone production in animal adrenals in the laboratory. Studies have been undertaken to see if calcium channel blockers also have effects on aldosterone production in man. This is the main hormone responsible for salt metabolism. If such effects exist, it will be possible to recommend the use of additional drugs to optimise the effects of calcium channel blockers.

RESEARCH PROJECT
Name of consultant: Walter McNicholas

Studies on the control of breathing and respiratory physiology during sleep. These studies are aimed principally at identifying the mechanisms of nocturnal asthma and sleep apnoea, with the particular aim of identifying effective treatment modalities.

RESEARCH PROJECT
Name of consultant: Alan J. McShane

ACID REFLUX AND ACID ASPIRATION STUDIES IN THE OPERATING ROOM AND INTENSIVE CARE

These involve placing fine catheters in patients' gullets and windpipes under anaesthesia to determine the incidence of and risk factors for acid regulation and the development of aspiration pneumonia—a condition associated with a high morbidity and mortality.

RESEARCH PROJECTS
Name of consultant: Dr James Masterson

1. Evaluation of risk factors for hip fractures in women, including measurement of bone density in the lumbar spine by CT Bone Densitometry as an index of the presence of osteoporosis.

2. Assessment of the value of high resolution CT imaging of the lungs of patients with cystic fibrosis to delineate the extent of disease and identify features of prognostic value.

RESEARCH PROJECT
Name of consultant: Dr Brian Maurer

In 1983 we developed permanent dual chamber pacing of the heart as a treatment for a relatively rare disease called hypertrophic cardiomyopathy. Over twenty patients who had failed to respond to other treatments have been significantly helped. The results of our research and ongoing studies have been published in international journals and confirmed by other centres. Two major multi-centre trials in the United States and in Europe have been started to evaluate further this mode of treatment and identify those patients who might be helped. We are participating in the European study.

RESEARCH PROJECT
Name of consultant: F.P. Muldowney

The metabolic and renal unit at the hospital is currently undertaking an active project in connection with kidney stone patients.

It has emerged that most people with kidney stones can be helped by a diet designed to reduce the amount of calcium appearing in the urine. Oddly enough this diet is based not on calcium restriction but on salt restriction which appears to control the amount of calcium appearing in the urine.

Most recently we have been defining the relative roles of sodium versus chloride in the salt molecule and the pattern of results has enabled us to define dietary management of stone disease.

RESEARCH PROJECT
Name of consultant: Niall O'Higgins

An international collaborative study on the epidemiology of breast and colorectal cancer is being conducted in Ireland and in fifteen other European countries. St Vincent's Hospital is the centre for this case control study at which various lifestyle and dietary factors will be taken into account in an effort to understand some of the factors responsible for the high incidence of breast cancer in Western Europe. In addition extensive basic science investigations and research is being conducted into the fundamental biochemical and biological processes which underlie the development of benign and malignant breast disease.

RESEARCH PROJECTS
Name of consultant: N.A. Parfrey

CURRENT FUNDED RESEARCH PROJECTS

Molecular Mechanisms in Acute Graft Versus Host Disease (funded by the Health Research Board).

Genetic Changes in Post-Transplant Lymphoproliferative Disease (funded by the Health Research Board).

Molecular Pathogenesis of Post-Transplant Accelerated Coronary Artery Disease (funded by the Irish Heart Foundation).

Molecular Pathology of Autoimmune Diabetes (funded by the President's Research Award—UCD).

THE GUSSY MEHIGAN MEMORIAL SCHOLARSHIP
1982 David McAvinchey
1983 Michael K. Glynn
1984 Alex Blayney
1985 Anthony O. Browne
1986 T.E.D. McDermott
1987 Ronald Grainger
1988 Enda McDermott
1989 John Thornhill
1990 Not Awarded

AUGUSTINE MEHIGAN AWARD FOR TEACHING EXCELLENCE
1982 Enda McDermott F.R.C.S.I.
1983 Paul Flanagan F.R.C.S.I.
1984 T. McDonnell M.R.C.P.I.
1985 Paul Flanagan F.R.C.S.I.
1986 Kenneth McDonald M.R.C.P.I.
1987 John Sheehan M.R.C.P.I.
1988 Michael Fitzpatrick
1989 William Boyd F.R.C.S.I., M.R.C.P.I.

PRIZE MEDAL IN ANAESTHESIA
1984 Dr Mary Peyton
1985 Dr William Casey
Dr Vincent Hannon Ex-Aequo
1990 Dr Brendan O'Hare

Appendix 14

SISTER OF CHARITY
(Published 22 August 1846 in the Nation*)*

1.

Sister of Charity! gentle and dutiful
Loving as seraphim, tender and mild
In humbleness strong and in purity beautiful
In spirit heroic, in manner a child
Even thy love like an angel reposes
With hovering wings o'er the sufferer here
Till the arrows of death are half hidden in roses
And hope speaking prophecy smiles on the bier
When life like a vapour is slowly retiring
As clouds in the dawning to heaven uprolled
Thy prayer like a herald precedes him expiring
And the cross on thy bosom his last looks behold
And oh as the Spouse to thy words of love listen
What hundred fold blessings descend on thee then!
Thus the flower-absorbed dew in the bright iris glistens
And returns to the lilies more richly again

2.

Sister of Charity child of the Holiest
Oh for thy loving soul ardent as pure
Mother of orphans and friend of the lowliest
Stay of the wretched, the guilty, the poor
The embrace of the God head so plainly enfolds thee
Sanctity's halo so shrines thee around
Daring the eye that unshrinking beholds thee
Nor droops in thy presence abashed to the ground
Dim is the fire of the sunniest blushes
Burning the breast of the maidenly rose
To the exquisite bloom that thy pale beauty flushes
When the incense ascends and the sanctuary glows
And the music that seems heaven's language is pealing—
Adoration has bowed him in silence and sighs
And man intermingled with angels is feeling
The passionless rapture that comes from the skies
Oh that this heart whose unspeakable treasure

Of love hath been wasted so vainly on clay
Like thine unallured by the phantom of pleasure
Could end every earthly affection away

3.

And yet in thy presence the billows subsiding
Obey the strong effort of reason and will;
And my soul in her pristine tranquillity gliding
As calm as when God bade the ocean be still!
Thy soothing how gentle! Thy pity how tender!
Choir-music thy face is, thy step angel-grace
And thy union with Deity shines in a splendour
Subdued but unearthly thy spiritual face

4.

When the frail chains are broken a captive that bound thee
Afar from thy home in the prison of clay
Bride of the Lamb! and earth's shadows around thee
Disperse in the blaze of eternity's day;
Still mindful as now of the sufferer's story
Arresting the thunder's of wrath e'er they role
Intervene as a cloud between us and his glory
And shield from his lightnings the shuddering soul
And mild as the moonbeams in Autumn descending
That lighting extinguished by mercy shall fall
While he hears with the wail of a penitent blending
Thy prayer holy daughter of Vincent de Paul

Richard Dalton Williams

REFERENCES

PROLOGUE
1. Henry D. Inglis, *A Journey throughout Ireland during the Spring, Summer and Autumn of 1834*

CHAPTER 1
1. R.F. Foster, *Modern Ireland*, p. 289
2. F.O.C. Meenan, 'Georgian Squares of Dublin and the Professions', *Studies* (Winter 1969), p. 405
3. J. Warburton, J. Whitelaw and R. Walsh, *History of the City of Dublin*, vol. 2, p. 738
4. Ibid. vol. 1, p. 459
5. M.D. Daly, *Dublin, the Deposed Capital*, p. 241
6. H. Burke, *People and the Poor Law in 19th Century Ireland*, p. 4

CHAPTER 2
Many of the details of this chapter have been taken from the life of Mary Aikenhead by Sarah Atkinson. Atkinson was the wife of a Dublin doctor, and a great friend and supporter of the Sisters of Charity.

CHAPTER 3
1. Sarah Atkinson, *Mary Aikenhead*, p. 228
2. T.C.J. O'Connell in Annual 1970, p. 13
3. E.D. Mapother, *Dub. J. Med. Sci.* (1877), LXIV, pp. 461–69
4. Atkinson, op. cit. p. 233
5. Georgian Society Records, *Eighteenth Century Domestic Architecture and Decoration in Dublin*, vol. 2, p. 72
6. D. Guinness in Annual 1964, p. 9
7. Atkinson, op. cit. p. 234
8. Atkinson, op. cit. p. 238
9. W. Doolin, 'The Third Hurdle', *J. Ir. Med. Ass.* (1957), XL 237, p. 70

10. F.F. Cartwright, 'Antiseptic surgery' in F.N.L. Poynter (ed.), *Medicine and Science in the 1860s*, pp. 85–87

11. P. Scanlan, *The Irish Nurse*, pp. 15–19

Chapter 4

1. Sarah Atkinson, *Mary Aikenhead*, p. 240
2. E.D. Mapother, *Dub. J. Med. Sci.* (1877), LXIV, pp. 461–75
3. H. Burke, *People and the Poor Law in 19th Century Ireland*, p. 4
4. Georgian Society Records, *Eighteenth Century Domestic Architecture and Decoration in Dublin*, vol. 2, p. 73
5. Atkinson, op. cit. p. 241
6. Atkinson, op. cit. p. 405
7. *Freeman's Journal*, 30 October 1869
8. D.J. Hickey and J.E. Doherty, *A Dictionary of Irish History*, p. 607
9. S. Leslie, *Dublin Review* (July 1917), pp. 179–98
10. C. Woodham-Smith, *Florence Nightingale* (1982), p. 103
11. Atkinson, op. cit. p. 427

Chapter 5

1. J.M. O'Ferrall, *Hosp. Gaz.*, 1 January 1859, pp. 1–18
2. A fuller account may be found in F.O.C. Meenan, *Cecilia Street*, chapters 3 and 4.

Chapter 6

1. K.D. Keele, 'Clinical medicine in the 1860s' in F.N.L. Poynter (ed.), *Medicine and Science in the 1860s*, p. 1
2. E.D. Mapother, *Dub. J. Med. Sci.* (1877), LXIV, pp. 461–75
3. D.J. Hickey and J.E. Doherty, *A Dictionary of Irish History*, pp. 427–28
4. *A Century of Service*, pp. 67–70
5. E.D. Mapother, 'Lectures in public health' in *Dublin Builder* (1864), vol. 6, p. 173
6. E.D. Mapother, *The Medical Profession* (1868), p. 122
7. E.D. Mapother, 'Dublin Hospitals', *J. Stat. and Soc. Inq. Soc. Ire.* (1869), pp. 134–42
8. E.D. Mapother, *Dub. J. Med. Sci.* (1888), LXXV, pp. 110–22
9. C. Cameron, *History of the Royal College of Surgeons in Ireland*, p. 645
10. The Queen v. Robert Kelly 1871
11. James Collins, *Life in Old Dublin*, p. 192
12. W. Doolin in *A Century of Service*, p. 69
13. J.A. Byrne, *Dub. J. Med. Sci.* (1882), LXXIII CXXI, pp. 57–58
14. Sarah Atkinson, *Mary Aikenhead*, pp. 478–80

Chapter 7

1. Minutes of Medical Board
2. Ibid.

3. Ibid.
4. C. Cameron, *History of the Royal College of Surgeons in Ireland*, p. 557
5. Ibid. p. 650
6. F.O.C. Meenan, *Cecilia Street*, chapter 8
7. Minutes of Medical Board
8. Ibid.
9. T.T. O'Farrell in *A Century of Service*, pp. 88–89
10. Minutes of Medical Board

CHAPTER 8
1. *Irish Monthly* (1884), vol. 12, pp. 143–45
2. F.O.C. Meenan in Annual 1970, p. 88
3. R. Ellmann, *James Joyce*, p. 375
4. F.O.C. Meenan in *Studies* (Winter 1969), p. 405
5. *The Irish Times*, 19 April 1900

CHAPTER 9
1. M.F. O'Hea in *A Century of Service*, p. 120
2. St Vincent's Hospital Report and Prospectus 1933, p. 4
3. A. Fagan in Annual 1962, p. 10
4. T.T. O'Farrell in Annual 1964, p. 69
5. T.J. Morrissey, *Towards a National University*, p. 299
6. R. Tobin, *Dub. J. Med. Sci.*, p. 352
7. Ian S. Uys, *For Valour*, chapter 9, p. 138
8. F.J. Morrin in Annual 1964, p. 60
9. P.T. O'Farrell in *A Century of Service*, pp. 136–45

CHAPTER 10
1. F.O.C. Meenan, *Cecilia Street*, p. 72
2. Ibid. p. 92
3. S. O'Casey, *Drums Under the Windows*, pp. 626–39
4. A.D. (Louis) Courtney, *Reminiscences of Easter Rising 1916*. Courtney had qualified in 1915 and was subsequently M.O. in Nenagh Hospital. He died in 1985.
5. *Irish Independent*, 24 August 1922
6. Dillie Fallon (*née* Corcoran) in Annual 1971, p. 106

CHAPTER 11
1. A. Fagan in Annual 1962, p. 11
2. F.O.C. Meenan in Annual 1968, pp. 86–89
3. R. White in *A Century of Service*, pp. 78–86
4. Annals
5. R. Barrington, *Health, Medicine and Politics*, pp. 108–17
6. Annals

7. *Irish Hospitals 1956–1971*
8. Tony Farmar, *Ordinary Lives*, chapter 11, pp. 137–45
9. *Irish Independent*, 31 May 1932

CHAPTER 12
1. L. Abrahamson, *Ir. J. Med. Sci* (January 1934), pp. 1–11
2. Annals
3. G.F. Stokes, 'Antiquities from Kingstown to Dublin', *J. Roy. Soc. Antiq. Ire.* (1895), vol. 5, 5th series, pp. 10–15

CHAPTER 13
1. Annals
2. Ibid.
3. T.C.J. O'Connell, *J. Ir. Free State Med. Union* (1941), 8–43, p. 2
4. Annals
5. D.K. O'Donovan in Annual 1978, p. 21
6. T.C.J. O'Connell in Annual 1968, p. 226
7. T.C.J. O'Connell, *J. Ir. Med. Ass.* (1974), 67–5, p. 142
8. J.A. Mehigan in Annual 1973, p. 77

CHAPTER 14
1. Annals
2. E.J. Cullen in *A Century of Service*, pp. 40–44
3. Annals
4. Ibid.
5. Ibid.
6. P.T. O'Farrell in *A Century of Service*, p. 145

CHAPTER 15
1. A.E. Pavey, *The Growth of Nursing*, p. 242
2. M. McNeill in *A Century of Service*, p. 127
3. J. Mowbray, ibid. pp. 167–71
4. D. Mitchell, *A 'Peculiar' Place*, p. 86
5. T.P.C. KirkPatrick, *The History of Dr Steevens' Hospital Dublin*, p. 281
6. T. Laffan, *The Medical Profession*, p. 190
7. Minutes of Medical Board
8. Pavey, op. cit. p. 242
9. Annals
10. Ibid.
11. G. McSweeney in St Vincent's Hospital Anniversary Year Book 1834–1984, pp. 34–42. McSweeney is nurse tutor in the Mary Aikenhead school of nursing.
12. M.F. Egan in *A Century of Service*, p. 160
13. P. Cannon in Annual 1971, p. 141
14. Moira Lysaght practised as a Public Health Nurse.

CHAPTER 16

1. R.J. Rowlette in *Irish Free State Hospital and Year Book* (1937), p. 42
2. R. Barrington, *Health, Medicine and Politics*, p. 265
3. Ibid. p. 189
4. Ibid. p. 204
5. Ibid. p. 246
6. Ibid. p. 246
7. Ibid. p. 267
8. Ibid. p. 272
9. *J. Ir. Med. Ass.* (1953), 33:195, p. 82
10. T. Murphy, *J. Ir. Med. Ass.* (1958), 42:248, pp. 58–59
11. D.K. O'Donovan, *J. Ir. Med. Ass.* (1956), 38:224, pp. 33–37

CHAPTER 17

1. Minutes of Medical Board
2. Library, Royal College of Surgeons in Ireland
3. Edythe Lutzker, *Women Gain A Place in Medicine*, p. 147
4. W. Rivington, *The Medical Profession*, pp. 135–37
5. T. Laffan, *The Medical Profession*, p. 46
6. E.D. Mapother, *The Medical Profession and its Educational and Licensing Bodies*, p. 83
7. Reports of the President, University College Dublin

CHAPTER 18

1. Report of the President, University College Dublin, 1957–58
2. D.K. O'Donovan, *Ir. J. Med. Sci.* (1986), vol. 155, pp. 311–16
3. *Irish Independent*, 13 October 1961
4. *J. Ir. Med. Ass.* (1965), 57:338:55

CHAPTER 19

1. J.K. Feeney, *Catholic Standard*, 1 August 1975
2. Minutes of Medical Board 1935
3. T.C.J. O'Connell in Annual 1971, p. 27
4. C. Stanford in *A Century of Service*, pp. 179–80
5. Morgan Crowe, personal communication. Dr Crowe is consultant physician to the hospital.
6. John FitzPatrick, personal communication
7. T.C.J. O'Connell in Annual 1971, p. 33

CHAPTER 20

I am indebted to J.P. McMullin for valuable assistance in the preparation of this chapter.
1. T.D. O'Farrell in Annual 1971, pp. 18–19
2. J.P. McMullin in Annual 1971, p. 20

3. Annals
4. J.P. McMullin in Annual 1971, p. 21
5. J.P. McMullin, personal communication
6. J.P. McMullin in Annual 1971, p. 21
7. J.N. McHugh in Annual 1968, pp. 7–9
8. Sean Galvin, personal communication
9. Annals
10. J.N. McHugh in Annual 1968, pp. 8–9
11. Annals
12. J.N. McHugh in Annual 1968, p. 9
13. Annals
14. Ibid.
15. Ibid.
16. Ibid.

Chapter 21
1. K. Connolly in Annual 1971, pp. 35–36
2. Sister Paula Mary in Annual 1971, pp. 23–26
3. This account is based on I.M. King's comprehensive account of the official opening of the hospital. King was a member of the Commissioning Executive Group. She was of tremendous assistance to the hospital in the introduction and implementation of new methods of keeping medical records.

John Bugler was medical registrar. John O'Sullivan was surgical registrar. Joe Linnane was a well-known RTE broadcaster.

Chapter 22
Many of the details of this chapter have been taken from the Hospital Report to the Board of Management 1975.
1. Annals

Chapter 23
Hospital Reports to the Board of Management 1975–80
1. Sister M. Baptist in Annual 1984, pp. 76–78

Chapter 24
Hospital Reports to the Board of Management 1980–90
1. Annual 1984, p. 90

Chapter 25
1. Helen Burke, *The Royal Hospital Donnybrook*, pp. 275–81
2. Gearoid Crookes, *Dublin's Eye & Ear*, pp. 174–76
3. T.J. McKenna, endocrinologist, first director, Education and Research Centre

4. M.X. FitzGerald in Hospital Report to the Board of Management 1993, p. 9
5. Ibid. p. 9
6. Davis Coakley, *Irish Masters of Medicine*, pp. 315–20
7. M.X. FitzGerald in Hospital Report to the Board of Management 1992, p. 7

BIBLIOGRAPHY

HOSPITAL REFERENCES

A Century of Service—The Record of 100 Years (ed. Alice Curtayne and William Doolin), published for the centenary of St Vincent's Hospital, 23 January 1934

Annals of St Vincent's Hospital

Hospital Annuals

Moira Lysaght, 'Reminiscences of Nursing School', unpublished

Minutes of Medical Board

Hospital Reports to the Board of Management 1975–93

Reports of the President, University College Dublin

St Vincent's Hospital Anniversary Year Book 1834–1984

Patient Records—St Vincent's Hospital Report and Prospectus 1933

BOOKS

Atkinson, Sarah, *Mary Aikenhead, Her Life, Her Work and Her Friends* (1879)

Barrington, R., Health, *Medicine and Politics in Ireland 1900–1970* (Dublin 1987)

Burke, Helen, *People and the Poor Law in 19th Century Ireland* (Dublin 1987)
—— *The Royal Hospital Donnybrook—A Heritage of Caring 1743–1993* (Dublin 1993)

Cameron, C., *History of the Royal College of Surgeons in Ireland* (2nd ed., 1916)

Coakley, Davis, *Irish Masters of Medicine* (Dublin 1992)

Collins, J., *Life in Old Dublin* (1913)

Courtney, A.D. (Louis), *Reminiscences of Easter Rising 1916*, private circulation

Crookes, Gearoid, *Dublin's Eye & Ear—The Making of a Monument* (Dublin 1993)

Daly, M.D., *Dublin, the Deposed Capital—A Social and Economic History 1860–1914* (Cork 1984)

Ellmann, R., *James Joyce* (Oxford 1982)

Farmar, Tony, *Ordinary Lives, Three Generations of Irish Middle Class Experience* (Dublin 1991)

Foster, R.F., *Modern Ireland 1600–1972* (Harmondsworth 1989)

Georgian Society Records, *Eighteenth Century Architecture and Decoration in Dublin*, two volumes

Hickey, D.J. and J.E. Doherty, *A Dictionary of Irish History since 1800* (Dublin 1980)

Inglis, Henry D., *A Journey throughout Ireland during the Spring, Summer and Autumn of 1834*, two volumes (London 1834)

Irish Hospitals 1956–1971, Hospitals Trust, Ballsbridge, Dublin 4

KirkPatrick, T.P.C., *The History of Dr Steevens' Hospital Dublin 1720–1920* (Dublin 1924)

Laffan, T., *The Medical Profession in the Three Kingdoms in 1879* (1879)

Lutzker, E., *Women Gain a Place in Medicine* (London 1969)

Mapother, E.D., *The Medical Profession and its Educational and Licensing Bodies* (Dublin 1868)

Meenan, F.O.C., *Cecilia Street—The Catholic University School of Medicine 1855–1931* (Dublin 1987)

Mitchell, D., *A 'Peculiar' Place—The Adelaide Hospital Dublin, Its Times, Places and Personalities* (Dublin 1989)

Morrissey, T.J., *Towards A National University, William Delany S.J. (1835–1924), An Era of Initiative in Irish Education* (Dublin 1983)

O'Casey, S., *Autobiographies* (London 1992)

Pavey, A.E., *The Story of the Growth of Nursing* (London 1938)

Poynter, F.N.L. (ed.), *Medicine and Science in the 1860s* (London 1968)

Report of the Trial of Robert Kelly for the Murder of Head Constable Talbot (1873)

Rivington, W., *The Medical Profession* (Dublin 1879)

Rowlette, R.J., *Irish Free State Hospital and Year Book* (Dublin 1937)

Scanlan, P., *The Irish Nurse—A Study of Nursing in Ireland: History and Education 1718–1981* (Manorhamilton 1991)

Uys, I.S., *For Valour: History of Southern Africa Victoria Cross Heroes* (Johannesburg 1973)

Warburton, J., J. Whitelaw and R. Walsh, *History of the City of Dublin*, two volumes (London 1818)

Woodham-Smith, Cecil, *Florence Nightingale 1820–1910* (London 1982)

JOURNALS

Dublin (subsequently Irish) *Journal of Medical Science*

Dublin Builder

Dublin Review

Hospital Gazette

Irish Monthly

Journal of the Irish Medical Association

Journal of the Irish Free State Medical Union

Journal of the Royal Society of Antiquaries of Ireland

Journal of the Statistical and Social Inquiry Society of Ireland

Studies

Contemporary newspaper reports

INDEX

Aberdeen, Lady, 75
Academy of Medicine, 164
accident and emergency department,
    79, 180, 188, 226, 227(p), 254
Act of Union, 3, 5, 15
Adelaide, Queen, 15
Adelaide Hospital, 43, 60, 82, 218, 223
    nursing school, 135, 137
administration, 170–71, 193, 209, 224,
    226, 233, 248
    staff, 252(p)
admissions, 23, 26–7, 38, 170
Agnes, Sr, 205(p)
Agnes Carmel, Sr, 189
agriculture, 3
Aikenhead, Dr David, 8
Aikenhead, Mother Mary, 9(p), 23, 26,
    27, 125, 199, 200, 201
    centenary, 158
    commemorative stamp, 237
    death of, 30–31
    early life, 8–12
    health of, 13, 30
    hospital foundation, 13–20
    hospital improvements, 24
    on insurance, 24, 26
    missionaries, 30
    staff appointments, 22
    and training, 32, 135, 253
air raid precautions, 116–17
Alexis, Sr, 124
Allen, Fr M., 106

almoners, 157
American Medical Association, 155
anaesthesia, 19, 97, 99, 120, 223, 238
    staff, 251(p)
Andrews, Emmet, 179(p)
Angela, Mother F., 108
angiography, 220
antisepsis, 19
Apothecary's Hall, 35–6
Ashe, Maureen, 247
Assaf, Richard, 223, 251(p)
Association of Surgeons of Great Britain
    and Ireland, 100, 165
Atkinson, Sarah, 11
Augustine, Sr Mary. *see* Aikenhead, Mary
Austin, Mother Joseph Ignatius, 127
Austin, Teresa, 185
Australia, 30, 41
Avila, Sr Teresa of, 146, 205(p)

Bahrain, 223
Ball, Fanny, 8, 10
Ball, Nicholas, 11
Ballsbridge, 12
Bannon, Christy, 184
Baptist, Sr, 205(p)
Bar Convent, York, 10, 15
Barlow, Brigid, 142
Barrett, Bridie, 238
Barrett, Monsignor, 204
Barrington, Ruth, 101, 152
Barry, A.P., 179(p)

315

Barry, Kevin, 95
Barry, P., 235, 249(p)
Barry-McKenna, Catherine M., 162
Bartholomew, Courtney, 237
Bartley, Josephine, 142, 144(p), 237
Beaumont Hospital, 142, 238
Beckett, Hylda, 235
Bellew, Ms M., 252(p)
Bellingham, Dr O'Bryen, 21–2, 27, 37,
    39, 78
Bellingham Gold Medal, 78
Bergspital, Berne, 186
Bernard, Sr M., 190
Berney, Sr Francis Borgia, 128, 154(p),
    224
Bertram, Rev. Canon Richard, 230, 248
Betagh, Fr Thomas, 8
Beveridge Report, 151
Bigger, Sir Edward Coey, 95
biochemistry, 220–21
Blake, John, 219, 246, 249(p)
Blanchardstown Hospital, 155, 248
blood transfusion, 117
Blood Transfusion Service, 165
Bloom, Marcus, 68, 97
Board of Management, 209–12, 239, 242
    list of members, 259–61
Boer War, 70
Boland, Dr Sylvester J., 118–19, 168, 169,
    192
Boland, Harry, 92
Bolton, Mr, 52
Bord Altranais, An, 140, 142
Borgia, Sr. see Berney
Bouchier-Hayes, David, 253
Bourke, Geoffrey, 219, 249(p), 253
Bourke, Sr Monica Joseph, 124
Bowater, Sr Magdalen Alphonsus, 124
Boyd-Barrett, Surgeon, 81
Boylan, John, 247, 251(p)
Brady, F., 224
Brady, Fr, 180
Brady, Ita, 162
Brady, Michael, 253
Brady, Val, 240
Bramwell, Miss, 135

Brennan, Philip, 119, 166–8, 172, 209,
    210(p), 216, 220, 237
Brereton, Annie, 162
Brereton, Gerry, 238
Bresnihan, Barry, 223–4, 239, 246,
    249(p), 250, 253
Brien, P., 224
British Medical Association, 46, 118
British Society for Colposcopy and
    Cervical Pathology, 248
Brodie, Sir Benjamin, 41
Brophy, Dr David, 179(p)
Browne, Alfred Carroll, 70–71
Browne, Barry, 179(p)
Browne, Loreto, 143(p), 247
Browne, Dr Noël, 152–3
Browne, Miss Wogan, 70
Bugler, Dr John, 194, 196
Burke, Barney, 176(p), 182
Burke, Carol, 150
Burke, Mrs J., 143(p)
Burke, Rena, 142
Burns, Brian, 179(p)
Butcher, Dr, 48
Butler, Paget, 178
Butler, Sr Fidelis, 125
Butler, Sr Louis Gonzaga, 82, 111
Butt, Isaac, 46, 48
Byrne, Sr Agnes Ursula, 127, 192
Byrne, Alfred, 108, 109(p)
Byrne, Beatrice, 146
Byrne, Dr, Archbishop of Dublin, 92, 95,
    106, 107(p)
Byrne, Fr, 70
Byrne, Dr John A., 48–9, 53–4, 68, 178
Byrne, Ralph, 185
Byrne, Miss S., 143(p)

Cahill, Fr Joseph, 230, 248
Campbell, Deirdre, 231
Campbell, Miss, 108, 137, 138
Campbell, Sr Pauline, 144(p), 237
Canisius, Mother. see O'Keeffe
Cannon, Mrs Pansy, 146–7
Cantwell, Dermot, 166, 168, 195, 210(p),
    221

cardiology, 216, 250
Carew, Mother Bernard, 62(p), 75, 120, 125, 126, 130(p), 147, 148, 177
  Easter Rising, 87–8
  hospital centenary, 108
Carey, John, 179(p)
Carlisle, Earl of, 124
Carmel Mary, Sr, 167(p)
Carmel Teresa, Sr, 144(p)
Carmichael, Richard, 14, 43
Carmichael Prize, 161
Carmichael School, 43
Carroll, Elizabeth, 212, 252(p)
Cassidy, Noel, 226
Castlebar Hospital, 142
CAT scanner, 232
Catherina, Sr, 167(p)
Catherine, Sr Mary. see Walsh, Alicia
Catholic Emancipation Act, 1829, 3
Catholic University, 35
  School of Medicine. see Cecilia Street Medical School
Cecil, Lord William, 71
Cecilia, Sr, 205(p)
Cecilia Street Medical School, 41, 46, 48, 55, 56, 68, 72, 81, 99–100, 161
  established, 35–6
  Professor of Midwifery, 53
  Professor of Surgery, 75
  transfers to NUI, 77
Century of Service, A (Curtayne and Doolin), 111, 133, 135, 145
chapel, 106, 129(p)
  Elm Park, 129(p), 192
chaplaincy, 180, 193, 230, 247–8
Charitable Infirmary, Jervis St, 6, 37, 218
Charity, Srs of. see Irish Srs of Charity
Chavasse, Judith, 247
Childers, Erskine, 203(p), 204, 206
Childers, Rita, 204
children, 38, 55
Children's Hospital, Temple St, 55, 73, 162, 250
Christmas, 130(p), 131, 132(p), 190, 229
'chronics', 181
Civil War, 90, 94

Clare, Anthony, 254
Clarke, Rosie, 146
Clifford, Sr Lucy, 23, 124
Clinical Association, 122, 154(p), 171
clinics, 77
Clongowes Wood College, 10, 61, 72, 76
Cloonan, Fr, C.Ss.P., 230
Coakley, Davis, 254
Cochrane, Miss, 71
Coffey, Dr, 108
Colbert, Gretta, 231
Coleman, Sr Alcantara, 124–5, 128, 135
Colette, Sr C., 205(p)
College of Commerce, Rathmines, 201
Collins, James, 48
Collins, General Michael, 90, 91(p), 92–3
Collum, L., 254
Columbiere, Sr. see Meehan
Comhairle na nOspideal, 155, 208
Conlon, Dr T.J., 103(p)
Connolly, Blanche, 146
Connolly, Isobel, 28
Connolly, James, 88
Connolly, Kevin, 194–5
consultant intensivist, 242, 248
consultants, 44, 46, 68–9, 212, 223–4, 249(p)
  knighthoods, 76
  state funding, 153
  women, 162
Conway, Fr Brendan O.S.Cam., 230
Cooke, Jessie N., 162
Coombe Hospital, 120, 165, 168, 224
Coppinger, Francis, 26
Corbett, Edward, 97
Corcoran, Dillie, 92–3
Corish, Brendan, 219
Cork, 11
Cork Street Fever Hospital, 6, 78
Cosgrave, W.T., 92
Costello, J.A., 158
Coughlan, David, 169
County Dublin Infirmary, 6
Courtney, A.D., 86–9, 91(p)
Couse, Eimear, 212, 252(p)

Cox, Arthur, 186, 188, 192
Cox, Bridget, 192
Cox, Michael F., 55–6, 57(p), 69, 70, 75–6, 79, 82, 91(p), 97, 136, 138, 155, 159, 160, 178, 192
Cox, Mrs, 70
Coyle, Charles, 120, 168
Crampton, Sir Philip, 22
Crawley, Miss L., 143
Crean, T.J., 76, 178
Cremin, Fr Tom, O.S.Cam., 230
Crimean War, 19
Crowe, Morgan, 179(p), 241, 249(p)
Crowley, Denis, 212
Crowley, Kieran, 242, 248, 251(p)
Crown, John, 242, 249(p)
Cryan, Robert, 48–9, 51, 52, 55, 209
Cuddihy, Mrs P., 252(p)
Cullen, B., 179(p)
Cullen, Mother Canisius, 62(p), 70, 71, 75, 125–6, 136–7, 154(p), 160
Cullen, Cardinal, 36, 125
Cullen, Michael, 253
Cullen, R.J., 98(p)
Cullen, Sr Teresa Paul, 190
Cullinan, Sr Francis Jude, 190
Cummins, T.C., 178
Cunningham, A., 235
Cunningham, Catherine, 162
Cunningham, John F., 97, 119–20, 164, 167(p), 174, 186, 188, 235
Cunningham, Roseanne, 142
Curley, Sr Margaret Cecilia, 128, 231
Curran, D.J., 179(p)
Curran, Michael, 73
Curry, Sr A., 143(p)
Curtayne, Alice, 111
Cyril, Sr J., 205(p)

Daly, Sr Manus, 226
Darby, Mary, 223, 250
Dargan, William, 70, 79, 91(p), 103(p), 107(p)
  appointment, 68
  hospital centenary, 108
  nurses' dance, 148

physician, 73
retirement, 119
Davys, G. Raymond, 120, 165, 168, 193, 209, 210(p), 235
de Chantal, Mother, 12, 13
de Valera, Eamon, 89, 108, 109(p), 158, 191(p), 204
Dease, Sir Gerald and Lady, 70, 71
Deasy, D., 103(p)
Deegan, Marjorie, 142
Deegan, Tessie, 145
Deering, Fr, 180
Delany, Fr William, SJ, 159–60
Dennis, A.R., 220
dentistry, 97, 120, 216
dermatology, 120, 216, 250
Desmond, Barry, 236
Devlin, Michael, 192
diagnostic committee, 251(p)
Dickens, Charles, 134
dietetics, 118, 238
Dinn, John J., 220
diseases, 37–8, 60–61, 75, 123
Diseases of the Heart (O'Bryen Bellingham), 22
dispensary system, 68
Disraeli, Benjamin, 48
Dockery, Sr Margaret Vincent, 144(p), 237
doll exhibition, 171
Dolores, Sr, 205(p)
Donnellan, W., 91(p)
Donnelly, Most Rev Dr, 70
Donnelly, Sr Nuala, 228
Donnybrook, 11
Donovan, Fergus, 156, 166, 168, 218, 235, 238
Donovan, Mrs, 176(p), 182
Donovan, Sr Loyola, 125
Dooley, Fr, 180
Doolin, Marian, 220–21, 242
Doolin, William, 19, 43, 48, 83(p), 91(p), 95, 103(p), 107(p), 109(p), 138, 154(p), 164, 179(p)

appointment, 82
career, 100
A Century of Service, 111
Dorrian, G., 235, 238
Dowdall, Jenny, 142
Downes, J.V., 186, 188
Downes, Meehan and Robinson, 189, 204
Doyle, H.A., 179(p)
Doyle, J. Stephen, 253–4
Doyle, Pauline, 143(p), 247
Doyle, Sr Asicus, 124
Dublin
  changes in Stephen's Green, 256–7
  development of, 3–4
  disease in, 12
  poverty in, 5–6, 12
  Unions, 7
Dublin Builder, 43
Dublin Corporation, 44, 50, 60, 116
Dublin Evening Post, 41
Dublin Hospitals' Football Union, 178
Dublin Journal of Medical Science, 18–19, 60
Duff, Frank A., 119, 120, 166, 167(p), 168, 209, 210(p), 218, 224, 235
Duffy, Gavan, 92
Duffy, George, 219, 251(p)
Duggan, Richard, 102
Duignan, Niall, 235, 248, 253
Duncan's Map, 1821, 115
Dungannon Club, 81
Dunne, Aggie, 145
Dunne, Emma, 76
Dunne, Ned, 182
Dwyer, Patrick, 41

Early, Michael, 248
ears, noses, throats, 119
Easter Rising, 1916, 86–90, 97
Eastern Health Board, 241
Edinburgh Royal Infirmary, 19
Education, Department of, 245
Education and Research Centre, 243(p), 244–6, 248
Ellis, Professor Andrew, 36–7

Ellis, Francis, 185
Elm Park, 26, 100, 116, 122, 142, 150, 166, 169, 171, 210(p)
  chapel, 129(p)
  commissioning, 188–90
  community, 205(p)
  community moves in, 190
  construction, 185–93
  description of, 200–201
  first patients, 192–3
  funding for, 188
  grounds, 190, 239–40
  move completed, 194–206
  opening ceremony, 191(p), 201–6
  purchase of, 111, 114–15, 126
  in the 1980s, 232–40
  in the 1990s, 241–55
  site blessed, 187(p)
  size of staff, 214–15
  social life, 229–30
  150th anniversary, 236–7
Elm Park Golf Club, 185
Elpis Hospital, 89
Emergency, the, 116–22, 151, 152, 186
Emmet, Robert, 14
endocrinology, 216
entertainment, 61, 63, 65, 69, 148, 229–30
Ericsen, Dr, 19
Esch, Sr Mercedes, 123
'Evening of the Stars', 236

Fagan, Albert, 94, 95, 103(p), 148, 168
Fagan, Patrick, 68, 70, 75, 79, 95
Fagan, Sean, 224, 226, 233
Fahy, Sr Francis Ignatius, 9(p)
Fallon, Dillie, 92–3
famine, 6
Farmar, Tony, 104
Farnan, Fr, 180
Farrell, Mona, 212
Farrell, Sr Philomena, 143(p)
Farrington, Mary, 162
Federated Dublin Voluntary Hospitals, 216
Feehan, Valerie, 143(p)

Feeney, Kevin, 118, 120, 168, 209, 218, 235, 237
Fellowship in Nursing RCSI, 144(p)
Fenelon, Lynda, 238, 249(p)
Fennelly, James J., 166, 216, 218, 237, 242, 250, 253
Ferris, B., 237, 251(p)
fever, 6, 11
Fianna Fáil, 87, 102, 152, 153
finances, 60, 101–2, 104, 171, 245
  costs, Elm Park, 226
  shortages, 232–3
Finnegan, Sr Pelagia, 124
fires, 24–5, 135
First World War, 81, 82, 94, 151, 178
FitzGerald, Dr Garret, 236
Fitzgerald, Garret, 253
FitzGerald, John, 176(p), 182, 206
FitzGerald, Mrs, 193
FitzGerald, Muiris X., 216, 217(p), 220, 224, 237, 249(p), 250, 254
FitzGerald, Oliver, 167(p), 168, 204, 209, 210(p), 216, 217(p), 236
  appointment, 119
  death of, 237
  Elm Park committee, 186
  gastroenterology, 218
  NDAB, 165–6
  retirement, 235
  VHI negotiations, 153
FitzGerald, Oliver Jnr, 239, 249(p), 250
FitzGerald, Patrick, 109(p), 166, 167(p), 168, 209, 216, 217(p), 224
  appointment, 119
  Elm Park committee, 186
  FitzGerald Report, 155
  vascular surgery, 164–5, 220
FitzGerald Report, 155
Fitzgibbon, John, 23
Fitzpatrick, John, 253, 257
Fitzpatrick, Mary, 238
Fitzpatrick, Mr, 181, 257
Fitzpatrick, Mrs, 193
Fitzsimons, Fr, 186
Fitzsimons, Fr Patrick, 158, 180
Flanagan, Sean, 155

Fleming, Lil, 144(p), 145, 231
Fletcher, P., 252(p)
Foley, Sr Rosaleen, 128, 231
Ford, R.A.W., 98(p)
Fortune, Josephine, 135, 173
Fortune, Mother Joseph Cyril, 144(p), 225(p), 233, 237
Foskin, Sr Mary Concepta, 226, 237
Foundling Hospital, 7
Fox, Fr Thomas, C.Ss.P., 193, 230
Fox, Michael, 224, 233
Francis de Sales, Sr M., 14
Francis Ignatius, Mother, 236
Freeman, Spencer, 102
Freeman's Journal, 49–50
Fulham, Eilish, 142

Gaffney, C. Burke, 121, 178
Gaffney, Fr Matthew, 248
Gallagher, Edward, 238, 251(p)
Gallagher, E.J., 98(p)
Gallagher, Joseph, 166, 168, 210(p), 219
Galvin, Sir John, 189, 190, 191(p), 209
Ganly, Arthur, 239–40
Garda Siochána, 111
Gardiner Street Upper, 11
gastroenterology, 218, 248, 250
General Medical Council, 33, 54
General Nursing Council, 138, 140
genito-urinary surgery, 218
Geoghegan, F., 226
George VI, King, 254
geriatric medicine, 219, 241–2
Gibney, Noel, 235
Gill, Ms K., 252(p)
Glasgow Royal Infirmary, 19
Gleeson, Hester, 146
Gleeson, Mother Paula, 146, 148, 167(p), 189, 198(p), 202(p), 204, 209
  memories of Stephen's Green, 199–200
  Reverend Mother, 127
  transfer to Elm Park, 192, 195, 196
Gogarty, Dr Oliver St John, 90
Gonzaga, Sr. see Butler
Gordon, Sr Jerome, 125
Graham, Alice, 184

Grangegorman Hospital, 6, 12
Graves, Robert, 18, 32
Great Famine, 6, 22, 55
Greenan, Mrs A., 252(p)
Greevy, Bernadette, 236
Griffin, Blanche J.C., 161–2
Griffin, Dr B., 98(p)
Griffin, Eddie, 240
Griffin, Gerald, 27
Griffin, J., 235
Griffin, James, 251(p)
Griffith, Arthur, 90, 92
Guerin, Sr Pascal, 128
Guinan, Philomena, 120, 162, 168, 219, 235
Guiney, E.J., 254
Gunn, Molly, 83(p), 164
gynaecology, 95, 97, 218

haematology, 221, 250
Halbert, Angela, 138, 147, 150
Hall, Miss H.A., 161
Hall, Mr, 257
Halligan, Maeve, 162
Hanly, Michael, 173, 178, 180, 198(p), 240
Hannan, Mary Josephine, 159–60
Hannon, Robert, 179(p)
Hannon, Sr Padua, 127, 130(p), 146
Hannon, Vincent, 238, 251(p)
Hardwicke Hospital, 41
Hargadon, Mr, 188
Harman, John, 166, 167(p)
Harold's Cross convent, 30
Harrington, Finola, 142
Harrington, Sr Otteran, 190
Hatch, Louis, 257
Hayes, Irene, 144(p), 146
Hayes, P.J., 75
Health, Department of, 170, 186, 188, 190, 219, 223, 226, 232, 238, 242, 245
Health Act, 1953, 153
Health Act, 1970, 155
health insurance, 153
health visitors, 157
Healy, P.A., 235, 237, 251(p)

Heaney, A., 235
Heffernan, Andrew, 216
Heffernan, Margaret, 245
Hegarty, John, 235, 247, 249(p)
Hennessy, Mary, 22
Hennigan, Miss K., 238
Henry of Battenberg, Princess, 70–71
Hickey, G., 178, 179(p)
Hickey, Noel, 219, 240, 245, 247
Hilary, Sr, 205(p)
Hillary, Dr, 52
Hillery, Dr Patrick, 236, 244
Hippocrates, 165
Hipwell, Rev. Trevor, 230
histopathology, 220
Hoban, Mary, 231
Hogan, Patrick, 92
Home Rule, 81
Hooper, A., 254
Horgan, John H., 254
Hospitalières of St Thomas of Villanova, 14, 17
hospitals, 10–11
   development of, 6–7
   duties and responsibilities of, 157–8
   essentials of, 43–4
   financial difficulties, 232–3
   fund-raising, 102, 104, 117, 152
   independence being lost, 155
   medical treatment in, 18–20
   regional, 155
   specialisation, 208, 221–2
   state support, 151–3
   training in, 35–6
Hospitals Commission, 102, 117, 152
Hospitals' Rugby Cup, 174, 177–8, 179(p)
Hospitals Sweepstakes, Irish, 102, 104, 105, 117, 152–3
Houlihan, J.F., 179(p)
Hourihane, J.B., 221
Howard, Bertha, 238
Hughes, Niall, 179(p)
hunger strikes, 93
Hurson, Brian, 248
Hussey, Gemma, 237

Hutchinson, Michael, 223, 238, 249(p), 250
hydrocephalus, 22
Hyland, John, 235, 241, 248, 249(p)

Ignatius, Sr, 205(p)
Ignatius, Sr M., 14
Income Tax Commissioners, 56
industry, 3
infection, 19, 123
Inglis, Henry, 1–2, 5, 256
Institute of Hospital Administrators, 223
Institute of Public Administration, 224
insurance, 24, 26
intensive care, 242, 248
International College of Angiology, 165
Iraq, 223
Irish Conjoint Board, 54
Irish Guild of Catholic Nurses, 247
Irish Hospitals Sweepstakes, 102, 104
Irish Journal of Medical Science, 97, 100, 105, 166
Irish Medical Association, 118, 153
  AGM, 1965, 171–2
Irish Srs of Charity, 22, 26, 61, 145, 223.
  see also St Vincent's Hospital
  established, 10–12
  hospital community, 113(p), 123–33
  missionaries, 30
  Mothers General, 258
  poem on, 28, 303–4
Irish Tribune, 27, 28, 41
Irish Universities Act, 1908, 77
Irish Volunteers, 86–90
Irishtown, 12
Ita, Sr, 205(p)

Jenner, Sir William, 160
Jermyn, Nicholas, 248, 252(p)
Jerome, Sr, 147
Jerrard, J.J., 178
Jervis Street Hospital, 43
Jones, Jack, 184
Jordan, Mother M. Aquin, 189
Joseph Ignatius, Sr. *see* Phelan
Joseph Miriam, Sr, 190

Josepha, Sr, 205(p)
Journal of the Irish Medical Association, 100
Joyce, James, 68, 97, 256
Joyce, Mr, 91(p)

Kavanagh, Bishop James, 229
Keane, A., 218
Keane, J.F., 237, 251(p)
Keane, W., 178
Kearney, Michael, 238
Kearns, T., 143(p)
Keating, Denis, 219, 241, 249(p)
Keating, Kevin, 238
Keaveny, T.V., 216, 220, 248, 249(p)
Kehoe, Matthew J., 55
Kelly, Annie, 110(p), 142, 144(p)
Kelly, Daniel, 166, 171, 179(p), 210(p), 218, 248
Kelly, Eamon, 238, 241
Kelly, Fr Edward S.J., 61
Kelly, Mary, 41
Kelly, Geraldine, 224
Kelly, Marcella B.M., 162
Kelly, porter, 78
Kelly, Robert, 46, 48
Kenna, Christy, 184
Kennedy, Denis, 75, 91(p), 103(p), 107(p), 119, 162, 175(p), 216
  appointment, 73
  'dry-wipes', 79
  Elm Park committee, 185
  Harry Boland, 92
  rugby club, 178
Kennedy, Eileen, 142, 162
Kennedy, Kathleen, 162
Kennedy, S., 250
Kenney, Fr Peter, S.J., 10, 11
Kenny, Fr F., 106, 107(p), 180
Kenny, Maisie, 183(p), 184, 206
Keogh, Brian, 235, 249(p), 253
Keogh, Des, 236
Keogh, P.J., 95, 103(p), 107(p), 148, 185
Kerley, Peter, 98(p), 254
Kettle, Tom, 256
Kevelighan, Miss H., 143(p)
Kiely, Fifi, 145

Kier, Sr Otteran, 124
Kilbride, Ronan, 179(p)
Killeen, Miss M., 143(p)
Killeen, Sr Ignatius. *see* Austin
King, Mary, 184
King, Richard Enda, 192
King, Fr William, 248
King and Queen's College of Physicians, 32
Kirby, A.J., 98(p)
KirkPatrick, T.P.C., 135
Kitchener, Lord, 81

laboratory, 52–3
ladies' committee, 171
Lady Presidents, 272
Laffan, student, 52
Laffan, Thomas, 136, 161
Lalor, Charles, 94
Lambe, Mrs, 193
Lancet, The, 44
Lang, Sr Francis Joseph, 209, 225(p), 233
Lavan, Sean, 178
Lavery, Frank, 166, 168, 209, 247
Lawn, Sr Frances Mary, 127, 146
Leahy, Christine, 257
Leahy, Pauline, 238
Lee, Anthony, 23
leeches, 80
Leinster, Duke of, 15
Lemass, Alice M., 162
Lemass, Sean, 162
Lenehan, Peter, 237, 248
Lennon, Michael, 89
Leonard, Thomas, 101
library, 169, 171, 235
lighting, 19
Linden convalescent home, 26–7, 44
Linnane, Joe, 195
liver transplants, 246–7
Llewelyn-Davies, Weeks, Forestier-Walker & Bor, Messrs, 190, 192
Local Government and Public Health, Department of, 117, 126
Lorcan, Sr, 205(p)

Loreto Order, 10
Lowry, Helen, 238
Lucey, Dr Mark, 179(p)
Luke, D.A., 237
Lynch, Jack, 191(p), 202(p), 204
Lynch, Kathleen M., 162
Lynch, Maureen, 202(p), 204
Lynch, Vincent, 220, 249(p)
Lyons, R.S.D., 36–7
Lysaght, Moira, 142, 147–8, 150

MacAlister, Professor, 43
McArdle, John S., 56, 57(p), 79, 91(p), 100
  career, 75
  death of, 99
  Medical Board, 160
  National Volunteers, 81
  royal visit, 69, 70–71
  rugby club, 178
McArdle, Joseph, 75
McArdle, Miss, 70
McArdle, Mr, 136
McArevey, J.B., 95, 185
Macaulay, G.B., 179(p)
McBride, Kitty, 146
McCabe, Cardinal, 61
McCabe, M., 250
McCabe, Mary, 220, 251(p)
McCambridge, Mr, 189
McCann, S., 253
McCarthy, Carmel, 146
McCarthy, Donal, 250
McCarthy, Mother Francis Magdalene, 22, 27, 39, 40(p), 125
McCarthy, Justine, 41
McCarthy, Misses, 257
McColgan, Maggie Josephine, 162
McCormac, Michael, 213(p), 237–8, 242
McCormack, B.L., 179(p)
McCormack, J., 103(p)
McCourt, Feargal, 179(p)
McCullen, Oliver, 120, 168, 219
MacDarby, Stephanie, 143(p)
McDermot, Sr Teresa, 228
McDermott, E., 249(p)

McDermott, Nancy, 145, 150
McDonagh, Joseph, 92
McDonagh, Sr Lorcan, 125
McDonagh, Tricia, 239
McDonald, A., 168
McDonald, Niall, 238
MacDonald, Sr M. Cephas, 190
McDonnell, Emma, 142, 144(p), 206, 233, 235
McDonnell, Sr Fidelma, 128
McDonnell, Robert, 72
McDonnell, T., 249(p)
McDonough, Ms T., 252(p)
McEntee, Gerry, 247
McEntee, Sean, 153, 167(p), 169, 188
MacErlaine, D.P., 221, 253
McGann, P., 178
McGovern, Josephine, 162
McGrath, Joe, 102
McGrath, John (Jock), 97, 99, 103(p), 165
McGucken, Sr Dolores, 128
McGuirk, Mr, 257
McHugh, James N., 189, 192, 202(p), 204, 206, 209
  Elm Park move, 194, 196
McHugh, Michael, 56, 58(p), 66, 68, 70, 79, 81
  rugby, 136, 178
McHugh, Roger, 48
McKeating, K., 251(p)
McKenna, M.J., 248, 249(p)
McKenna, T.J., 223, 242, 244–6, 248, 249(p), 253
McLaughlin, Francis, 120, 168, 235
McManus, Brian, 179(p)
McMullin, Joseph P., 166, 168, 193, 202(p), 209
  building committee, 186, 188, 216, 218
  Elm Park opening, 204, 206
  sesquicentenary, 236
McNamara, Mr, 91(p)
McNamara, Sr Marie Joan, 231
McNicholas, Walter, 235, 249(p), 250
McParlan, Sr Mary Magdalen, 225(p), 233, 248

McQuaid, Dr J.C., Archbishop of Dublin, 130(p), 167(p), 192, 193, 202(p), 203(p), 204, 206
McQuillan, Robert, 226
McShane, A., 251(p)
McSharry, Kitty, 184
McSweeney, Geraldine, 138, 140, 143(p), 144(p), 237, 247
MacSwiney, Terence, 93
Madden, Justice, 115
Magan, Mother Baptist, 127
Magennis, J.B., 81–2, 83(p), 90, 91(p), 103(p), 107(p)
  appointed physician, 97
  death of, 118
  Elm Park committee, 185
Magner, Siobhan, 150
Maguire, May, 144(p), 146
Maher, Bernadette, 171
Maher, Dr Brian, 179(p)
Maher, James, 120–21, 154(p), 167(p), 168, 171, 179(p), 209, 216, 224
Maher, Nora, 171
Maher, T.J., 171
Malachy, Sr, 205(p)
Mallin, Commdt Michael, 86
Malone, Mrs A., 143(p)
Mangan, James Clarence, 27
Manning, Cardinal Henry, 28–9
Manus, Sr, 205(p)
Mapother, Dr E.D., 21–2, 39, 41, 46, 51, 52, 63, 155, 159, 161, 209
  career, 43–6
Marchant, Miss H., 143(p)
Margaret, Sr, 205(p)
Margison, Mrs, 39, 52, 125
Marie, Sr A., 205(p)
Marie de Montfort, Sr, 205(p)
Marie Therese Claire, Sr, 167(p), 193, 230, 248
Marine, Department of the, 256–7
Markievicz, Countess, 86, 256
Marsh, Sir Henry, 22
Martin, Edward A., 218, 238, 242
Martin, Nicholas, 120, 168, 216, 237
Martin, Petronilla, 143(p), 144(p), 237

Mary, Sr F., 205(p)

Mary Aikenhead school of nursing. *see* nursing school

Mary Aikenhead ward, 174

Mason, Miss, 137

Masterson, James, 224, 251(p)

Mater Hospital, 30, 43, 99, 155, 216

Maume, Miss M., 143(p)

Maunsell, Dr, 18–19

Maunsell, Mother Theckla, 126–7

Maureen, Sr, 205(p)

Maurer, Brian, 216, 249(p), 250

Maxwell, Sr Benedict Joseph Constable, 124

Meade, Harry, 73, 74(p), 75, 82, 90, 92, 100, 103(p), 154(p), 164
  Elm Park committee, 186

Meagher, Declan, 162, 168, 224

Meagher, Mary Winifred, 162

Meath, Earl of, 2, 15, 61, 63, 192

Meath Hospital, 6, 18, 43, 46

Medical Act, 1858, 32–3

Medical Act, 1886, 54

Medical Board, 51–9, 111, 118, 119, 123, 174, 192–3, 206, 210(p), 246
  Centenary Dinner, 167(p)
  Chairmen, 262
  commissioning committee, 189–90, 196, 199
  Elm Park sub-committee, 185–6, 188
  and Emergency, 116
  female students, 159–61
  laboratory, 52–3
  members of Executive, 261
  and nursing school, 136–7
  re-organisation, 209, 211–12
  secretaries, 262
  structure, 121–2

medical education
  structural change, 1879, 54

Medical Profession, The (Rivington), 160–61

medical records department, 239

Medical Registration Council, 169

Medical Research Council, 164

medical science, 18–19, 72–3, 105, 120,
  170, 207–8
  specialisation, 221–2

Medical Society, UCD, 81

medical staff, 21–2, 39, 41–9, 55–9, 66, 68–9, 72, 73, 78
  1992, 141(p)
  and the community, 123–33
  decrease in, 232
  Elm Park, 215–21, 223–4, 233, 235, 237–8, 241, 248–50, 253–4
  Elm Park move, 194–5
  during Emergency, 117–21
  house surgeon, 52
  lecturing fees, 121–2
  list of, 263–70
  on Medical Board, 209
  method of appointment, 155–6
  relations with nurses, 145
  RMOs, 80
  1950s–1960s, 164–9
  salaries, 52, 55, 59
  specialists, 53–4, 55, 157, 168
  in the thirties, 103, 107, 111
  in the twenties, 95–100
  war service, 82
  women doctors, 120, 159–63

medical training, 32–6, 99–100, 174
  dispensaries, 77–8
  education and research, 242, 244–6
  Elm Park, 215
  established in St Vincent's, 36–7, 61, 72
  fees to Medical Board, 121–2
  female students, 159–63
  list of past students, 273–86
  Medical Board, 51–9
  O'Farrell's recollections, 78–80
  para-medical schools, 221
  prizewinners, 287–95
  supervision of, 212
  US committee report, 155–6

Meehan, Sr Claude de la Columbiere, 128, 193

Meehan, F.B., 186, 188, 204

Meenan, F.O.C., 120, 168, 195, 210(p), 216, 237, 250
  press officer, 214

Meenan, J.N., 74(p), 81, 91(p), 103(p), 107(p), 148, 154(p), 164, 178
  appointment, 72–3
  clinical association, 122
  psychiatry, 120
  as teacher, 99–100
Meenan, Livina, 171
Meenan, Mairead, 171
Meenan, P.N., 153, 165, 167(p), 168, 189, 192, 204, 206, 209, 210(p)
  microbiology, 220
  retirement, 242
Mehigan, Denis, 235, 241, 248
Mehigan, J.A., 166, 168, 192–3, 202(p), 209, 210(p), 216, 218
  death of, 233
  Elm Park move, 194–5, 196, 198(p)
Mercer's Hospital, 43, 46
Merrigan, Joan, 236
Merrion school for the blind, 61
metabolism, 218
microbiology, 220
Midwives Board, 140
Mills, James, 115
Minch, J.B., 178
Mitchell, Charles, 236
Mitchell, Jim, 237
Molloy, Michael, 179(p)
Molloy, Monsignor, 70
Moloney, Dan, 238
Moloney, J.J., 179(p)
Molony, J., 166, 220, 239, 242
Molyneux, D., 235
Monaghan, Mary, 237
Monahan, Eileen, 171
Mooney, A.J., 98(p)
Mooney, Herbert, 91(p), 95, 103(p), 107(p)
Moore, Sr Dismas, 124
Moore, Gretta, 212
Moore, Nan, 182(p), 184
Moore, Thomas, 14, 27
Morgan, Ross, 179(p)
Moriarty, A., 252(p)
Moriarty, Michael, 223

Morrin, F.J., 77, 82, 95, 103(p), 107(p), 118, 121, 168, 169, 175(p)
  Elm Park committee, 186
Morris, Sr Phillippa, 123
Morrissey, P.J., 179(p)
Morrissey, T.J., 76
Mother and Child scheme, 152
Mowbray, John, 135
MRI scanner, 231
Mulcahy, Risteard, 166, 168, 169, 209, 216, 237
  landscaping, 239–40
Muldowney, F.P., 166, 168, 169, 209, 210(p), 216, 218, 248
Mullen, Michael, 99, 107(p)
Mullins, Michael, 26
Mullins Convalescent Hospital, 26
Mulvey, Fr, 167(p), 171, 180
Murnaghan, Dr D., 98(p)
Murphy, Brendan, 218
Murphy, E.L., 103(p), 119, 166, 168
Murphy, James, 97, 103(p), 223, 248, 249(p)
Murphy, J.B., 75
Murphy, John F., 237, 248
Murphy, Margaret, 143(p)
Murphy, Mary, 143(p)
Murphy, O.J., 97, 103(p), 168, 169
Murphy, Sr Salome, 124
Murphy, Sr Stephanie, 128, 167(p), 226
Murphy, Thomas, 156
Murphy, Tom, 184
Murphy, William, 73, 83(p), 103(p), 107(p), 111
Murray, Daniel, Archbishop of Dublin, 4(p), 8, 10, 15, 17, 21, 23, 26
Murray, Mr, 188

Nash, Michael, 120, 168
Nation, the, 41
National Drugs Advisory Board, 165
National Health Service Act, 1948, 151
National Maternity Hospital, 97, 119, 120, 168, 224, 241
National University of Ireland, 76, 77, 82, 165, 237

National Volunteers, 81
nephrology, 218
neurology, 218, 250
neurosurgery, 168–9, 238
Newman, John Henry, 28, 35–7, 256
Nicell, Mrs M., 143(p)
Nightingale, Florence, 28–30, 135
'96 – From the One Who Got Away!', 146–7
Nolan, Niamh, 241, 251(p)
Nolan, Richard, 235
Norton, Dr, Bishop of Bathurst, 158
Norton, Ian, 179(p)
Notre Dame de Pitiè, Paris, 14–15
Nowlan, Dr F.B., 178
nuclear medicine, 219, 253
nurse attendants, 135
Nurses' Act, 1950, 140
nurses' home, 100–101, 138, 181, 183(p)
  Elm Park, 190, 192, 193
Nurses Registration (Ireland) Act, 1919, 138
nursing homes, 65–6, 125, 169, 196, 200, 230, 231
  96 Lower Leeson St, 66, 90, 101, 145–7
nursing school, 127, 134–50, 168, 169
  centenary, 247
  Elm Park, 190, 223
  list of staff, 271–2
  numbers training, 1974, 223
  prizewinners, 296–7
  schedule, 140
nursing staff, 127, 234(p)
  annual dance, 148
  hours of work, 140, 147–8
  relations with staff, 145
  salaries, 140, 147
  training of, 66, 68
  uniforms, 142, 148

O'Brien, Ann, 237, 241, 250
O'Brien, Brian, 119, 168, 179(p), 188, 209, 219, 224
O'Brien, Sr Catherina, 128, 146, 233
O'Brien, D., 179(p)
O'Brien, Fr, 230

O'Brien, Francis V., 254
O'Brien, Mrs John, 8, 10, 11, 18
O'Brien, Sr Joseph Rosario, 231
O'Brien, Michael, 179(p)
O'Brien, Paul, 179(p)
O'Casey, Sean, 82, 85–6
O'Connell, Daniel, 27
O'Connell, Daniel (patient), 23
O'Connell, Liam, 166, 168, 221, 250
O'Connell, T.C.J. (Bob), 114, 118, 119, 154(p), 164–5, 167(p), 168, 174, 177, 182, 202(p), 216
  appointment, 111
  blood transfusion, 117
  death of, 237
  Elm Park opening, 204, 206
  Medical Board, 209
  retirement, 235
  VHI negotiations, 153
O'Connor, Madame, 70, 71
ocupational therapy, 239
Odevaine, Ferdinand, 68, 70
O'Doherty, Kevin Izod, 27, 41
O'Doherty, William J., 41
O'Donnell, Brendan, 254
O'Donnell, James, 224
O'Donnell, Sr Mary Basil, 125
O'Donnell, Tess A., 103(p), 162
O'Donnell, Turlough, 179(p)
O'Donoghue, Carmel, 169
O'Donoghue, Dermot, 224, 248, 249(p), 250
O'Donoghue, Fr, 180
O'Donoghue, Rory, 179(p)
O'Donovan, D.K., 113(p), 118, 165, 166, 167(p), 168, 191(p), 202(p), 210(p), 216
  appointment, 111
  on duties of hospital, 157
  Elm Park committee, 186
  Elm Park opening, 204
  endocrine unit, 216
  honours, 164
  lecturer, 119, 120
  Medical Board, 209
  retirement, 224

O'Donovan, Fred, 236
O'Donovan, J.S., 98(p)
O'Donovan, Sr Vincent de Paul, 128
O'Driscoll, J.R., 93
O'Duffy, Eimear, 97
O'Duffy, General Eoin, 104, 108
O'Duffy, Kevin, 97
O'Duffy, Mr, 70
O'Duffy, Mrs, 70
O'Farrell, Fr Ambrose, O.P., 247
O'Farrell, Denis, 118–19, 168, 186, 224
O'Farrell, Sr Francis Teresa, 13
O'Farrell, Joy, 238
O'Farrell, P.T., 78–80, 82, 95, 98(p),118,
    133, 164
O'Farrell, T.D., 186, 209
O'Farrell, T.T., 73, 91(p), 95, 100,
    103(p), 111, 118, 165
  Elm Park committee, 185, 186
O'Ferrall, Joseph M., 4(p), 13–14, 32,
    33, 36–7, 39, 41
O'Ferrall Medal, 78
O'Flynn, Sr Frances Rose, 142, 223, 230
O'Grady, Geraldine, 236
O'Grady, John, 240
O'Hea, Dr M.F., 73, 83(p), 98(p),
    103(p), 109(p)
O'Higgins, Kevin, 102
O'Higgins, Niall, 217(p), 224, 237, 248,
    249(p)
O'Higgins, T.F., 153, 158
O'Keeffe, Declan, 238, 251(p)
O'Keeffe, Mother Canisius, 144(p), 146,
    209, 210(p), 229
  Elm Park opening, 204
  honorary degree, 237
  move to Elm Park, 188–92, 196
  Reverend Mother, 127
  school of nursing, 142
O'Kelly, B., 251(p)
O'Kelly, Sean T., 108
O'Leary, Conor, 179(p)
O'Leary, Denis, 120, 168, 210(p)
O'Leary, M., 98(p)
O'Leary, Dr William Hegarty, 46–8, 51,
    52, 54–5, 209

O'Malley, Donagh, 171
O'Malley, Mr, 189
O'Mathuna, Fr Ciaran, 248
oncology, 218, 242, 250
O'Neill, Ann, 142
O'Neill, Sr Anthony M., 190
O'Neill, Dick, 182
O'Neill, Mary, 231
O'Neill, Paddy, 240
operating theatres, 73, 75, 79, 95, 118
  Elm Park, 188
  ophthalmology, 95, 219, 242, 246
oratory, 235
O'Reilly, Miss C., 143(p)
O'Reilly, Joseph, 257
O'Reilly, Pat, 182
O'Riain, Seamus, 166, 220, 248
O'Riordan, J.P., 179(p)
O'Rourke, Kieran, 238, 241
orthopaedics, 219
Orwell, George, 235
Osborne, Frances, 146
O'Shaughnessy, Justice, 95
O'Shea, June, 238
O'Sullivan, J.E., 98(p)
O'Sullivan, John, 194
otorhinolaryngology, 95, 120, 219–20
Our Lady's Choral Society, 236
Our Lady's Hospice, 220, 238, 242
Our Lady's Hospital for Sick Children,
    Crumlin, 246
Our Lady's ward, 234(p)
out-patients' department, 77, 80, 82,
    124–5, 128, 157, 181
  Christmas party, 130(p)
  Elm Park, 188, 226, 227(p), 228, 254
  enlargement, 94–5
Owens, Anthony, 235, 251(p)

Pacelli, Cardinal, 106, 107
Palmer, Bert, 184
paramedical staff, 252(p)
Parfrey, N., 250, 253
Paris, 14–15, 134
Parkinson, Billy, 184

Parnell, C.S., 69, 76
parrot, 18
pathology, 95, 97, 100, 156, 182, 250
  Elm Park, 190, 220
patients
  children, 38, 55
  numbers of, 23, 26–7, 38, 60–61
  origins of, 38, 60
  referral of, 37
  state funding, 170
Patrick, St, 115
Patterson, Frank, 236
Patterson, Glasgow, 121
Paul, Sr, 85–6, 92
Paula, Mother. see Gleeson
Pavey, Agnes E., 134, 137
Peel, Sir Robert, 33
Pembroke Nursing Home, 127, 128, 146,
  169, 182
penicillin, 117–18
Petrie, Dr George, 115
pharmaceuticals, 117–18
pharmacy, 97, 181, 188, 193, 238, 257
Phelan, Betty, 223
Phelan, Sr Joseph Ignatius (Pearl), 145,
  167(p), 193
Phelan, T.D., 103(p), 178
Philomena, Sr, 205(p)
physiotherapy, 118, 238
Pidgeon, Christopher, 224, 238
piggeries, 177
Pigot, Chief Baron, 24
Pius IX, Pope, 33, 35
Pius XII, Pope, 106, 107
plastic surgery, 220, 248
Plunkett, W.R., 189
Polding, Archbishop, 30
Poor Law, 7, 68
porters, 125, 164, 173, 176(p), 182, 240
Portley, Catherine, 162
Potter, John I., 97
Potter, Maureen, 236
Potter, S.B., 103(p)
Powell, Jenny, 146
Power to Heal, The, 149(p), 150

Prendergast, T.J., 98(p)
Prendiville, Dr E.J., 103(p)
Prentice Hall Press, 150
press officer, 214
preventive medicine, 219
psychiatry, 120, 218–19, 250
Public Charitable Hospitals Temporary
  Provision Act, 1930, 102
Purcell, Catherine, 162
Purcell, Mr, 91(p)
Pusey, Dr Edward, 28

Queen v. Kelly, 46, 48
Queen's Colleges, 33, 35, 43
Quigley, Peter, 238, 249(p), 250
Quinlan, David, 238, 248, 249(p)
Quinlan, F.B., 26–7, 41, 42(p), 51, 52,
  55, 66, 159, 160, 161, 209
Quinlan, Harold, 95, 103(p), 118, 166,
  167(p), 168, 203(p), 206, 209, 224
  rugby club, 178
Quinlan, John, 179(p)
Quinlan, Mrs, 70
Quinlan, William, 224, 241, 248, 249(p)
Quinn, Larry, 240

Radio Éireann, 195
radiography, school of, 190, 221, 253
radiology department, 72–3, 83(p), 111,
  118, 119, 166, 183(p)
  Elm Park, 221
Reddin, Dr Kerry, 116
Redmond, Denis, 53–4, 68, 178
Redmond, Sr Ibar, 128, 130(p), 131, 147
Redmond, Janice, 250
Redmond, John, 69, 76
Reeves, Oswald, 111
Reidy, Sr Elizabeth, 123
religion, 135
religious orders, 208
research projects, 298–303
residency, 63, 162, 174, 177
respiratory unit, 220
Reynolds, Sr Agnes, 143(p), 225(p), 247
Reynolds, Annie, 184

Reynolds, Bridie, 184
rheumatology, 220, 250
Rice, Edmund, 27
Rice, Marian, 216, 223, 237
Richmond Asylum, 6, 7
Richmond Hospital, 14, 41, 43, 46
'riding the franchise', 115
Rigby, Oran, 179(p)
Ringsend, 12
Riordan, Sr Ann, 233
Rising, 1848, 28
Rita, Sr C., 205(p)
Rivington, Dr Walter, 160–61
Robin, Mr, 178
Robinson, Fr J., 106, 180
Robinson, Miss, 137
Robinson, President Mary, 162
Robinson Keefe and Devane, 230
Roche, Alistair, 240
Roche, J.W., 103(p)
Roche, Kevin, 226, 252(p)
Rogers, S., 224, 249(p), 250
Rorke, Mary and John, 8
Rosario, Sr, 205(p)
Rotunda Lying-In Hospital, 6, 53
Rouse, Molly, 145
Rowlette, R.J., 151
Royal City of Dublin Hospital, 43, 89,
    220
Royal College of Physicians, 14, 43–4, 48,
    53–4, 95, 118
  national training scheme, 215
Royal College of Physicians of London,
    164
Royal College of Science, 53
Royal College of Surgeons, 14, 21, 41,
    43, 46, 48, 66, 166
  fees, 44
  Fellowship of Nursing, 237
  Meade President, 100
  national training scheme, 215
  and Royal University, 54
  St Vincent's recognised by, 32
  women students, 160–61
Royal Hospital, Donnybrook, 241–2

Royal Hospital for Incurables, 6
Royal University, 54, 68, 256
Royal Victoria Eye and Ear Hospital,
    219, 242, 246
RTE Symphony Orchestra, 236
rugby, 177–8
Ruigrok, June, 238
Russell, G., 252(p)
Ryan, Connie, 184, 193, 206
Ryan, D., 178
Ryan, Dr Dermot, Archbishop of Dublin,
    229, 236
Ryan, F.P., 103(p)
Ryan, Dr James, 87, 152, 153
Ryan, student, 52

St Agnes's ward, 180
St Anne's Hospital, 218, 241
St Anne's ward, 37, 70, 128, 180, 192,
    250
St Anthony's Rehabilitation Centre, 220,
    239
St Benedict's ward, 180
St Bridget's ward, 70
St Brigid's ward, 108, 111, 127, 180
St Camillus's ward, 37, 70, 180
St Charles's ward, 94, 100, 108, 127, 180,
    193
St Columcille's Hospital, Loughlinstown,
    241
St Elizabeth's ward, 70, 180
St Gabriel's ward, 180
St George, Usher, 15
St James's Hospital, 242, 250
St John of God, Srs of, 65
St Joseph's Rehabilitation Centre, 220
St Joseph's ward, 15, 18, 37, 70, 84(p),
    95, 128, 147, 178, 180, 200
St Kevin's Hospital, 155
St Laurence's Hospital, 142, 152
St Laurence's ward, 24, 38, 55, 70, 80,
    84(p), 108, 125, 127, 128, 147, 180
  O'Casey in, 82, 85–6
St Leger, Fr, S.J., 10
St Luke's Hospital, 218, 241
St Mary's College, Dundalk, 56

St Mary's Hospital, Cappagh, 219
St Mary's ward, 37
St Michael's Hospital, 237, 241
St Michael's ward, 180
St Patrick's College, Maynooth, 75, 99
St Patrick's Hospital, 6
St Patrick's ward, 21, 38, 93, 96(p), 127, 147, 180
St Peter and Paul's, 169
St Raphael's ward, 96(p), 127, 128, 180
St Rita's Staff Hostel, 193
St Stephen's, 72, 162
St Stephen's Green, 5–6, 15, 256–7
St Teresa's ward, 100, 180
St Vincent de Paul, Society of, 97
St Vincent's Hospital, 10, 112(p). *see also* Elm Park
  atmosphere of, 228–9
  centenary year, 105–15
  door closes for last time, 198(p)
  enlargements, 21, 23–4, 26, 63–6, 94–5, 100–101, 127, 152, 168–9
  established, 13–20
  first prospectus, 16(p), 17–18
  Freeman's Journal article, 49–50
  Golden Jubilee, 60, 61, 63
  Leeson Lane building, 167(p), 169
  memories, 173–84
  non-sectarian, 50
  number of beds, 21, 68
  preparing to move, 164–72
  in 1860s, 44
  Superiors of, 258–9
  university departments, 156, 166
  visitors, 27–30, 70–71
St Vincent's Hospital, Sydney, 30
St Vincent's Hospital Pools, 169
St Vincent's Private Hospital, 205(p), 230–31
St Vincent's ward, 70, 127, 128, 180
St Winifred's, 66
St Patrick's ward, 55
Sallinave, Sr Camillus, 14, 15, 22, 40(p), 134–5
Sandymount, 11, 12, 24

Saunders, C.M., 98(p)
Savage, Matthew B., 121
Scratton, secretary, 36–7
Scully, Annie, 162
Seagrave, Mrs, 56, 125
Second World War. *see* Emergency, the
secretary managers, 261
Securicor, 199
Sexton, Sr Marie John, 127, 144(p), 237, 247
Shaw, Keith, 220, 237
Shaw, Mrs, 70
Shaw, Dr Richard, 68, 91(p)
Sheahan, Kieran, 251(p)
Sheehan, D.K., 250
Sheehan, J.M., 219
Sheehan, Nuala, 162
Sheehan, R.A., 179(p)
Sheeran, Kate, 142
Sheridan, Richard Brinsley, 14
Sherry, V.F., 179(p)
Shiel, Dr John, 97, 103(p), 181
Shortall, Christopher, 103(p), 121
Shortall, Sr Josepha, 125
Sigerson, Dr George, 56
Silke, J.J., 98(p)
Simpson, Thomas Trant, 15
Sinn Féin, 81
Sir Patrick Dun's Hospital, 46, 89, 137
Sisk, Messrs John, 188, 204, 230
Srs of Mercy, 30
Skin and Cancer Hospital, Hume St, 241
Slazenger, M., 224
Smart, Maura, 146, 231
Smith, Mother A. Joseph, 108
Smith, Alfred, 68, 70, 91(p), 95
Smith, Fr, 230
Smith, Gerard, 189
Smith, Maureen, 231
Smith, Walter, 60
Smyth, Leo, 97
Smyth, M., 91(p), 103(p)
social work, 157, 238
Society of Jesus, 10
Somers, Sr Baptist, 231

Spanish flu, 93
speech therapy, 238
Stacpole, Mary, 8
staff. *see* medical staff; nursing staff
Stanhope Street, 11
State of Irish Poor, Commission of
  Enquiry on, 12
Statistical and Social Inquiry Society of
  Ireland, 44
Staunton, Fr, S.M., 180
Stephanie, Sr. *see* Murphy
Stillorgan, 26
Stokes, G.T., 115
Stokes, William, 14
Storr, Paul, 178
Sullivan, Ann, 162
Sullivan, Fr Donal, 248
Sullivan, Mary, 231
Sun Insurance Office, 24
Sutton, Miss, 108, 110(p), 138
Swift, Dean Jonathan, 6
Switzerland, 186

Talbot, Head Constable, 46, 48
Tanham, Peter, 224
Taylor's Map, 1816, 115
Teach Ultan, 142
Telefís Éireann, 193
telephone, 55
telephonists, 170–71, 184
Teresa Anthony, Mother, 130(p), 196,
  198(p), 199
Teresa Augustine, Sr, 124
Teresa of Avila, Sr, 146, 205(p)
Teresita, Sr, 205(p)
Therese, Sr M., 205(p)
Thompson, Sir William, 75, 95
thoracic surgery, 220
Tierney, Bridin, 142
Tierney, Gerald, 73, 97, 103(p), 118
Tobin, Ellen, 46
Tobin, Mrs, 70
Tobin, Richard, 58(p), 69, 70, 75, 88,
  91(p), 136, 160, 181
  anaesthesia, 80

appointment, 56
career, 76–7
classes, 78–9
rugby club, 178
son killed, 82, 85
Todd, C.H., 14
Towers, R.P., 166, 168, 210(p), 220
trade, 3
Traynor, Oscar, 237, 247, 248, 249(p)
Trinity College Dublin, 41, 53, 54, 56,
  238, 239, 253
Trotter, L., 192, 193, 195, 204
Troy, Dr, Archbishop of Dublin, 10
Tuohy, Lil, 145, 231
Tyndall, Fiona, 143(p)

Ullathorne, Dr, 30
University College Dublin, 72, 211
  Cecilia St transfers to, 77
  dental school, 97
  Medical School
    appointments, 119–20, 164–5, 168,
      224, 237–8
    chairs, 253
    control over appointments, 155–6
    and Elm Park, 206, 207
    medical oncology, 242
    President's Report, 162
    relations with hospital, 127
    and research centre, 244–5
    social work training, 238
    Woodview, 215, 218
  urology, 248
Ursula, Sr, 205(p)
Ursuline Convent, Cork, 10

vaccination, 19
Van Boven, Victor, 190
vascular surgery, 220
Verner, Mrs R., 189
Victoria, Queen, 69–71, 75, 160
Violet Day, 101, 125, 132(p)
Voluntary Health Insurance Board, 153,
  165

waiting lists, 226
Wall, Dr, Bishop of Thasos, 106
Wall Brothers, Messrs, 186
Wallace, George, 182
Wallace, Miss, 145
Walsh, Alicia, 10, 11
Walsh, Bishop Eamon, 229
Walsh, Justice Brian, 212, 213(p), 236, 237
Walsh, Dr W.J., Archbishop of Dublin, 136–7
Walsh, J., 103(p)
Walsh, Noel, 218, 250, 253
Walshe, May, 146
War of Independence, 92
Watson, A., 249(p)
Watters, Canon, 89
Wellesley, Marchioness of, 15, 18

Wellington, Duke of, 14
Wesley Female Institution and Magdalene Asylum, 18–19
Westmeath, Earl of, 23
Whelan, Fr, 13
Whelan, Noel, 213(p), 242
White, Dr Reginald, 95, 97, 103(p), 109(p), 120, 178, 188
    Elm Park committee, 185
White, V.J., 98(p)
Whitworth Hospital, 41
Whyte, Samuel, 14
William IV, King, 15
Williams, Bishop Desmond, 229
Williams, Richard Dalton, 27–8, 41, 63
Wiseman, Cardinal, 22, 27
Woodham-Smith, Cecil, 30
workhouses, 7